title

S0-CFB-706

APHASIA

A CLINICAL APPROACH

1/14 p 53+54 ✓   1/28 Chap 3 ✓

2/4 Rosenbeck (181 – 196 ✓   2/11 R
                 240 – 254 ✓)   142 – 151 ✓
                                          163 – 173 ✓

2/18 Read
      ~~Handouts~~
      ABSTRACT ✓

APHASIA

A CLINICAL APPROACH

John C. Rosenbek, Ph.D.

Chief, Audiology and Speech Pathology
William S. Middleton Memorial Hospital
Madison, Wisconsin

Adjunct Professor, Department
of Communicative Disorders
University of Wisconsin
Madison, Wisconsin

Adjunct Professor, Department of Neurology
University of Wisconsin Medical School
Madison, Wisconsin

Leonard L. LaPointe, Ph.D.

Professor and Chair
Department of Speech and Hearing Science
Arizona State University
Tempe, Arizona

Consultant, Audiology and Speech Pathology
Veterans Administration Medical Center
Phoenix, Arizona

Consultant, Audiology and Speech Pathology
Veterans Administration Outpatient Clinic
Los Angeles, California

Robert T. Wertz, Ph.D.

Chief, Audiology and Speech Pathology
Veterans Administration Medical Center
Martinez, California

Adjunct Professor, Department of Neurology
University of California
Davis School of Medicine
Davis, California

pro·ed

8700 Shoal Creek Boulevard
Austin, Texas 78757

©1989 by PRO-ED, Inc.

Printed in the United States of America

Library of Congress Cataloging-in-Publication Data

Rosenbek, John C., 1940–
    Aphasia : a clinical approach / John Rosenbek, Leonard L.
LaPointe, Robert T. Wertz.
      p.   cm.
    Reprint. Originally published: Boston : Little, Brown, ©1989.
    Includes bibliographical references and index.
    ISBN 0-89079-270-4
    1. Aphasia. I. Lapointe, Leonard L. II. Wertz, Robert T.
III. Title.
    [DNLM: 1. Aphasia. WL 340.5 R813a 1989a]
RC425.R66 1989
616.85'52 — dc20
DLC
for Library of Congress   90-52763
                             CIP

pro·ed

8700 Shoal Creek Boulevard
Austin, Texas 78757

5 6 7 8 9 10   98 97 96 95

CONTENTS

Preface   vii

Dedication   ix

Chapter 1   An Introduction to Clinical Aphasiology   1

Chapter 2   Neurological Bases of Aphasia   15

Chapter 3   Nosology: What Aphasia Is and What It Is Not   34

Chapter 4   Appraisal, Diagnosis, and Prognosis   55

Chapter 5   Aphasia Treatment: Its Efficacy   104

Chapter 6   Principles in Clinical Aphasiology   131

Chapter 7   Treating Auditory Comprehension Deficit   142

Chapter 8   Acquired Dyslexia: Treating Reading Problems
             Associated with Aphasia   163

Chapter 9   Treating Naming   181

Chapter 10   Treating Aspects of Verbal Expression   211

Chapter 11   Treating Aphasic Writing Deficits   240

Chapter 12   In Recognition   276

References   277

Subject Index   305

PREFACE

We are clinical aphasiologists. When we decided to write this book, we agreed it would be about our work in a variety of university and hospital clinics during the 60 years of our combined practice and about clinical aphasiology in general. For us, aphasia is to be measured, judged, and treated, and if it is poked, prodded, and stared at under the harsh, sometimes unkind light of experimentation, the result should contain at least a meager dividend for the person with aphasia. People with aphasia are to be helped, not handled. This is not to denigrate research nor the professionals who do it. Research is at or near the heart of every chapter in this book, just as it is in each of our clinical sessions and publications. The difference between the research of neuropsychologists, neurolinguists, and psycholinguists, and that of clinical aphasiologists, including ourselves, however, is that the clinician's practice rather than the patient's aphasia is under the lights.

Clinical aphasiology is a speciality within speech–language pathology. Generalists in speech pathology try to know something about most things so they can treat a great many disorders. Clinical aphasiologists try to know a great deal about a few things so they can treat a few disorders. In Chapter 1, "An Introduction to Clinical Aphasiology," we describe the fields of knowledge we consider essential to the successful treatment of people with aphasia, namely, linguistics; medicine, especially behavioral neurology; experimental

design; business; and speech–language pathology. By specifying these areas of expertise, we have defined the boundaries of clinical aphasiology, at least for us.

The nervous system has been reviewed in the majority of books about aphasia, dysarthria, and dementia. Like the groom's grandparents at a wedding whom we meet early in the festivities and never thereafter, these reviews of the nervous system often appear early and then disappear. Our Chapter 2, "Neurological Bases of Aphasia," aspires to be different. Neuroanatomy and physiology appear in proportion to their importance to aphasia management, as does information on the nervous system's blood supply. In addition, major portions of the chapter are devoted to the neurosciences, such as brain imaging, that contribute to how people with aphasia are evaluated and treated.

The debate about whether aphasia is one entity or more than one has turned otherwise friendly professionals into adversaries since the first days of aphasia research. Chapter 3, "Nosology: What Aphasia Is and What It Is Not," is an essay written by neutrals more concerned with exploring the issues than with converting the opposition. In practice, the authors classify each aphasic patient when the patient allows it. They do so in the same way they listen to cello music—naturally but without any assumptions about the essential rightness of the activity.

Clinical aphasiology has never been able to

settle upon the essentials of an aphasia examination. New tests, analyses, and interpretations are ubiquitous. Woe unto the professional who argues for standardization. Creativity rather than consistency seems to be the sine qua non in aphasiology. Sometimes we find ourselves wondering how neurology ever did it. Perhaps, however, aphasiology really does have an aphasia examination, at least in the sense that most tests sample listening, speaking, reading, and writing; and most clinicians write reports describing performance in each of these modalities. Chapter 4, "Appraisal, Diagnosis, and Prognosis," is written as a guide to systematic aphasia testing and interpretation. One of the chapter's goals is to compare and contrast selected aphasia tests. A second is to provide a framework for creative test selection that will be useful to clinical aphasiologists and people with aphasia, none of whom have the time, energy, or money for exhaustive testing. Prognosis is included in the chapter as well, because testing is as much to predict the future as it is to describe the present.

Clinical aphasiologists, like all other members of the health care team, have been and continue to be challenged to demonstrate their worth. Like other team members, they have collected and continue to collect the group and within-subject data that contribute to that demonstration. Chapter 5, "Aphasia Treatment: Its Efficacy," begins with a summary of the extant data. This section makes it clear that the issue no longer is, Does aphasia therapy do good? The answer is, Of course. The issues are (1) Which treatments do the most good for the most aphasic people most efficiently? (2) When should treatment be changed or stopped? and (3) Which patients need to be spared treatment? Ways of confronting these and related issues and data from some of our own patients are also discussed in Chapter 5.

Courses in speech–language pathology almost universally have been long on concepts and short on methods. This may partly explain the popularity of continuing education in speech–language pathology and the lust for clinical relevance. We sympathize. Treatment cannot be atheoretical, but neither can it rest on arcane concepts. In Chapter 6, "Principles in Clinical Aphasiology," we summarize our attitudes about what aphasia management should be, and the criterion of clinical relevance is applied to each.

Chapters 7, 8, 9, 10, and 11 are about treatment. We have divided the chapters traditionally—auditory comprehension, reading, naming, other aspects of verbal expression, and writing. We recognize the wholeness of each patient's and even each clinic's treatment for aphasia. We also recognize that other writers separate treatment along other seams—semantics, syntax, phonology; auditory–verbal, auditory–graphic, auditory–gestural, visual–verbal. We created the pieces we did because when techniques from each chapter are ordered and combined the product is comfortable and—we hope—durable. The emphasis in these chapters is on specific methods, their experimental underpinnings, and on how to select and apply them. The short last chapter, Chapter 12, is an overview of the criteria that guided our writing.

DEDICATION

For Debra Shimon and John Tracy

For my parents, Lyell and Eileen (Dupont and Ossie) and
For my Uncle Jimmy, who lived with it all those years.

For the folks, Mary V. and Robert C.

1

AN INTRODUCTION TO
CLINICAL APHASIOLOGY

Speech-language pathologists specializing in the evaluation and management of aphasic speakers have been dubbed clinical aphasiologists (Porch, 1969), and their activity—clinical aphasiology. Generalists, trained in speech-language pathology but without special training in aphasiology, can treat aphasic speakers, but unless they are special people, not nearly as well as can clinical aphasiologists. The reasons are (1) the aphasias are not merely language disorders, (2) aphasic speakers are not merely people who talk worse than they once did, (3) assessment and diagnosis in aphasia are more than test administration and scoring, and (4) aphasia management is more than the selecting and ordering of language stimuli and the liberal slathering of emotional balm.

This chapter briefly surveys the disciplines whose activities and literature we think clinical aphasiologists should be familiar with. The survey is tendentious rather than inclusive. It was shaped by our clinical experience. The lessons of good teachers—our patients—provided that experience. They may have been better teachers than we were students. Fortunately, our educations will continue. For now, this is what we believe is important.

LINGUISTICS

Aphasia is, in part, a language disorder. Linguistics is, in part, the study of normal and abnormal language. It was inevitable that linguists would study aphasia, and beginning in the mid–twentieth century they flocked to the disorder. Lesser (1978) ably reviewed several decades of the linguistic literature. She stated, "Linguistics has achieved a revolution in aphasiology in two unobtrusive ways" (p. 23). The first way, she said, sprang from the linguistic notion "that language is not a uniform mass from which any sample is as good as any other of the same size" (p. 27). The second resulted from the idea "that language can be described in terms of different levels of organization" (p. 24). The levels she identified are phonology, syntax, semantics, and communication.

It must be humbling to have won a revolution unobtrusively. Revolutions and revolutionaries usually seize the airwaves and the headlines. Perhaps it is more accurate to say that linguistics has contributed to an evolution. What one calls the outcome, at least in this instance, however, is less important than that it occurred at all. Linguistics and aphasiology have both been enhanced by decades of research.

Practice in aphasiolgy has unquestionably been enriched by data and hypotheses from linguistics. The notion that language is not a uniform mass has given rise to greater sophistication in selection and ordering of test and treatment stimuli and to the measurement and interpretation of aphasic responses. Reliance upon a controlled array of linguistically sophisticated speaking tasks, including imitation of a variety of stimuli and spontaneous speaking in a variety of conditions—interview, picture description, narration, process description, at home—is now commonplace. Traditional, global judgments about the fluency of spontaneous speech and the difference between imitative and spontaneous speech are still being made. These judgments, however, are being supplemented by sophisticated (in some cases computer-based) analyses of discourse and of other characteristics of speech as it is used by people talking about and to each other.

What Lesser identified as language's "levels of organization" have been especially useful to clinical practice. Breakdown at different levels of organization helps to differentiate Alzheimer's disease, Broca's aphasia, and Wernicke's aphasia. Concepts from phonology have guided comparative studies of conduction aphasia, Broca's aphasia, and apraxia of speech. And so on.

Two subspecialties of linguistics with special interest in aphasia—psycholinguistics and neurolinguistics—have appeared. Green (1970) wrote an early summary of the influence psycholinguistics and aphasia have had on one another. Goodglass and Blumstein's book, *Psycholinguistics and Aphasia* (1973), features selections of the major studies. Lebrun (1976) wrote a short history of neurolinguistics, a term he said appeared originally in 1935, a long time after the appearance of the first aphasic person, but at about the same time as the first clinical aphasiologist's appearance. Collections of relevant neurolinguistic data appear in books edited by Whitaker and Whitaker (1976a, 1976b, 1977, 1979).

Aphasiology and aphasia have contributed to linguistics as well. Studying how language breaks down and how particular patients with particular sites of lesions communicate helps inform linguists about language's organization and neural substrates. Response to treatment can be equally informative.

Our own reliance upon linguistic data—admittedly filtered by our primarily clinical and process-oriented training and activity—is reflected throughout this book. One can treat aphasic people without linguistic information, but that treatment may be less sophisticated, orderly, insightful, and efficient than treatment influenced by such information.

BEHAVIORAL NEUROLOGY

Aphasia results from brain damage, and people with aphasia do best if their recovery begins in a hospital under a neurologist's care. Aphasiologists do best if they spend some time in a medical library and in a neurologist's company. The goal of that study time and companionship is not to become a junior-grade neurologist nor to learn enough jargon to hold up one end of a hallway conversation about the prospects of an individual with aphasia. The goal is knowledge about behavioral neurology which can then be melded with knowledge from a variety of other sources to form a durable basis for decisions about the appropriateness, timing, type, and expectation of aphasia evaluation and treatment. Virtually all aspects of behavioral neurology influence aphasiology.

MEDICAL DIAGNOSIS

Behavioral neurologists establish the etiology of each person's aphasia. Etiology can influence the onset, progress, and type of aphasia symptoms and is therefore of concern to the aphasiologist. Most of these influences are prosaic but worth exemplifying. The onset of symptoms is likely to be insidious in tumor and abrupt in stroke. Improvement is more likely after stroke than tumor, depending, of course, on the type of tumor and its response to medical/surgical management. These guidelines, coupled with a healthy skepticism about cherished notions, however, alert the aphasiologist to exceptions: the acute onset of aphasia when a tumor reaches a crucial size, the insidious onset of aphasia secondary to a rare degenerative process involving the perisylvian region of the left hemisphere (Mesulam, 1982), the staggered onset of aphasia in an evolving cerebrovascular accident (CVA).

Etiology may also govern the pattern of aphasic deficit. Symptoms are not the same regardless of whether the brain is pressed, starved, or torn. In our experience, for example, patients with tumors may have surprising differences in severity of deficit across the modalities. Extravagant differences among the modalities—reading, writing, listening, speaking—are less likely from a stroke unless it is confined to the distribution of either the anterior or posterior cerebral arteries. As but one more example, an aphasia resulting from trauma is likely to be accompanied by a greater variety of cognitive deficits than is an aphasia resulting from stroke.

OTHER SEQUELAE

Behavioral neurologists also know about the entire array of sequelae from brain injury. Benson (1979a) created a list of common neurobehavioral sequelae, which are displayed in Table 1-1.

The speech pathologist's goal in knowing about and noting such coexisting abnormalities is not to catalog them. Their presence or absence is important diagnostically, first of all, because aphasia and the aphasic person are lawful. This is not to deny that each aphasic person is unique. It is only to reaffirm our belief that the nonpareil diagnostician anticipates and recognizes patterns and unique appearances and responds to observations of total—not only speech-language—behavior. For example, the typical globally aphasic person has a right hemiplegia. Profound deficits across all language modalities in the absence of hemiplegia signal the possibility of an atypical lesion and perhaps an atypical future. Similarly, the Wernicke's aphasic person with an accompanying hemiplegia is atypical especially if the lesion is cortical. The

TABLE 1-1.
Neurobehavioral Sequelae of Brain Damage

Hemiplegia
Pseudobulbar palsy
Hemisensory loss
Visual field defect
Unilateral inattention
Disorders of extraocular movement
Seizures, epilepsy
Mutism, hypophonia
Dysarthria
Acquired stuttering
Scanning speech
Palilalia
Confusional state
Amnesia
Dementia
Gerstmann syndrome
Visual agnosia
Auditory agnosia
Tactile agnosia
Apraxia

future of such an aphasic person may be startling as well. Atypical appearing aphasic people require repeat and expanded evaluations and cautious predictions. Expectations are to be confirmed, and surprises are to be pursued.

Aphasia is also influenced by these other sequelae of brain damage. Depressed and happy people talk differently whether or not they are aphasic. Hurting and comfortable people do too. Diagnostically, the aphasiologist tries to separate the core of aphasia from the effects of these sequelae. Therapeutically, the clinician decides whether the sequelae are to be ignored, accommodated, or modified. We seldom ignore them because patient performance will not allow it. We usually accommodate them with our scheduling, stimulus selection and ordering, goals, and reinforcements. Sometimes we join with other members of the treatment team in modifying them.

TYPE AND EXPECTATIONS OF MEDICAL MANAGEMENT

Aphasiologists also benefit from knowing about the type and expectations of medical managements. This is not to imply that aphasiologists should memorize specific drugs, dosages, and effects, nor criteria for using one drug rather than another. It is to remind them that medications can influence alertness, mood, and performance; and that toxicity may make performance impossible. The *Physician's Desk Reference* (PDR) is an appropriate addition to the aphasiologist's library as is any general discussion of drug effects on behavior. We also suggest making it standard practice to read or inquire about each patient's medication list, the length of time each drug has been taken, and the present effectiveness or future expectations for these medications.

EPILEPSY

Because epilepsy is seldom discussed in the aphasiology literature and because it is a relatively common treatable consequence of brain damage, we have decided to feature it in this discussion. Epilepsy, medications for its control, and the adequacy of that control probably are critical influences, especially on how the aphasic patient appears and does in speech therapy. Epilepsy even in the absence

of an aphasia-producing lesion can result in disturbed language (McKeever, Holmes, & Russman, 1983). In addition, epilepsy may increase the aphasia in someone who is already aphasic. One of our patients attempted to write as soon after a seizure as he could lift a pencil. His attempts to describe how he felt immediately after and two hours after a seizure appear in Figure 1-1. A sentence from one of his letters to a politician written during a long seizure-free period appears in Figure 1-2. These samples suggest what long experience with this man confirmed: his language was better when his seizures were controlled.

Epilepsy or its management may have other influences as well. They may, for example, influence the amount and speed of recovery with aphasia. In addition, epileptic aphasic people whose seizures are controlled by medication may do better than those whose seizures are not. Aphasic people with certain kinds of seizures may do better than those with other kinds. Certain medications may be less threatening to language and language recovery than others. Subsequent group and single-case studies of aphasic people probably should

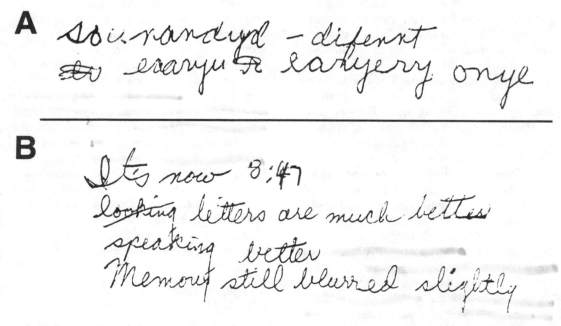

Figure 1-1. An aphasic person's attempt to write immediately after a seizure (A) and again after approximately two hours (B).

Such services should be equivalent to those recieved by others who have developmental disabilities -- namely, people with mental retardation, cerebral palsy, epilepsy and autism.

Figure 1-2. A typewritten example of the same patient's writing during a seizure-free period.

include data on their seizures (if any), on the adequacy of control, and on the medications responsible for that control. Complex-partial seizures may be a more important part of the history than being a 55 year old, right-handed man with eight years of education.

The basics of behavioral neurology are available in a variety of books. *Principles of Neurology* by Adams and Victor (1981) is typical of those intended for the practicing neurologist. A number of other references are complete enough to give the clinical aphasiologist a quick overview of a variety of topics and the insight to know when more complete or different references are advisable. These include *Neurology for the House Officer* (Weiner & Levitt, 1978), *Neurology for Non-Neurologists* (Wiederholt, 1982), and *Quick Reference to Clinical Neurology* (Gunderson, 1982).

NEUROSCIENCE

Somewhere there exists a person confident about neuroscience's rigorous definition. We must content ourselves with a popular definition. Neuroscience is the study of nervous system structures and functions. Anatomists, physiologists, chemists, bioengineers, psychologists, and a host of other professionals have contributed to neuroscience. The aphasiologist interested in a scholarly survey of selected hypotheses and data can read *Principles of Neural Science*, edited by Kandel and Schwartz (1981). Kandel and Schwartz acknowledged that neurology and psychiatry have profited from research in the neurosciences but that findings with no or only potential clinical relevance are equally valuable and intriguing. And so they are. The majority of clinical aphasiologists, however, are understandably most interested in those

hypotheses and data that improve their practices. A selected number of these will be surveyed here.

IMAGING THE BRAIN

LaPointe (1983) lamented the decadeslong search for an answer to the query, "Lesion, lesion, where's the lesion?" to the neglect of the equally important question, "How do we treat aphasia?" The search for lesions, if not its dominance over the search for treatments, was understandable. Neuroscientists, probably from the first day of their interest in central nervous system function, have pursued what some fear may be the mythological correlations of structures and functions. The threats to establishing these correlations reliably and validly, including the difficulty of collecting valid localization data, have been identified by Kertesz (1983). Early localization methods, including the neurological examination, the electroencephalogram, and the brain scan, were adequate within narrow limits. Modern methods of brain imaging—computerized tomography (CT), positron emission tomography (PET), magnetic resonance imaging (MRI)—although imperfect, do, as a group, expand the limits of adequacy. These methods, especially as they have contributed to aphasiology, have been ably reviewed by Metter and Hanson (1985) and are also outlined in Chapter 2. Other reviews that place modern imaging techniques in a historical context and describe particular methods have been done by Ackerman (1980), Oldendorf (1978), Brownell, Budinger, Lauterbur, and McGeer (1982), and Baker and colleagues (1985). Kertesz and his colleagues (Kertesz, Black, Nicholson, & Carr, 1987) updated the contribution of magnetic resonance imaging to the understanding of stroke.

In the 1970s, the CT scan provided scientists and clinicians alike with the best-yet views of normal and abnormal structures. The literature reporting correlations of lesion site and aphasic type exploded. In 1985, MRI's superiority over CT in identifying the presence and extent of structural lesions was "confirmed" in a large series at the Mayo Clinic (Baker et al., 1985). PET's images of disturbed metabolic activity made it a popular additional tool for studying aphasic people. Comparisons of structural lesions as measured by CT and MRI and of functional lesions as measured by PET were a natural development. CT and MRI images of the subcortical lesion suffered by an aphasic, dysarthric, apraxic, dysphagic man who made an excellent recovery of communication appear in Figure 1-3. A PET for the same patient (Figure 1-4) suggests that the

lesion was not limited to the subcortex but involved the cortex as well.

Metter has been leading the way in studies correlating images of structural and functional abnormality. At the conclusion of an early study, he and his colleagues (Metter et al., 1984) made the understandably cautious statement that "[18F]" FDG tomography and CT demonstrate different aspects of the pathophysiologic state of the brain following stroke... and... current anatomic theory based on structural damage needs modification to account for observed metabolic changes" (p. 205).

Researchers are listening. Two relatively new notions, that of the basal ganglia's importance to language comprehension-use and of the reality of one or more basal ganglia aphasias are already being revised. Olsen,

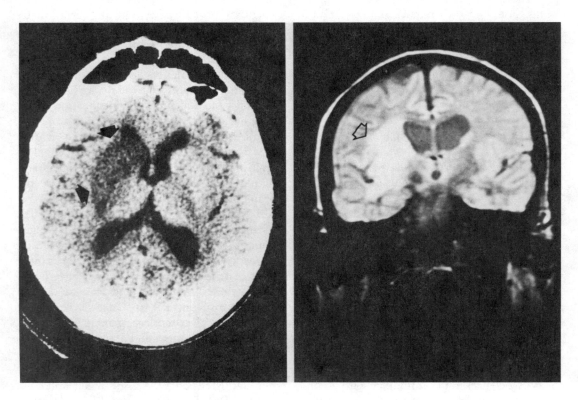

Figure 1-3. Cranial radiographic imaging of a 63-year-old man with a large subcortical hemispheric infarction in the left cerebral hemisphere. Plain CT imaging (A) reveals that the ischemic infarction involves the deep irrigation zone of the left internal carotid artery. An MRI (B) confirms the area of infarction and shows the cortex's structural integrity. (Courtesy of R. Levine, M.D.).

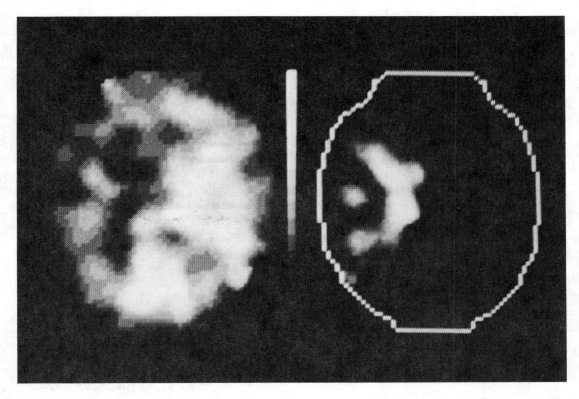

Figure 1-4. PET image of cerebral blood flow (A) for the same patient using fluoromethane shows a disturbance of both subcortical and cortical regions. An interhemispheric subtraction technique (B) highlights the area of blood flow (and presumed functional) deficit. (Courtesy of R. Levine, M.D.).

Bruhn, and Oberg (1986), for example, suggested that the aphasia following a "structural" lesion to the basal ganglia on the left actually results from "cortical hypoperfusion." PET data, in other words, suggest that structural lesions to the basal ganglia are accompanied by functional disruptions of cortical language areas in those patients whose aphasia persists.

Further revisions in anatomic theory are likely as better methods for localization appear, but only if researchers attend as carefully to their speech, language, and cognitive testing as they do to their localization procedures. A report by Fromm, Holland, Swindell, and Reinmuth (1985) is one possible model for such testing. Those authors think it is premature to identify a subcortical aphasia, primarily because they did careful and complete speech, language, and cognitive testing. Other researchers should be as thorough.

This book was written when the literature appeared—at least superficially—to offer no simple answer to the "lesion, lesion" question. We agree with Metter and Hanson (1985) that even now, however, it is safe to conclude that "language requires the interaction of a number of highly integrated systems of the brain. This interaction involves both hemispheres as well as cortical and subcortical structures" (p. 199). This conclusion, however tentative and general, looms large for clinical aphasiologists. Differences in the relative amounts of cortical and subcortical and left and right hemisphere involvement may influence (1) prognosis for recovery with aphasia, (2) type and underlying reason for the linguistic and cognitive deficits following brain damage, and (3) type and focus of communication therapy.

Speech pathologists need not fear advances in imaging nor threats to tired but assumed to be true notions. Better images must be accompanied by better clinical examination, including clinical speech-language examination. Without such data, increasingly sophisticated images will be increasingly hard to interpret. Exhaustive clinical examinations are essential if neuroradiologists are to separate normal and abnormal variance. Nor will images become the nonpareil or sole data bases for prognosis. They will not, that is, if aphasiologists stay abreast of developments in imaging and if they simultaneously develop a convincing case for the use of learning and retention data to support decisions not only about how long a patient is to be treated but about whether any speech-language treatment at all is to be administered. Finally, among the best tests of many notions in neuroscience is how particular patients respond to treatment. Just as clinicians need to read what scientists write, so too do scientists need to read the clinical literature.

ANATOMY AND PHYSIOLOGY

Clinical aphasiologists, if one can judge from the extant speech anatomy and physiology textbooks, learn more about the neuron than they do about the arcuate fasciculus, more about the corticospinal system than about the corticobulbar, and as much about the parietal bones as about the parietal lobes. Writers try, however. Broca's and Wernicke's areas are ineluctably mentioned, as are the carotid system, the ventricles, the supramarginal gyrus, and even the insula. A complication for readers, however, is that most anatomy and physiology for the aphasiologist is flat stuff unleavened by modern data from neuroscience and too meagerly spiced with clinical experience. Practicing clinicians require more and better nourishment if their daily activities are to be more than a technician's repetition of tasks. Certainly there are notions a plenty to leaven one's practice. Some were alluded to in the section on imaging; others will be described next and in Chapter 2.

Aphasiologists need to know more about the brain's vascular supply than is discussed in the typical textbook. Kertesz and Black (1985) stated, "Strokes do not occur randomly in different locations within the brain but rather in a predictable pattern that reflects the anatomy of the cerebral vasculature" (p. 83). Poeck (1983) suggested that types of aphasia are but useful "artifacts" of the nervous system's vascular supply.

The correlations of aphasia type with specific cortical divisions of the anterior (Rubens, 1976), middle (Albert, Goodglass, Helm, Rubens, & Alexander, 1981), and posterior cerebral arteries (Rosenbek, Robbins, & Levine, 1985) are being discussed with increasing frequency. Mohr and colleagues (1978) even suggested the middle superior artery syndrome as a synonym for Broca's aphasia. Likewise, the correlation of aphasia type with occlusion of a particular artery supplying subcortical structures has been attempted by any number of researchers. Typical of the reports are those by Wallesch and colleagues (1983), Tanridag and Kirshner (1985), and Mohr and colleagues (1978).

Nor are the typical textbooks helpful enough in describing modern notions of the neural substrates of speech and language, although recent books by Perkins and Kent (1986) and Love and Webb (1986) showed an awareness of the issues. Aphasiology, however, is not alone in its ignorance. Standard neurology textbooks are little better. It appears that speech pathology and medical students generally are provided a simple notion of neural organization for higher cortical functions that emphasizes centers and pathways. The comprehension center is Wernicke's area. The production center is Broca's area. The pathway connecting these two centers is the arcuate fasciculus. What works well for the cartographer works less well for the aphasiologist or the neurologist, however, If today's students write tomorrow's textbooks, alternatives to the traditional centers-pathways model will probably be featured.

Alternative models are already abundant. Luria (1970) posited that behavior results from the interaction of "analyzers" or functional units of cortical tissue. In Luria's scheme, the motor analyzer, for example, interacts with visual, tactile, auditory, and other analyzers to produce normal verbal expression. Brown (1972) and colleagues (Brown & Perecman, 1985) have elaborated a microgenetic view of neural organization. Brown and Perecman described it best: "1) language processing is conceived as an event that emerges over evolutionary sequential brain levels rather than across cortical areas; 2) language is processed simultaneously by complementary systems in the anterior and posterior division of the brain; and 3) pathways serve to maintain in phase different regions of the brain rather than to connect language units" (p. 56–57). The interaction of cognitive (Segalowitz, 1983) and affective (Kent, 1984) processes and the structures supporting them with language are also increasingly important influences on language research and treatment.

Until textbooks catch up with modern developments, good clinicians will have to rely on primary sources. We have tried to provide a sampling. The motivation for most clinicians to search out these and other sources is weak, however. Knowledge of vascularization is hard to gain and harder to retain. Myriad communicative disorders programs have survived even though their curricula are entirely uninfluenced by even a centers and pathways notion of cortical organization. One can treat aphasic people for years and be ignorant of arteries and even cortical organization. Hard work and robust concepts, however, help aphasiologists break free of technicianship's powerful pull. Aphasiologists who have never felt that pull must do everything possible to keep it that way. Those who have been pulled into the technician's orbit around some greater force, usually a physician's, must escape. Neuroscience, the data and the concepts, will help.

COGNITIVE SCIENCE

Gardner (1985) defined cognitive science as "a contemporary, empirically based effort to answer long-standing epistemological questions—particularly those concerned with the nature of knowledge, its components, its sources, its development, and its deployment (p. 6). Because of language's importance to knowledge's development and use, it is inevitable that cognitive scientists and aphasiologists brush against one another in the laboratory and in the literature. For political and clinical-academic reasons it is crucial that aphasiologists stay abreast of developments in the relatively new intramural discipline called cognitive science.

Some aphasiologists, of course, have long been aware of cognitive science. Wepman (1972, 1976), on the way toward a revised notion of aphasia therapeutics, raised the issue of language's relationship to thought. He concluded "that language usage is inextricably related to thought but is not identical with it, that language is a product of thought; that thought is man's highest mental process and language its maid servant" (1976, p. 13). Therefore aphasia, according to Wepman (1976), is a "cognitive-linguistic impairment" (p. 134) with certain forms of aphasia reflecting more cognitive than linguistic deficit and other forms of aphasia showing the reverse. He stated, "When cortical impairment produces an observable linguistic deficiency, the disturbance may be in the language structure and form of expression or it may be in the limitation of the underlying thought processes thereby affecting the linguistic expression" (p. 131). Girders to support the pragmatic therapies that predominated in aphasiology in the 1980s are clearly visible in Wepman's notions.

An American Speech-Language-Hearing Association position paper (1987) featured Neisser's (1967) description of cognition as involving "the processes by which sensory input is transformed, reduced, elaborated, stored, recovered, and used" (p. 4). Thus defined, language comprehension-use can be included alongside other cognitive processes such as attention, memory, and perception. In turn, these processes, including language comprehension-use, can be conceived of as acting on or depending on systems of images or mental representations, including language. Thus conceived, language and language comprehension-use, are part of cognition. A language disorder such as aphasia is, by definition, a cognitive disorder. McNeil's (1982) definition of aphasia as "a multimodality physiological inefficiency" (p. 693) and the research it is spawning (McNeil & Hagemen, 1979) make enlightening reading against this background. This portrayal of language's relationship to cognition is also especially felicitous for those who would legitimize the speech-language pathologist's role in cognitive rehabilitation. It is equally useful to those, like Martin (1981c), who would have aphasiologists spurn specific drills of specific linguistic stimuli.

Fodor's *The Modularity of Mind* (1983) is especially rich in ideas for the clinical aphasiologist. In Fodor's view, language comprehension-use is one of several modules, the others being perceptual, that serve cognitive activity. These modules "serve to get information about the world into a format appropriate for access by such central processes as mediate the fixation of belief" (p. 46). Fodor graciously permits us to consider the modules, including language comprehension-use, as vertical and the central processes as horizontal. He included among the characteristics of modules that they are domain specific, fast, and informationally encapsulated; exhibit characteristic patterns of impairment; and are subserved by specific neural substrates. He admitted to ignorance about most of the central, horizontal processes, but posited that they are none of those things. Gardner (1985) summarized and evaluated both modularity (like Fodor's) and centralist notions of cortical organization for the interested reader.

Fodor (1983) said that the "aphasias constitute patterned failures of functioning—i.e., they cannot be explained by mere quantitative decrements in global, horizontal capacities like memory, attention, or problem-solving" (p. 99). Even taken alone this idea offers much to savor. The monograph, however, contains more. For example, he described the mental lexicon as an hierarchically organized, integrated pattern. Once a word is elicited, other words in the pattern are also more accessible. The relative closeness of words in the lexicon and their position in various hierarchies can be predicted from certain criteria that he also specified. Despite or because of its simplicity, this notion may explain why priming or deblocking work and why aphasic errors are so often within-class substitutions.

At a time when the forces to put hyphens rather than commas between words (cognitive-linguistic rather than cognitive, linguistic) are so powerful, oversimplification, especially of ideas about the relationship of language and other higher cognitive functions, is a danger. Fodor's notion of the "cognitive impenetrability" of the language module offers a substantial counterforce. He argued that many language activities can occur quite independently of central, horizontal processes. If he is correct, one cannot help but wonder about the therapeutic uses of simple elicitation and facilitation, especially in chronic aphasia. Using cloze techniques, for example, may simply activate the damaged module without otherwise affecting it, and certainly without contributing to its repair. Lack of generalization is inevitable. Successful treatment, which is to say, treatment that makes a response, once elicited, more likely to reappear, may require activities that enhance cognitive penetration. Drill and slow, volitional rather than fast, automatic responses may be important. Problem-solving rather than some other kind of response may be crucial.

Salvatore (1982), Wertz (1986a), Gardner, Zurif, Berry, and Baker (1976), and Glass, Gazzaniga, and Premack (1973) are among the clinical scientists who have suggested that alternative symbols or symbol systems may be crucial to the treatment of some—usually severe—aphasic people. Gardner and colleagues (1976) called their system of geometric and representational forms VIC, for visual communication system. They reported that selected severely aphasic patients learned to use the system for at least limited communication; Wertz (1986a) also reported this. Fodor's modularity idea gives us another way to think about their findings (Hixon, personal communication, October 10, 1986). It may be that a system such as VIC accesses central processes through the visual module and makes communication possible. Because modules are independent, it can be hypothesized that verbal expression would be unchanged after such treatment. The data seem to support this hypothesis.

Programs such as VIC are not failures because speech is not improved. Their limited effects are predictable from the theory. Perhaps one of the soundest contributions of the modularity notion is that it supplies the traces to slow aphasiology's breakneck lunge toward generalization as the ultimate treatment goal. Generalization across types of performance may sometimes be impossible. Perhaps knowing when not to expect generalization is as important a part of the clinical art as is knowing how to measure it.

Regardless of one's specific definitions of models it is increasingly popular to say that cognition and communication are inextricably linked. Although focal brain damage and even more generalized dysfunction such as occurs in Alzheimer's disease may dissociate aspects of cognition from aspects of communication, aphasiologists cannot concentrate either their reading or their practice solely on language. The issue is not domain—who should do what kind of cognitive retraining. The issue is appropriate evaluation and treatment of brain damaged people, including those with aphasia, appropriateness that is likely to be enhanced by knowledge of developments in cognitive science.

Books by Fodor (1983) and Gardner (1985) are good introductions to specific and general notions. Brown (1977), Kreindler and Fradis (1968), and Bayles and Kaszniak (1987) are among those who have already made clinically useful translations of cognitive science's hypotheses and data into aphasiology's terms.

RESEARCH

Brookshire (1985) reviewed the aphasiology literature, and concluded that few clinical aphasiologists publish and that much of the aphasia literature has limited clinical relevance.

For those whose clinical spirits sink at such public exposés, Brookshire's review also offers buoyancy. He said disciplined, professional, creative clinical aphasiologists can change these conditions. He thinks many such practitioners are out there. We agree. We also think they have been out there for decades. Why then are there not more clinically relevant studies by more clinicians?

The question is a hard one. One answer may be that clinically relevant research is difficult to do reliably and validly. Fortunately, experienced clinicians such as McReynolds and Kearns (1983) have begun favoring the profession with book-length discussions of one type of research methodology—single-subject designs—within the reach of most aphasiologists, even those with more patients than time. The length of the required reach was further shortened by the appearance of three tutorial articles in the *Journal of Speech and Hearing Disorders* (Connell & Thompson, 1986; Kearns, 1986; McReynolds & Thompson, 1986). Useful data, too, are appearing, primarily in the *Proceedings of the Clinical Aphasiology Conference.* Those *Proceedings* are a valuable resource for clinicians interested in becoming clinical researchers and better practitioners. This mention of single-subject designs, however, is not meant to be an exclusive endorsement of that research for clinical aphasiologists. Wertz and Rosenbek (1978) advocated both single-case and group designs and highlighted strengths and contributions of both, contributions that are extensively reviewed in Chapter 5.

The relatively late arrival of a research technology that makes it easier for clinicians with more patients than time or colleague support to become clinical researchers is not the sole potential explanation for the scanty treatment literature, however. An equally or more important reason is that many clinical aphasiologists, because of their educations, are unprepared to complete research even with a single patient. The majority of clinic aphasiologists do not have a research degree nor much sophistication about how to ask and answer questions. This is not a criticism of practitioners. Many try research by writing a thesis on the way to the masters degree. The typical thesis, however, is more likely to hone one's telephone skills as part of the desperate attempt to find subjects than it is to develop one's research skills. It is, however, a lament about some training—the kind that produces technicians. One does not become a researcher solely by formulating questions and collecting and interpreting data, but those activities help. One must also come to cherish research for what it contributes to personal and professional growth. Many programs seem to feel that there is nurture enough in a range of coursework and a few hundred hours spent in a treatment suite. The leaders of such programs ought to be forced to subsist on such a meager diet.

A third answer may be that most clinical practitioners see research and clinical activities and the people doing them as separate. Siegel and Spradlin (1985) said, "The goals, the requirements, and the tastes for research often differ from those for therapy" (p. 229). That may be true for "therapy" but it is an exaggeration of the differences between research and clinical aphasiology. Clinical aphasiology's goals include the answering of questions, especially about each method's effectiveness. Clinical requirements dictate that practitioners be systematic. Finally, biting off a clinical question or two can leave a wonderful taste in one's mouth, especially the mouth of one whose palate has been cleansed by postdoctoral research.

Maybe clinicians do not contribute to the data base nor worry about its limitations because they assume that therapy is good and that clinical practice is a good thing to do. No procedure is inherently above suspicion, however. Indeed, treatments are as likely to be bad or neutral as to be good. Our nominee for the universal clinical assumption to be taught by all programs is this: untested treatments are immoral, therefore clinical practice must include clinical experimentation.

Clinical aphasiology need not be the domain solely of the clinical researcher, but it does need some researchers. It also needs a substantial majority of practitioners who can evaluate and use research even if they are not

contributing to it. In addition to literature already listed, potential and present clinical researchers may want to read Kent and Fair (1985), Kent (1985), and Barlow, Hayes, and Nelson (1984). Without an expanded data base, clinical aphasiology will eventually become a union of technicians punching someone else's clock.

ECONOMICS

Clinical aphasiologists need to understand the economics of health care. This discussion, however, is not about money for salaries, larger staffs, more instrumentation, or larger lengths of stay so much as it is about prognosis, new skills, and hard decisions. Health care is changing: clinical aphasiology must change too. What follows is our view of why and how.

In the 1970s, medical expenses threatened the economy of the United States. A variety of reimbursement models, including diagnosis related groups or DRGs which specified the resources available for the management of illnesses and their various complications, was one national response. Among the outcomes were (1) doctors began making fewer referrals, and (2) patients began spending a shorter time in acute care facilities. Money to support chronic care became increasingly tight as well. As this book was being written, aphasiologists, like all other members of the health care team, were having to consider adjustments in the way they practiced their profession. The following paragraphs are written in the future tense because they appeared before most adjustments had been made.

A critical change for the average aphasiologist will be to spend as much time and energy in ordering patients according to whether or not they can benefit from treatment as is presently spent devising strategies to evaluate and treat all aphasic patients. One way to accomplish such an ordering would be to divide patients among the three large groups that constitute the average caseload. One group profits from task-oriented drills and counseling. Another profits from stimulation and counseling. A third group can be spared treatment's rigors, and they and their families or other caregivers can be provided with guidance about how to make communication the best that it can be. These groups can be further divided. Some need only a little therapy of whatever sort and some need a lot. Some can be treated at home, some cannot; some can be treated by aides, some cannot.

Decreasing resources not only require tough decisions, they force a redefinition of treatment. In speech pathology, a traditional, albeit tacit, definition is that treatment is the orderly flow of clinician stimuli and patient response, usually in the privacy of a clinic suite. That definition is too narrow. For us, aphasia treatment is anything that enhances an aphasic person's communication and the aphasic person and families' adjustment to the language disability. This definition makes legitimate group and individual treatment, clinic and extra-clinic treatment, treatment by professionals and by people trained by professionals, counseling, education, and support. It makes spaced treatments, spaced follow-up visits, and short bursts of intensive treatment appropriate as well. It even allows us to change the way we talk about the previously mentioned subgroup three. That group is not denied treatment,it is only spared direct drills and stimulation.

Shrinking resources and increased restraints, therefore, do not dictate that treatments be denied. They do dictate that the full range of treatments be matched to the full range of patients. Money may talk; hard, humane decisions shout.

Clinicians also need to know about the economics of their practices. Naïveté about what it costs to turn on the lights in a speech clinic is too risky. Clinicians need to know how much it costs to see a patient for an hour. They need to know how to charge appropriately and collect accounts, and traverse the sometimes tricky courses to third party payments.

Accountable aphasiology is good aphasiology. Books for private practitioners, including one by Wood (1986), are good sources of information about the eocnomics of practice. We cannot wail at the darkness until we have done everything possible to keep the lights plugged in.

PSYCHOLOGY

To say that psychology is important to the aphasiologist is about as useful as saying music is important to the educated. Nonetheless, we are compelled to label this section psychology, because the term, despite, or because of, its inclusiveness, focuses practitioners on all the things aphasic people are and need. It also focuses practitioners on the aphasic family. The aphasiologist who treats only the language and only the patient is a tuneless whistler. A nervous flurry of pats and murmured reassurances about how it will all get better if we can only be strong are as deadening as a tape loop of an amateur rendition of "Pomp and Circumstance."

Eisenson (1984), Schuell, Jenkins, Jimenéz-Pabón (1964), and Benson (1979a) are among the writers to include in discussions of psychology in aphasiology. Most such published discussions contain little that is new to the experienced clinician. Aphasic patients and their families have been educating us for years. Nonetheless, the literature is mandatory reading because it is likely to include observations and data from groups that make the individual clinician's interpretations of the individual patient's depression or catastrophic reaction more confident. Pamphlets for the patient's family such as the one by Sarno (1983) make useful reading as well. Accounts by recovering aphasic people also intensify the portrait of what illness and aphasia produce. McKenzie Buck (1968) was an aphasic speech pathologist. Moss (1972) was a psychiatrist at the time of his stroke and was subsequently treated by Joseph Wepman. Moss wrote *Recovery with Aphasia*, a title, contrasting as it does with Wepman's *Recovery from Aphasia* (1951), that reveals both his spirit and insight. Nor did he exhaust his supply of either by coming up with the title—the text is equally rich. For example, he said, "Quite unintentionally they (neurosurgical residents) imparted the feeling that they were only interested in my neurological impairment, and didn't respond to me as a whole human being, one filled with psychological reaction at having suffered a catastrophic accident" (p. 4). Aphasiologists should never be guilty of the same charge.

A discussion of psychology—as we are tacitly defining the term here—so easily deteriorates into the self-evident and banal. This short discussion may as well; we hope not. Treating the aphasic person "as a whole human being" is the toughest part of the job. Some whole aphasic humans are obnoxious, hard to like, and a chore to treat. Some whole aphasic human beings have specific additional needs, some of which existed long before the aphasia, some of which arrived with it. Recognizing the duration of each need, the degree to which each will influence specific aphasia treatment procedures and outcomes, and the advisability of referral requires good vision. The clinical aphasiologist with vision blurred by the smoke of "We spend more time with them than anyone else. We know how to communicate with them. After all, no one else will handle these problems unless I do" will probably fail.

Knowledge of aphasiology's limits is among the lessons that training in psychology brings. It may also bring awareness that some aphasic people—even if they want to but cannot drive, or make love, or control their bitterness—require (even demand) only communication therapy from their aphasiologists. The ability to provide that therapy, and that therapy only, unless something more or something else is appropriate characterizes clinical competence and maturity.

Some parts of the aphasiologist's job can be done by a technician or speech aide. These include the parts that computers are increasingly being used to perform. The aphasic person who gets only those parts gets therapy, but therapy is not treatment. Treatment requires creativity, spirit, and scholarship. In this first chapter we have identified the kinds of knowledge we think aphasiologists need.

2

NEUROLOGICAL BASES
OF APHASIA

Many blood moons and generations passed before the brain was recognized with the awe it deserved. Early stories merely hinted at the connection between broken brains and broken behavior, but the strong interdependence was not appreciated for centuries. The first associations between nervous system and behavior were in animals. The ancient poet Homer described the rotary movements of a horse which had been wounded in the head by an arrow (McHenry, 1969). In another ancient reference, the Assyrian masterpiece *The Dying Lioness* (circa 750 B.C.) depicts the animal's spinal cord severed by arrows as the stricken creature crawled toward her tormentors, snarling and dragging her paralyzed hind limbs (McHenry, 1969).

At first, the emphasis was on the heart. The thumping pump was thought to be the seat of everything. Even such an astute thinker as Aristotle believed that the heart was the center of intelligence, of the emotions, and the origin of the nerves. To Aristotle, the brain was merely an organ for cooling the heat and fervor of the heart. Next, the pineal gland was physiologically beknighted. This tiny gland was thought to be the locus of the soul. To this day, the role of the pineal gland in humans is obscure, though certain visual functions have been assigned to it in salamanders, lizards, and lampreys.

Subsequently, though slowly, it became apparent that neither the heart nor the pineal gland but rather the brain was the master organizer and integrater of all human behavior. In the brain, the only organ capable of studying itself, we find not only the embodiment of all human failure, fear, bitterness, and irascibility, but also compassion, delight, fantasy, and love. Our brain permits the use of reason, the ability to plan what is to come, and to review the past and revel in it. It also allows us to become immersed in the learning and living of the moment. Most importantly, the brain enables us to engage in communication, the medium not only essential for the transaction of the daily trivialities of our business, but for the development and nurture of the intimate relationships with those who brush against us. When the brain and communication are compromised, quality of life can be profoundly altered; relationships deteriorate, delights seep away. All of these changes are *possible* with the catastrophe of brain damage, but not inevitable. Rehabilitation provides the hope and medium for turning things around.

For a long time, scientists accepted a few general principles in the quest for understanding the brain's operation, but many thought the challenge so formidable that the complicated organ might forever defy analysis. To

15

this day, neuroscience is viewed as a great challenge and the study of the brain-behavior relationship is viewed as one of the great scientific frontiers. But tremendous strides have been made, and it is vital that the clinical aphasiologist have an intimate appreciation of the brain and its function.

This chapter will not catalogue all that is known about the brain, but it will synthesize those bits of knowledge about structure and function that relate to aphasia and particularly relate to the task of clinical management of the disorder. The objective is not simply to learn enough to avoid looking dumb to other members of the health care team, but to learn enough to enable us to call upon and integrate principles of neurophysiology into our clinical management decisions. As a by-product of this knowledge, we should be able to communicate more efficiently with our professional colleagues. This chapter will provide the basics for clinical aphasiologists. Many other sources are available for immersion in neuroanatomy, the study of nervous system structure, and neurophysiology, the study of nervous system function.

FUNCTIONAL ORGANIZATION– COMPOSITION

The simplest and most stylized expression of a nervous system is a chain of structures necessary to transmit signals from the environment to the organism and from one part of the organism to another. The components needed in this chain of structures is a signal receiving unit, the *receptor*; a *conductor*, which conveys the signal from the receptor; the *synapse*, an interrupted union between nerve cell conductors (neurons); and the final unit, the *effector*, which activates a responding part, usually a muscle or organ (Minckler, 1972).

It seems contradictory to mention the miracles and complexities of the nervous system in one breath and then reduce it to the simplest expression of a signal-carrying chain of structures as depicted in Figure 2-1. Within this chain of structures, however, an intricacy emerges that to this day has defied complete understanding.

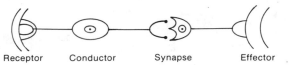

Receptor   Conductor   Synapse   Effector

Figure 2-1. Simplest version of a nervous system.

CENTRAL AND PERIPHERAL NERVOUS SYSTEMS

Very often, complex issues and systems must be segmented and separated into morphological units purely for the convenience of getting a more convenient grasp of the subject. So it is with the nervous system. Traditionally, it has been divided into two principal divisions, *central* and *peripheral*. Though variations are encountered in different books, the *central* nervous system (CNS) in this text includes the brain, or more accurately, the cerebrum, cerebellum, brain stem, and spinal cord plus a few structures located between the cerebrum and brain stem; the diencephalon (including everything with the name *thalamus*; namely, thalamus, hypothalamus, epithalamus, and subthalamus), and the basal ganglia (a group of structures including the caudate nucleus, globus pallidus, putamen, claustrum, and amygdala). A detailed understanding of the connections of the diencephalon and basal ganglia is not as important in aphasia as it is in understanding certain motor speech disorders and neurogenic disruptions of speech flow, though some language disruption has been attributed to these subcortical structures. Figure 2-2 is a simplified version, after Goldberg (1979), of the major portions of the CNS.

As Minkler (1972) emphasized, the central and peripheral nervous systems are structurally continuous and cannot function independently. The CNS is composed of the masses of nerve cells or neurons (perhaps 15 to 20 billion) that lie within the bony coverings of the skull and the vertebral canal. If all of these neurons were placed end to end, this chain would extend from the Ernest Hemingway Memorial in Key West, Florida to just outside the parking lot of the Oak Creek Tavern in Sedona, Arizona.

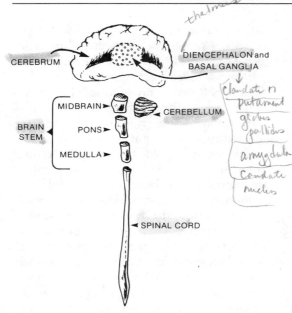

(handwritten annotations: thalmus; Caudate n, putament, globus pallidus, amygdala, Caudate nucleus)

CEREBRUM

DIENCEPHALON and BASAL GANGLIA

MIDBRAIN

CEREBELLUM

BRAIN STEM

PONS

MEDULLA

SPINAL CORD

Figure 2-2. The central nervous system (CNS). Adapted from Goldberg (1979).

The *peripheral* nervous system (PNS) is the collection of afferent neurons (impulses directed toward the CNS) and the receptors from which they conduct, plus the efferent neurons (impulses directed away from the CNS) and their associated effectors (muscles and glands). The PNS lies almost totally outside the skull and vertebral canal.

COMPOSITION

The brain itself (cerebrum) is a pinkish-white approximately three pound mass of nerve cells, glial cells (which support, separate, and may nourish nerve cells), arteries, and veins of the vascular (blood) system. Estimates vary, but the most frequently encountered guess is that the brain itself contains about 10 billion nerve cells. Twenty percent of the body's total blood supply can be found in the brain at any given moment, and the CNS is a voracious consumer of oxygen, requiring upward of 25 percent of the body's total oxygen requirement.

CENTRAL NERVOUS SYSTEM (CNS)

Neuroanatomy refers to nervous system structure and neurophysiology to nervous system function. As Minckler (1972) indicated,

structure and function are difficult to separate, and are frequently studied simultaneously. One way of viewing the nervous system is according to units that appear to serve distinctive functions, such as motor or sensory. This provides a basis for studying neuroanatomy as it relates to functional systems, such as vision, hearing, motor acts, and pain. These systems usually are segregated into specific anatomic portions that contribute to a particular function. Often these units are oriented to the long axis of the nervous system and are designated as *pathways* for a specific function. In addition to this longitudinally oriented division according to function, scholars have viewed the nervous system with a transverse or segmental orientation, but as Minckler (1972) pointed out, this orientation also carries some degree of functional distinction, as each higher segment adds greater and greater complexity to the neural activity. Other ways of dividing the nervous system are based on embryonic, developmental, gross anatomic and biochemical grounds.

PROTECTION: COVERINGS AND FLUID

COVERINGS. The brain and spinal cord need protection. Because they are so delicate and susceptible to jostling, they are afforded an ingenious, though not impenetrable, protection and support system. The brain is covered by three membranes, floated in a clear fluid, and encased in the bony vault of the skull. The most external covering, beneath the skull, is dense connective tissue called the *dura mater*. The innermost connective tissue membrane is the *pia mater*, a thin, see-through membrane which adheres to the surface of the brain and spinal cord and accurately follows every convolution and contour. In between these membranes is a delicate layer of fibers that form a weblike membrane called the *arachnoid*. Collectively, these coverings are called the *meninges*.

FLUID. The internal spaces within the brain are called the *ventricles*, and the subarachnoid spaces surrounding the brain and cord contain about 140 ml of cerebrospinal fluid (CSF). This fluid is a clear,

(handwritten at bottom: bathed)

colorless liquid composed mostly of water, but also containing small quantities of protein, glucose, potassium, and sodium chloride. In addition to supportive functions, CSF has been suggested to have certain nutritive functions as well that serve to remove waste products of neuronal metabolism (Carpenter, 1978). The composition and measured pressure of CSF plays an important role in the riddle of neurodiagnostics. Many times the neurological examination reports of aphasic patients will indicate the status of CSF.

CEREBRUM

Some writers have remarked on the resemblance of the nervous system to a tree (Cotman & McGaugh, 1980). The paired cranial and spinal nerves serve as the roots and lead to the trunk—the spinal cord and brain. The most dramatic feature of this tree-like structure is uppermost, the *cerebrum*. This is the highest communication center of all, and enables the rest of the body to be integrated and evaluated. Analysis of environmental features (both internal and external) and synthesis of response patterns are overseen with a complexity of detail that is unmatched in other parts of the nervous system. With flexibility, instantaneous speed, and reliability, signals are generated and evaluated in relation to both current and past environmental events. The most prominent features of the cerebrum are the right and left *cerebral hemispheres*, and these hemispheres are composed primarily of deeply grooved and convoluted gray matter known as the *cerebral cortex*. The striking convolutions and fissures of the cerebral cortex allow mammals to pile huge populations of neurons (10 to 15 billion in humans) in a very restricted space (Cotman & McGaugh, 1980). In addition to specialized sensorimotor functions, this great mass of cortical tissue at the very top of the nervous system tree permits the higher mental processes of learning, memory, thought, communication, music-making, calculation, daydreaming, planning, and the whole gamut of abstract functions enjoyed by the human species.

About 90 percent of the gray, wrinkled mantle that lies draped over the cerebrum is classified as neocortex, as it contains six layers of cells. The folds or convolutions are called *gyri* (singular: *gyrus*) and the intervening grooves are called *sulci* (singular; *sulcus*). This folding is for economy of space. Just as it is easier to get a large tablecloth into a small linen cabinet drawer if we fold and refold it, more cortex can be put in the small skull if it is folded and refolded (J. Menges, personal communication, 1983). About two-thirds of the cortex forms the walls of the sulci and fissures and therefore is hidden from view if one just peruses the brain's surface. Most of the major gyri are constant features of the cerebral surface from person to person, though individual variability dictates that differences may be noted even between the two hemispheres of the same brain. In some cases, the variability from brain to brain makes it difficult even to identify major landmarks.

By using three principal fissures and sulci that usually can be fairly reliably identified, the brain had been divided into four paired lobes, the *frontal, temporal, parietal,* and *occipital.* The gyri within these lobes can be identified by a numbering system derived by the German neuroscientist Karl Brodmann in 1909. Brodmann's system is an attempt to locate areas on the surface of the cortex more precisely than simply by lobe division (Figure 2-3).

The frontal lobe includes all of the cortex from the *central fissure* (fissure of Rolando) forward. The parietal lobe extends from the

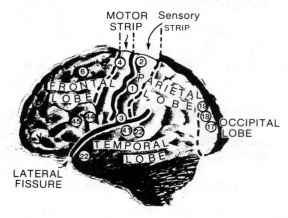

Figure 2-3. Lobes of the cerebral cortex with representative Brodmann's system numbers.

central fissure toward the back (posteriorly) to approximately the border of the posterior end of the *lateral fissure* (Sylvian fissure). The temporal lobe is lateral and ventral to the lateral fissure, whereas the occipital lobe is a poorly defined area, usually demarcated with imaginary lines, at the back of the brain. Generally speaking, the lobes subserve different functional roles, which will be considered in greater detail subsequently.

CONNECTIONS

The cortex is not an island. The gray matter of the cerebral center and much of the nervous system can be appreciated as a complex system of chains of interrelated neurons. The simplest chain, a two neuron arc, involves a connection (synapse) between a simple sensory or afferent fiber and a neuron whose axon becomes a motor or efferent neuron. However, interposed within these simple chains are any number of internuncial neurons. The interrelations of neurons involved in cortical activity can be vast and extremely complicated; the activity of any given cortical area depends on the integration of impulses arriving from the thalamus and other subcortical or lower levels, from other cortical areas, and from neurons in the immediate neighborhood (Peele, 1977).

CORTEX-TO-CORTEX CONNECTIONS

ASSOCIATION FIBERS. Fibers within the cortex may connect areas within the same or opposite hemisphere. These cortex-to-cortex connections may be limited to a course within the gray matter, or they may cross subcortical white matter. Intracortical association fibers may be short and may interconnect adjacent regions or simply run from sulcus to sulcus. These are called *U association fibers* (Peele, 1977). A good example of these are those that pass beneath the central fissure and connect the precentral (motor) and postcentral (sensory) gyri. Other association fibers are longer and connect remote parts of the same hemisphere or homologous regions of the two hemispheres by way of one of several major

hemispheric bridges or commissures. There are five or six major bundles of long unihemispheric association fibers, but the most important for those interested in speech and language functions may be the bundle called the *superior longitudinal* or *arcuate fasciculus*. This bundle runs just below the surface of the cortex and arches posteriorly from the lower portion of the frontal lobe and ends in the posterior superior temporal region. Many view it as an important association system that interconnects the sensory and motor speech areas (Wernicke's and Broca's areas). Figure 2-4 depicts the approximate course of the arcuate fasciculus.

COMMISSURE FIBERS. What the Golden Gate is to bridges, the *corpus callosum* is to nervous system commissures. Both are huge, important, and create impressive spans. This bundle of fibers can be viewed best on the medial side of the hemisphere of a brain sectioned through the large fissure (longitudinal) that separates the right and left hemispheres. Generally, it is divided into the *genu* (front portion), *rostrum* (middle) and *splenium* (posterior).

Both physiological and psychological so-called split-brain studies have aided in establishing not only the functions of the corpus callosum but also the nature of behavior when the left and right hemispheres are disconnected and isolated from each other's influence.

In addition to the corpus callosum, other

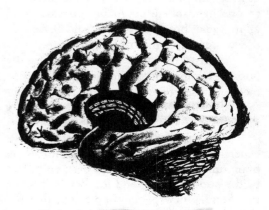

Figure 2-4. The arcuate fasciculus.

bridges between the hemispheres include the *anterior commissure* and the *hippocampal commissure.*

THE SPLIT BRAIN

During the 1940s when the authors of this book were schoolboys mastering the art of catching a ground ball without closing the eyes, the corpus callosum was still poorly understood and considered a puzzle. Neurologists and neurosurgeons generally were of the belief that this "great cerebral commissure" could be cut or destroyed without much harm (Gazzaniga & LeDoux, 1978).

Early experiments that disproved this attitude were conducted at the University of Chicago by Ronald Myers and Roger Sperry. Early work on splitting the brain was done on the visual systems of cats, with the result that discrimination trained to one half of the brain left the other side naïve to the previous training.

In 1960, this line of research was extended to humans when Dr. Joseph Bogen suggested that the spread of epilepsy could be controlled by splitting the corpus callosum. Bogen's first patient, W. J., was studied extensively and a variety of dramatic behavioral effects were observed.

One of the most striking behavioral aftereffects of brain bisection was the observation that exchange of information between the left and right hemispheres could be totally disrupted. This disruption affected the systems involved in vision, touch, proprioception, hearing, and smell; and information presented to one hemisphere could be processed and appreciated, but apparently would be outside the awareness of the other half-brain.

Because the left hemisphere usually possesses dominance for language and speech mechanisms, it became dramatically apparent that only stimuli projected to the left half-brain could be verbally described by patients.

The split-brain studies of the 1960s generated a great deal of popular interest in brain function. The topic has been embraced by the popular press, and for awhile it was a rare Sunday newspaper supplement that did not have an article on strategies for determining whether the reader was "right-brained" or "left-brained." The generalizations about hemispheric function usually associated the left hemisphere with such descriptors as "linguistic," "logical," "analytic," and viewed it as a processor of "temporal" or "sequential" stimuli. The right hemisphere, on the other hand, was associated with the more mystic qualities of "emotion," "intuition," "holistic analysis," and processed stimuli that were "nonverbal," "visual-spatial," "simultaneous," or "parallel" (Davis, 1983).

Recent work suggests that the accumulation of a list of specialized functions for each hemisphere may be an oversimplification of the complexity of hemispheric integration. Recent studies of regional cerebral flow (rCBF) have offered evidence that both hemispheres activate to some degree for both verbal and nonverbal tasks. Some stimuli or tasks produce much more activity on one side than the other but evidence mounts for the contention that the right and left hemispheres interact in a variety of ways depending on the task and/or idiosyncracies across individuals. Certainly, we are beyond the belief that for any given task one hemisphere is totally dominant while the other remains inhibited or silent. Time and further research will allow a better understanding of interhemispheric relationships and this information will be vital to explanations of the nature and course of recovery of aphasia. Additionally, it may well guide the development of treatment strategies that capitalize on utilization of the nondamaged hemisphere.

LEFT HEMISPHERE FUNCTIONS

The left hemisphere rose to prominence in the mid-1800s with the advocacy of the French scientists Bouillaud and Auburtin. They argued, presented evidence, and insisted that the frontal lobe of the left cerebral hemisphere was a special place; a place that subserved and controlled the production of speech. Paul Broca subsequently received most of the credit for focusing on the third frontal convolution as the "seat of articulate speech," and with the further elaboration of Karl Wernicke in 1874 of the association of "sensory" or auditory comprehension functions with the first temporal gyrus, the role of the left hemisphere in both the production and reception of language became secure (LaPointe, 1983).

Although controversy exists to this day on the nature of aphasia and on the existence of reliably identifiable aphasic syndromes (see Chapter 3), the process of anatomical mapping of the aphasias continued to gain refinement and followers. Geschwind (1970) probably is most responsible for advocating and perpetrating the modern view of localization of the aphasia syndromes. The Boston Aphasia Research Center's classification system is widely used and a host of researchers have shed light on the relationship between clusters of characteristics and site of neuropathology. Benson and his colleagues (1967) advanced the idea of consistent association between amount and degree of speech fluency and cerebral location of lesions. Through the use of brain scan technology, these researchers suggested a consistent relationship between halting, nonfluent speech and pre-Rolandic lesions, and between fluent, paraphasic speech and post-Rolandic damage.

The nonfluent aphasias were those of the Broca and transcortical motor varieties (correlated with left frontal lobe damage) and the fluent aphasias included those labeled Wernicke's, conduction, and transcortical sensory, which were associated with the left posterior regions of the hemisphere. Recent work with computerized tomography (CT) has reinforced some of these earlier ideas on the conformity of aphasia type to classical localizations (Naeser & Haywood, 1978). Damasio (1981) presented a cogent review of cerebral localization of the aphasia syndromes, whereas Darley's view (1982) lent perspective to the issue by presenting the opinions of those less taken with the idea that distinct aphasia types can be reliably associated with specific sites of cerebral damage.

Figure 2-5 outlines the broadly conceived "language areas" of the left hemisphere. Figure 2-6 associates some traditionally regarded important areas of the left cerebral hemisphere with certain aphasic syndromes.

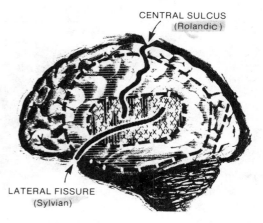

Figure 2-5. Left hemisphere and language function. Damage to area of "x's" almost invariably leads to aphasia. Damage to shaded area may or may not produce aphasia. Damage to outermost unshaded area is rarely asociated with aphasia. Adapted from Benson (1979).

SUBCORTICAL STRUCTURES AND APHASIA

The role of subcortical structures, and particularly the thalamus, has received a great deal of recent attention. Early work by Penfield and Roberts (1959) suggested that certain "subcortical integration" takes place via cortico-subcortical connections. Penfield and Roberts proposed that the functions of "all three cortical speech areas in man be coordinated by projections of each to parts of the thalamus, and that by means of these circuits the elaboration of speech is somehow carried out" (p. 208).

Subsequently, the possibility of a so-called thalamic aphasia was investigated by Ojemann (1975). Evidence that the thalamus plays a role in speech and language function was derived from studies of deficits after thalamic tumor, stereotaxic stimulation, precisely placed surgical lesions to remedy motor impairment, and electrical stimulation of portions of the left thalamus. Additional investigation and review of the thalamic role in aphasia has tempered some of the early conclusions. As Davis (1983) has pointed out, Luria (1977) concluded that the communication behavior resulting from thalamic lesions

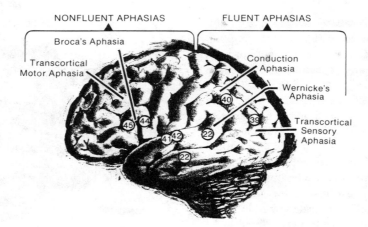

Figure 2-6. Lesion sites associated with principal types of aphasia (44-45 = Broca's area. 22 = Wernicke's area. 39 = angular gyrus. 40 = supramarginal gyrus. 41-42 = primary auditory cortex). Adapted from Damasio (1981).

is very different from aphasia. The processes attributed to the thalamus appear to be more basic than specific linguistic processes, and more related to attention, arousal, and vigilance.

Studies in the *Archives of Neurology* have described aphasia with predominantly subcortical lesion sites (Naeser et al., 1982; Damasio, Damasio, Rizzo, Varney, & Gersh, 1982). In the study by Naeser and her colleagues, nine cases of subcortical aphasia with lesions in the region of the internal capsule and putamen are described. Although these cases of capsular-putamen (C/P) subcortical aphasia shared certain features of Broca's and Wernicke's cortical aphasia syndromes, they did not completely resemble cases of either Broca's, Wernicke's, global, or thalamic aphasia in neurological findings, CT scan lesion sites, or language behavior.

Damasio and his colleagues (1982) described six cases of "atypical aphasia" which they suggested were associated with circumscribed nonhemorrhagic damage to the anterior limb of the internal capsule and of the striatum in the dominant hemisphere. None of the cases could be classified in terms of the classic cortical syndromes, nor did they correspond to the description of aphasia produced by hemorrhage in the putamen or thalamus. The Damasio study suggested that

there is a powerful association between aphasia and a well-circumscribed anatomic region: the anterior limb of the internal capsule and both the head of the caudate nucleus and the anterior aspect of the putamen. At this point, further research is needed to clarify those subcortical structures that are important in aphasia and those that have no role. The interdependence of cortical and subcortical areas and their relative importance to language function awaits further elucidation. There can be no doubt, however, that the pioneering work of Penfield and Roberts was a harbinger of what is now a mushrooming interest in the relationship of subcortical structures to language integrity.

NEUROPATHOLOGY AND EPIDEMIOLOGY: CAUSES AND NUMBERS

Unlike high country backpackers who carry small emergency packets of life-sustaining freeze-dried food in case they get in trouble, the CNS has no metabolic or nutritional reserves and is completely dependent on its blood supply for life-sustaining oxygen, glucose, and other metabolic sources of nutrition. If the blood supply to the brain is interrupted, consciousness is lost in about 10 seconds, and if no blood reaches the brain for about four minutes, permanent brain damage can occur. A variety of causes can result in this damage and this section outlines those that are major. This section also provides some statistics on neuropathology and aphasia. Numbers, cold facts, and droning recitations of figures sometimes can give the impression of dehumanization of the problems of a disorder. We take that risk in order to present a case for the scope of the problem of aphasia. Generally, we feel the cost, extent, and degree of suffering caused by this disorder is not fully appreciated in this country. We hope this relative neglect of a major health problem will be changed both within the health care community and with the general public.

CEREBROVASCULAR ACCIDENTS

The old term for cerebrovascular accident (CVA) was *apoplexy*. Today the term *stroke* is most used among lay persons and it is increasingly acceptable among health care personnel as well. CVA is associated with disease of the blood supply system or vascular tree within the cranium or skull. According to many sources, including Chusid (1979), the main types of spontaneous CVAs include (1) cerebral thrombosis, (2) cerebral hemorrhage, (3) cerebral embolism, and (4) subarachnoid hemorrhage.

Cerebral thrombosis is highly associated with arteriosclerosis (disease of the blood vessels) and is believed to follow clotting of the blood site where its flow is impeded by a bit of plaque on a blood vessel wall. Ischemia (reduction in nerve cell efficiency caused by reduced blood supply) and infarction (damage or death of brain tissue) in the area supplied may follow plugging or occlusion of a cerebral artery. A CVA may cause swelling (edema) of cerebral tissue, but after a few days the edema lessens. The ischemic brain tissue may undergo necrosis (cell death), and eventually necrotic brain tissue is liquified and dissolves away. A glial and vascular scar usually replace the destroyed brain tissue (Chusid, 1979).

Two primary suppliers of nourishment to the brain are the carotid and vertebral arterial systems. The vertebral system supplies primarily the deep cortical structures and areas of the brain stem and the internal carotid system branches into the cerebral arteries that nourish the cerebral hemispheres. One of these paired branches, the middle cerebral artery serves most of the dorsolateral surface of the hemisphere and if affected on the dominant side, is most frequently associated with aphasia.

Cerebral hemorrhage into the brain or meninges is caused by a bursting or rupture of one of the cerebral blood vessels. Other causes of hemorrhage include the bursting of aneurysms (ballooning or bulging of weakened vessel wall) or direct trauma to portions of the arterial system. The blood clot produced by hemorrhage destroys and replaces adjacent brain tissue, and neighboring areas of brain tissue usually are softened. The most common site for simple hemorrhages is the basal ganglia with extension into the internal capsule. These deep, less severe hemorrhages may be responsible for some of the so-called subcortical aphasia syndromes that have attracted so much recent attention. Hemorrhage produces a high mortality rate. However, if death does not occur, eventually the blood is replaced by connective tissue and glial cells, producing a shrunken, fluid-filled area (Chusid, 1979).

Cerebral embolism is the plugging of a cerebral vessel by a small piece of blood clot, tumor, fat, air, or clump of bacteria. An embolism is merely a thrombosis that traveled and eventually lodged in an area too small for its passage. Most cerebral emboli are noninfectious, although the emboli of patients with lung infections or infectious cardiac disease may contain bacteria that then lead to encephalitis, abscess, or meningitis.

The most common source of cerebral embolism is heart disease, but "throwing a clot" can occur from thrombotic or supportive conditions from the lungs, legs, or any other part of the body. Emboli to the brain frequently occur in series, and there may be simultaneous embolic infarcts to lungs, spleen, kidneys, and other viscera and peripheral organs.

CLINICAL SIGNS AND SYMPTOMS

The overall clinical picture of strokes of various causes can be similar. Onset is usually sudden, and maximum intensity is reached within a few hours. Headache is common and stupor or coma may be present during the very early phase. Vomiting and convulsions may occur as well as focal neurological signs such as paralysis, sensory loss, confusion, memory loss, or speech-language abnormalities. The onset of CVA may cause the person to fall to the ground or the floor, and lie inert as if in deep sleep with flushed face, altered respiration, full and slow pulse, and one arm and leg usually flaccid. Slighter strokes may cause slight derangement of speech or language, thought, motion, sensation, or vision. (Chusid, 1979).

Blockage or occlusion of the main trunk of the middle cerebral artery (MCA) may cause coma, contralateral flaccid hemiplegia, hemisensory loss, and profound aphasia affecting both comprehension and production of language. Damage or blockage to the various branches may result in a variety of aphasic syndromes. Generally, if anterior branches are involved speech will be nonfluent and agrammatic with phonological impairment and relatively good comprehension. If the posterior branches are involved, impaired comprehension, reading deficit, fluent-empty speech, and verbal paraphasias are more likely to occur.

The posterior cerebral artery nourishes the posterior pole and the posterior one-third of the medial portion of the cerebral hemisphere and the lower portion of the temporal lobe. Occlusion of the main trunk or branches of this artery may cause contralateral hemiplegia (usually transient), sensory loss on the opposite side, contralateral homonymous hemianopsia (visual field defect in the right quandrant or half of each eye), and fluent aphasia with comprehension impairment, if the dominant hemisphere is involved. Visual agnosia and reading deficit, sometimes with the dramatic syndrome of alexia without agraphia, that rare condition where writing is spared but reading comprehension is affected, may occur. In alexia without agraphia a patient may be able to write and be unable to read what was just written.

CEREBRAL TRAUMA

Rocks, ski poles, knives, shrapnel, bullets, car dashboards, bridge abutments, guardrails, stairs, and the ground are all capable of inflicting craniocerebral traumatic injuries. Closed head injuries (CHI) are those that do not penetrate, fracture, or displace the skull. Open or penetrating head injuries involve fracture and penetration of the skull along with underlying cerebral damage. Cerebral tissue may be damaged by contusion or bruising either at the direct point of impact or directly contralateral to the zone of impact (contrecoup injury). Because of the nature of the surrounding skull bone configurations, contusions frequently occur along the base of the posterior frontal lobes and the adjacent temporal lobe tips.

Brain laceration (a tearing of the substance of the brain) usually occurs at the point of greatest force. Lacerations at the base of the brain usually result in death in a short time. Lacerations of the brain and meninges may cause extensive intracranial hemorrhage, leading to necrosis (cell death) of areas of the cortex, subcortical white matter, or brain stem.

Clinical signs and symptoms include loss of consciousness, lasting from seconds in mild brain concussion to days or weeks with extensive damage. After regaining consciousness, residual impairment is related to the severity and site of brain injury. Hemiplegia, aphasia, cranial nerve pathologies, and other focal neurological signs may be evident, depending on nature and extent of damage. Loss of memory for the period immediately after recovery of consciousness (posttraumatic amnesia) is common, as is memory loss for the period immediately preceding the injury (pretraumatic or retrograde amnesia).

In the recovery phase, and sometimes persisting for months after the injury, the injured person may complain of headaches, dizziness, and personality changes (posttraumatic cerebral syndrome) (Chusid, 1979).

The speech-language pathologist charged with evaluation of a person with traumatic cerebral injury has a difficult task that must be meticulously undertaken, because such an array of language, motor speech, cognitive, perceptual, personality, memory, and other deficits may be seen.

OTHER NEUROPATHOLOGIES

The nervous system is susceptible to a variety of other agents or diseases that can cause aphasia and associated behavioral deficits. Tumors, both benign and cancerous, can begin in the brain. Cancerous neoplasms or tumors also can result from infiltration of the CNS by cancerous cells from primary sites in other parts of the body. This process of movement of cancerous growth from one site to another is called *metastasis*.

As tumors grow, progressively greater destruction or displacement of healthy brain tissue may occur, causing focal neurological signs that involve the hemispheres, brain stem, or cranial nerves. Medical treatment includes surgical removal followed frequently by x-ray irradiation, and the prognosis for recovery varies widely depending on individual differences in tumor type, site, and size.

In addition to CVAs, trauma, and tumors, the CNS is vulnerable to other pathologies, including poisonous or toxic damage, and infectious diseases, such as meningitis, viral encephalitis, brain abscess, and less frequently, neurosyphilis.

Additionally, an array of degenerative diseases may attack the nervous system. In these conditions the damage is usually diffuse, but focal deficits such as aphasia may be present even if masked by a more generalized dementia or intellectual and memory deterioration, as seen in Alzheimer's disease or Huntington's chorea. Another diffuse, chronic, slowly progressive disorder is multiple sclerosis, usually classified as a demyelinating disease. Aphasia is usually not a part of the picture in multiple sclerosis, which is characterized by fluctuating periods of exacerbation and remission, but nystagmus, motor speech impairment, weakness, ataxia, and tremor may be present (Chusid, 1979).

EPIDEMIOLOGY: SCOPE OF THE PROBLEM

The most frequent cause of damage to the nervous system is stroke, or cerebrovascular accident (CVA). The term stroke is well chosen, for in most cases an individual is suddenly struck down, as if by lightning, and may be robbed of movement, memory, and meaning. Some episodes are not sudden, however, and signs and symptoms may come on gradually in stairstep fashion in an evolving stroke or CVA-in-evolution. Others may be tiny, with fast, complete recovery as in transient ischemic attacks (TIAs).

The completed stroke constitutes a major cause of death and disability, especially among the elderly. Though there is some indication in recent years of a reduction in stroke incidence, it still ranks as the third leading cause of death in the United States, following coronary heart disease (CHD) and cancer. The relationship between age and stroke is logarithmic and only 20 percent occur in persons under age 65.

There are approximately 500,000 new strokes each year in the United States and strokes account for about 11 percent of total mortality (Wolf, Dawber, Thomas, Colton, & Kannel, 1977). Table 2-1 is adapted from

TABLE 2-1.
Recovery Levels for 100 Survivors of Acute Stroke.

For every 100 survivors of stroke:	10 return to work virtually without impairment
	40 retain mild residual disability
	40 remain so disabled they require special service
	10 will need institutional care

information presented by Sahs, Hartman, and Aronson (1979), and provides a rough guide to the distribution of severity of disability.

Incidence and prevalence figures on aphasia are difficult to come by and disparate reports are common in the literature. With the high incidence of central nervous system pathology (1 of every 70 persons in the general population has some form of neurological disease, and 1 in 130 of the general population is affected with neuropathology each year [Kurtzke & Kurland, 1973]), and particularly with the high incidence of middle cerebral artery stroke (which affects the language areas if it occurs in the dominant cerebral hemisphere), we can appreciate that aphasia is no small problem. To get some idea of the number of aphasic individuals in the United States, the following figures have been extrapolated from data presented by Sahs and colleagues (1979).

In each sample of 1,000,000 persons in the United States, we could expect 2,500 to experience stroke each year. Of these new strokes, approximately 1,175 will die within one month. In this sample of 1,000,000 people, one would find 12,500 living persons who suffered stroke sometime in the past. Therefore, based on a population total of 230,000,000 people in the United States, we could expect 2,875,000 living persons who had suffered a stroke. If we assume equal susceptibility of each of the cerebral hemispheres, the 1,437,500 people would be alive with left cerebral hemisphere damage. Not all who suffer left hemisphere damage become aphasic, so if we assume that 80 percent of left hemisphere damaged persons suffer residual aphasia, then we could extrapolate a figure of 1,150,000 living aphasic persons in the United States.

Another way of viewing the epidemiology of the problem is to attempt to determine the number of expected new cases of aphasia each year. These figures, too, are extrapolated from statistics by Sahs and colleagues (1979). If the number of new strokes per million population is 2,500, then for 230,000,000 people in the United States we could expect 270,250 new strokes per year. Again assuming equal vulnerability of the hemispheres, that would result in 135,125 new left hemisphere damaged patients per year. Because we assumed that 80 percent of these would be left with residual aphasia, that would leave 108,000 new aphasic patients per year in the United States.

These figures are extrapolated and not based on an actual census, so their validity awaits epidemiological verification. What is readily apparent, though, is that the problem of aphasia is widespread and has the potential to affect nearly every family. When the cold statistics are translated to the suffering of mothers and grandfathers and friends, the statistics lose their chill and can be appreciated on a level we are all better able to appreciate. Aphasia is a horrible, costly, widespread health problem, twisting the lives of millions of Americans, and it needs as much support, research, and rehabilitation effort as we can muster.

NEURODIAGNOSTICS AND APHASIA

The search for the telltale lesion has been a consuming passion for aphasiologists since Broca's time. Localization of damage in the CNS was and is driven primarily by the clinical need to find and treat diseases and neuropathologies. Early on, scientists realized that an additional impetus for studying loss of function and location of damage would be the furthering of our understanding of neuroanatomic correlates of behavior. Our knowledge of aphasia and its relation to portions of the brain that might be affected has relied for over 100 years on a handful of well-established techniques.

Kertesz (1983) compiled a useful review of localization of brain damage and loss of function. He traced the progress made over the years by the only means available to reveal brain-behavioral relationships. Autopsy findings, observation of loss following head injuries, neurosurgical resection, and cortical stimulation during surgery provided most of what we knew about cerebral localization until relatively recently. Advances in brain imaging technology greatly expanded clinical neuroscience in the 1970s, and breakthroughs in and refinements of neurodiagnostic procedures nearly outstrip our ability to keep up with them.

At the Clinical Aphasiology Conference in 1984, a symposium was convened on recent advances in the application of special neurodiagnostic techniques to aphasiology. Papers were presented on computerized axial tomography (Rosenbek & Shimon, 1984), nuclear magnetic resonance (Duffy, 1984), positron emission tomography (Hanson, Metter, Riege, Kuhl, & Phelps, 1984), cerebral blood flow (Horner & Chacko, 1984), and cortical evoked potentials (Selinger, 1984). A risk in writing about these techniques is that the state of the art may change even before the daisy wheel is silent, but a summary of basic methodology, advantages and limitations, and applications to aphasia is essential for those who would treat people with aphasia.

EEG AND EVOKED POTENTIALS

One of the oldest objective methods of measuring brain activity is the electro-encephalogram (EEG). This technique uses surface electrodes to pick up tiny electrical discharges generated by neurons. Distinctive wave patterns can be plotted for various locations and for a variety of activities, and areas of pathology generally result in a slowing of the expected wave frequency. Remote effects and movement can introduce artifacts into the EEG signal that make interpretation difficult.

The use of the signal averaging computer advanced this technique and allowed measurement of the brain's response to external sensory stimuli while averaging or negating the effect of random electrical activity. Both cortical and brain stem evoked potentials have been studied extensively, and a vast literature exists using evoked potentials to demonstrate abnormal sensory systems, lesion localization, and the distribution of disease processes.

As Selinger (1984) indicated, only a few studies have used the event-related potential (ERP) in investigations of aphasia. Most studies have attempted to relate ERPs to recovery or severity factors. Few used standardized methods for either aphasia measurement

or classification and, as stated by Selinger (1984), most studies used discrete stimuli, some of which had no relation to language. With sophisticated technology, some of the mysteries of hemispheric involvement in recovery may be clarified. Selinger (1982), for example, compared electrophysiological measures and aphasia test scores and concluded that a relationship existed between greater severity of aphasia and right hemisphere processing of language tasks.

ISOTOPE SCANNING

Isotope brain scans are widely available and have been in use for decades. Certain neuropathologies are susceptible to the "uptake" of radioisotopes, and it became apparent that tumors and vascular lesions could be outlined clearly if the procedure was carried out at the proper time. Acute lesions can be differentiated from chronic lesions, and the traditional "brain scan" remains superior to other methods for the detection of certain conditions (Kertesz, 1983). Although some see the traditional brain scan procedure as somewhat of a biplane in a space-age era, a continuing advantage is its availability in nearly every hospital and its relatively low cost.

COMPUTERIZED AXIAL TOMOGRAPHY   *density*

When it skyrocketed upon the scene of neurodiagnostics in the 1970s, many heralded computerized axial tomography as the most significant breakthrough in the history of medical science. At first, computerized axial tomography was referred to as a "CAT scan" but this terminology was soon dropped, perhaps because of feline or animal research connotations. CT scan is the current abbreviated term, and the procedure has lived up to a good deal of the early predictions, with some revision and tempering of early enthusiasm. CT scans utilize the computer and x-ray technology. A rotating x-ray beam circles the head rapidly along with a paired detector, and densities of the tissues being imaged are calculated by the computer. Typical CT scans

Early shows seizure when you have me

image the brain in 9 to 18 slices (8 to 100 mm thick) at a 15-degree transverse angle. Contrast enhancement with a radio-opaque material increases visualization of vascular structures. CT scans can show lesions earlier than radioisotope scans, but the early changes tend to be not as clear as those taken after three weeks. Hemorrhages and brain tumors are dramatically apparent on CT scans. Old infarcts are quite distinct with easily viewed margins, and an accurate measure of atrophy also can be seen readily (Kertesz, 1983). As Rosenbek and Shimon (1984) indicated, CT scans are not infallible, in that small lesions may go undetected, and large lesions may not be noticed if the scan is not taken at the proper time. In aphasia, the CT scan has been used to study locus of lesion and aphasia type (Hayward, Naeser, & Zatz, 1977), relative integrity of the right and left hemispheres (Naeser et al., 1981), extent of lesion in Broca's aphasia (Mazzocchi & Vignolo, 1979; Mohr et al., 1978), global aphasia (Poeck, DeBleser, & Graf von Keyserlingk, 1984), and evolution of the disorder (Selnes, Knopman, Niccum, Rubens, & Larson, 1983; Yarnell, Monroe, & Sobel, 1976). A comprehensive and more detailed review of the clinical study of aphasia using CT scan has been compiled by Rosenbek and Shimon (1984).

CEREBRAL BLOOD FLOW

Cerebral blood flow (CBF) research has been carried out since the 1940s, but in the last 15 years it has emerged as a powerful technique for advancing our understanding of neurobehavior. Because CBF reflects neuronal activity as a function of oxygen utilization, and blood flow varies across brain areas and tasks, it has allowed study of the activation of specific brain waves during selected tasks (speech, comprehension, reading, etc.) in both neurologically normal and brain damaged subjects. Horner and Chacko (1984) reviewed over 100 studies and presented a synthesis of this research along with 47 selected abstracts on CBF as it relates to normal brain-behavior relationships, stroke, and aphasia.

In CBF studies, a radioisotope (Xenon 133 is a popular choice) must be infused or

injected into the vascular system of the brain. Either injection or inhalation may be used, with inhalation used most frequently, as it is distributed to both hemispheres at the same time, is noninvasive, and clears rapidly. An apparatus must be positioned around the subject's head that will detect and monitor radiation uptake in the blood flow to the brain. Amount of blood flow is then measured and displayed graphically. Blood flow is measured in milliliter/gram/minute and typically is displayed by a computerized visual system that produces different colors for different blood flow rates.

Cerebral blood flow studies, particularly regional cerebral blood flow (rCBF) research, has contributed a great deal to our understanding of brain-behavior relationships, especially in the area of hemispheric activation during specific activities. Horner and Chacko (1984) summarized the limitations of this technique, related to: (1) amount of Xenon 133 inhaled; (2) artifacts caused by recirculation of the radioisotope; (3) contamination outside of the brain; and (4) methodological, task, and subject variables.

Despite these disadvantages, CBF retains great potential for advancing what we know about aphasia and the brain, especially in the area of the relative effects of different treatment approaches.

POSITRON EMISSION TOMOGRAPHY

The complicated methodology of positron emission tomography (PET) depends on the measurement of oxygen and glucose metabolism by utilizing a computerized tomographic scanner that is able to detect influences of a positron emitting isotope on metabolism. Brain metabolic activity is primarily attributed to neuronal metabolic demands. Changes in neuronal function correspond to changes in local cerebral metabolic rates of glucose (LCMRGlc). PET scans, then, reflect functional changes in the brain as measured by changes in the rate of glucose metabolism.

The major advantage of PET is that both nonneurologically damaged subjects and those with neurological disease can be studied. The

A phon... what's function... (handwritten)

major disadvantages include enormous expense, very limited availability, and artifacts created by unrelated cerebral activity (Kertesz, 1983). In speculating about the future, Hanson and colleages (1984), who have produced a good deal of research on PET with aphasic subjects, suggested that positron emission tomography should aid in the clinical management of persons with aphasia. Hanson and his colleagues predicted that the "black box" of the brain will become much less opaque, and the technique will allow us to learn much more about how the brain is reorganized following injury.

MAGNETIC RESONANCE IMAGING (MRI)

Magnetic resonance imaging (MRI) is the latest imaging modality, and some have remarked that it shows greater promise than all other techniques for the accurate localization of brain lesions without invasive radiation (Kertesz, 1983). MRI used to be referred to as NMR (nuclear magnetic resonance), but apparently the connotations of "nuclear" were sufficient to signal a terminological change as the technique became increasingly applied to clinical objectives. This complex technique uses the inherent magnetic properties of spinning nuclei of atoms in the brain. The structure to be imaged (the head) is placed within the field of a large magnet and shortwave radio frequency pulses are applied to produce a resonance signal that can be measured and computerized (Kertesz, 1983).

Various pulse sequences have been used to look at the metabolic and molecular environment of different regions of the brain. One pulse sequence is called *inversion recovery* and with it, differences in white and gray matter of the brain are emphasized to provide sharp anatomical detail. The second pulse sequence, *spin echo*, has been used to detect edema and other changes associated with disease or lesions (Kertesz, 1983).

In a comprehensive summary, Duffy (1984) traced the advantages and disadvantages of MRI and suggested several areas of potential future applications to our understanding of neurogenic disorders of com-

munication. Studies that apply MRI to problems of stroke and aphasia are beginning to appear in the literature, and no doubt significant conceptual revision about certain aspects of aphasia will ensue. For example, in a study of MRI and aphasia (DeWitt, Grek, Buoanno, Levine, & Kistler, 1985), an aphasic patient was described in which CT scan suggested that the lesion was entirely subcortical. MRI, however, demonstrated the considerable size of the lesion, including significant infiltration into the cortex. This case indicates that the CT scan may be insufficient for defining actual lesion extent, and the MRI may show that apparently subcortical lesions may actually involve the cortex.

In another clinical study of 1,000 consecutive patients examined at the Mayo Clinic, MRI was concluded to be equal or superior to other imaging techniques in most cases (Baker et al., 1985). Certain cerebral infarcts were well displayed at a considerably earlier time after damage by MRI than by CT scan; however, CT scan was more accurate than MRI in revealing fresh blood.

MRI and the other neurodiagnostic and brain imaging techniques described in this section have a vast potential for advancing what we know about aphasia and particularly about how to best treat the person with aphasia. In the future, reports of the results of sophisticated imaging strategies no doubt will be used on a routine basis by the aphasiologist to guide selection of treatment candidates to help determine type and duration of treatment, and to confirm that maximal physiological recovery has been reached.

GLOSSARY OF TERMS IN NEUROANATOMY AND NEUROPHYSIOLOGY

AMYGDALA (L. almond) Amygdaloid nucleus in the temporal lobe of the cerebral hemisphere.

Key: L. = Latin, GR. = Greek

ARACHNOID (GR. resembling spider's web) The delicate meningeal layer forming the outer boundary of the subarachnoid space.

ASTEREOGNOSIS (GR. a, neg + *stereos*, solid + *gnosis*, knowledge) Loss of ability to recognize objects or appreciate their form by touching or feeling them.

ASYNERGY (GR. a, neg + *syn*, with + *ergon*, work) Disturbance of the proper association in the contraction of muscles which assures that the different components of an act follow in proper sequence, at the proper moment, and of the proper degree, so that the act is executed accurately.

ATAXIA (GR. a, neg + *taxis*, order) A loss of muscle coordination with irregularity of muscle action.

ATHETOSIS (GR. *athetos*, without position or place) A movement disorder caused by degenerative changes in the corpus striatum and cerebral cortex, characterized by bizarre, writhing movements.

AXON (GR. *axon*, axis) Efferent process of a neuron conducting impulses to other neurons or to muscle fibers (striated and smooth) and gland cells.

BRACHIUM (L. from GR. *brachion*, arm) A large bundle of fibers connecting one part with another.

BRADYKINESIA (GR. *brady*, slow + *kinesis*, movement) Abnormal slowness of movement.

BRAIN STEM In the mature human brain, usually denotes the medulla, pons, and midbrain.

BULB Referred at one time to the medulla oblongata; in the context of *corticobulbar tract*, refers to the brain stem, in which motor nuclei of cranial nerves are located.

CAUDA EQUINA (L. horse's tail) The lumbar and sacral spinal nerve roots in the lower part of the spinal canal.

CAUDATE NUCLEUS Part of the corpus striatum; named because it has a long extension or tail.

CEREBELLUM (L. diminutive of *cerebrum*, brain) Part of the brain situated in the posterior cranial fossa, which regulates and controls movement and equilibrium.

CEREBRUM (L. brain) The principal portion of the brain, including the diencephalon and cerebral hemispheres, but not the brain stem and cerebellum.

CHOREA (L. from GR. *choros*, a dance) A disorder characterized by irregular, spasmodic, involuntary movements of the limbs or facial muscles.

CINGULUM (L. girdle) A bundle of association fibers in the white matter on the medial surface of the cerebral hemisphere.

COLLICULUS (L. a small elevation or mound) Superior and inferior colliculi located in the midbrain.

CORONA (L. from GR. *korone*, a crown) Corona radiata (fibers radiating from the internal capsule to various parts of the cerebral cortex).

CORPUS CALLOSUM (L. body + *callosus*, hard) The primary neocortical commissure of the cerebral hemispheres.

CORPUS STRIATUM (L. body + *striatus*, furrowed or striped) A mass of gray matter, with motor functions, at the base of each cerebral hemisphere.

CORTEX (L. bark) Outer layer of gray matter of the cerebral hemispheres and cerebellum.

CUNEUS (L. wedge) A gyrus on the medial surface of the cerebral hemisphere.

DENDRITE (GR. *dendrites*, related to a tree) A part of a nerve cell on which axons of other neurons terminate.

DIENCEPHALON (GR. *dia*, through + *enkephalos*, brain) Part of the cerebrum, consisting of the thalamus, epithalamus, subthalamus, and hypothalamus.

DURA (L. *durus*, hard) Dura mater (the thick external layer of the meninges).

DYSKINESIA (GR. *dys*, difficult or disordered + *kinesis*, movement) Abnormality of motor function, characterized by involuntary, purposeless movements.

DYSMETRIA (GR. *dys*, difficult or disordered + *metron*, measure) Disturbance of the power to control the range of movement in muscular action.

ENGRAM (GR. *en*, in + *gramma*, mark) Used by some to mean the lasting trace left by previous experience, a latent memory picture.

EPENDYMA (GR. *ependyma*, an upper garment) Lining epithelium of the ventricles of the brain and central canal of the spinal cord.

EPINEURIUM (GR. *epi*, upon + *neuron*, nerve) The connective tissue sheath surrounding a peripheral nerve.

EPITHALAMUS (GR. *epi*, upon + *thalamos*, inner chamber) A region of the diencephalon above the thalamus, including the pineal gland.

EXTEROCEPTOR (L. *exterus*, external + *receptor*, receiver) A sensory receptor which serves to acquaint the individual with the environment (exteroception).

EXTRAPYRAMIDAL SYSTEM In broadest terms, consists of all motor parts of the central nervous system except the pyramidal motor system.

FASCICULUS (L. diminutive of *fascis*, bundle) A bundle of nerve fibers.

FUNICULUS (L. diminutive of *funis*, cord) An area of white matter which may consist of several functionally different fasciculi, as in the lateral funiculus (column) of white matter of the spinal cord.

GANGLION (GR. knot or subcutaneous tumor) A group of nerve cell bodies, as in cerebrospinal and sympathetic ganglia. Also used inappropriately for certain regions of gray matter in the brain, e.g., basal ganglia of the cerebral hemisphere.

GLIA (GR. glue) Neuroglia, the interstitial or accessory cells of the central nervous system.

GLOBUS PALLIDUS (L. a *ball* + *pale*) Medial part of lenticular nucleus of corpus striatum.

HEMIBALLISMUS (GR. *hemi*, half + *ballismos*, jumping) A violent form of motor restlessness involving one side of the body, caused by a destructive lesion involving the subthalamic nucleus.

HEMIPARESIS (GR. *hemi*, half) Weakness of one side of the body.

HEMIPLEGIA (GR. *hemi*, half + *plege*, a stroke) Paralysis of one side of the body.

HIPPOCAMPUS (GR. *hippocampus*, sea horse) A gyrus that constitutes an important part of the limbic system.

HYDROCEPHALUS (GR. *hydro*, water + *kephale*, head) Excessive accumulation of cerebrospinal fluid.

HYPOTHALAMUS (GR. *hypo*, under + *thalamos*, inner chamber) A region of the diencephalon which serves as the main controlling center of the autonomic nervous system.

INSULA (L. island) Cerebral cortex concealed from surface view and lying at the bottom of the lateral fissure. Also called the island of Reil.

INTEROCEPTOR (L. *inter*, between + *receptor*, receiver) One of the sensory end organs within viscera (internal organs).

KINESTHESIA (GR. *kinesis*, movement + *aisthesis*, sensation) The sense of perception of movement.

LEMNISCUS (GR. *limniskos*, fillet [a ribbon or band]) A bundle of nerve fibers in the central nervous system, e.g., medial lemniscus and lateral lemniscus.

MAMMILLARY (L. *mammilla*, diminutive of *mamma*, breast [shaped like a nipple]) Mammillary bodies: small swellings on the central surface of the hypothalamus. Also spelled *mamillary.*

MASSA INTERMEDIA A bridge of gray matter connecting the thalmi of the two sides across the third ventricle; present in 70% of brains. Also called the *interthalamic adhesion.*

MEDULLA (L. marrow, from *medius*, middle) Medulla spinalis: spinal cord. Medulla oblongata: caudal portion of the brain stem. In current usage, *medulla* refers to the medulla oblongata.

MESENCEPHALON (GR. *mesos*, middle + *enkephalos*, brain) The midbrain.

METENCEPHALON (GR. *meta*, after + *enkephalos*, brain) Pons and cerebellum.

MYELENCEPHALON (GR. *myelos*, marrow + *enkephalos*, brain) Medulla oblongata.

MYELIN (GR. *myelos*, marrow) The layers of lipid and protein substances composing a sheath around nerve fibers.

NEOCEREBELLUM (GR. *neos*, new + diminutive of cerebrum) The phylogenetically newest part of the cerebellum, present in mammals and especially well developed in humans. Ensures smooth muscle action in finer voluntary movements.

NEOCORTEX (GR. *neos*, new + L. *cortex*, bark) Six-layered cortex, characteristic of mammals and constituting most of the cerebral cortex in man.

NEURON (GR. a nerve) The morphologic unit of the nervous system, consisting of the nerve cell body and its processes (dendrites and axon).

NYSTAGMUS (GR. *nystagmos*, nodding, from *nystazo*, to be sleepy) An involuntary oscillation of the eyes.

OLIVE (L. *oliva*) Oval bulging of the lateral area of the medulla. Inferior, accessory, and superior olivary nuclei.

OPERCULUM (L. cover or lid, from *opertus*, to cover) Frontal, parietal, and temporal opercula bound the lateral fissure of the cerebral hemisphere and conceal the insula.

PARAPLEGIA (GR. *para*, beside + *plege*, a stroke) Paralysis of both legs and lower part of the trunk.

PIA MATER (L. tender mother) The thin innermost layer of the meninges, attached to the surface of the brain and spinal cord; forms the inner boundary of the subarachnoid space.

PINEAL (L. *pineus*, relating to the pine) Shaped like a pine cone (pertaining to the pineal gland, also called the pineal body).

PNEUMOENCEPHALOGRAPHY (GR. *pneuma*, air + *enkephalos*, brain + *grapho*, to write) The replacement of cerebrospinal fluid by air, followed by x-ray examination (pneumoencephalogram); permits visualization of the ventricles and subarachnoid space. This technique has been replaced by computerized tomography (CT scan).

PONS (L. bridge) That part of the brain stem which lies between the medulla and the midbrain; appears to constitute a bridge between the right and left halves of the cerebellum.

PROPRIOCEPTOR (L. *proprious*, one's own + *receptor*, receiver) One of the sensory endings in muscles, tendons, and joints; provides information concerning position of body parts (proprioception).

PROSENCEPHALON (GR. *pros*, before + *enkephalos*, brain) The forebrain, consisting of the telencephalon (cerebral hemispheres) and diencephalon.

PUTAMEN (L. shell) The larger and lateral part of the lenticular nucleus of the corpus striatum.

PYRAMIDAL SYSTEM Corticospinal and corticobulbar tracts. So called because the corticospinal tracts occupy pyramid-shaped areas on the ventral surface of the medulla. The term *pyramidal tract* refers specifically to the corticospinal tract.

QUADRIPLEGIA (L. *quadri*, four + GR. *plege*, stroke) Paralysis affecting the four limbs. Also called *tetraplegia*.

RETICULAR (L. *reticularis*, pertaining to or resembling a net) Reticular formation of the brain stem responsible for attention, arousal, and wakefulness.

ROSTRUM (L. beak) Recurved portion of the corpus callosum.

SOMESTHETIC (GR. *soma*, body + *aisthesis*, perception) The consciousness of having a body. Somesthetic senses are the general senses of pain, temperature, touch, pressure, position, movement, and vibration. Also spelled *somatesthetic*.

SPLENIUM (GR. *splenion*, bandage) The thickened posterior extremity of the corpus callosum.

SUBSTANTIA NIGRA A large nucleus with motor functions in the midbrain; many of the constituent cells contain dark melanin pigment.

SYNAPSE (GR. *synapto*, to join) Word introduced by Sherrington in 1897 for the site of contact between neurons, at which site one neuron is excited or inhibited by another neuron.

TECTUM (L. roof) Roof of the midbrain consisting of the paired superior and inferior colliculi.

TELENCEPHALON (GR. *telos*, end + *enkephalos*, brain) Cerebral hemispheres.

THALAMUS (GR. *thalamos*, inner chamber) A major portion of the diencephalon with sensory and integrative functions.

TRAPEZOID BODY Transverse fibers of the auditory pathway situated at the junction of the dorsal and ventral portions of the pons.

UVULA (L. little grape) A portion of the inferior vermis of the cerebellum.

VENTRICLE (L. *ventriculus*, diminutive of *venter*, belly) Lateral, third, and fourth ventricles of the brain. Caverns containing cerebrospinal fluid.

(Adapted from Chusid, 1979, with permission)

3

NOSOLOGY:
WHAT APHASIA IS AND
WHAT IT IS NOT

Juliet Capulet asked, "What's in a name? That which we call a rose by any other name would smell as sweet." What's in a name? A lot. That which we call a rose by any other name would smell as sweet. Perhaps, but it may not be identified as a rose in neurology rounds. Had Juliet been ruled more by her cortex than by her glands, had she read the aphasia literature rather than trashy, Italian romantic novels, she would not have asked the question. She would have had a position. She would have specified an American Beauty rose as opposed to a John F. Kennedy rose, or she would have taken the position that "a rose is a rose."

The Juliet syndrome is represented in contemporary aphasiology, and clinicians, like their patients, have difficulty with naming. The clinicians' problem is not so much one of the names of things, but one with the name of the thing, aphasia. We seem to know what to call it, but we do not agree on how to describe it or whether to divide it. And, like Verona, we feud like Montagues and Capulets. Our problem is not one of finding names but of having found too many.

The difficulties, we believe, are three. First, most agree, if you rule out those with a prefix preference for dysphasia, that aphasia is good for openers. But, we begin to gather

into factions when we define the term. Differences in definition quickly render one person's aphasia another's dementia, or not aphasia, or something else. Second, we split on whether aphasia should stand alone or whether it requires adjectives that divide it into types. Some hold that the symptoms are the tie that binds, and the whole is greater than the sum of the parts. These eschew fractionating with adjectives that describe salient symptoms. Others advocate classifying to organize the poorly understood whole into its more easily understood parts. These utilize differences that they believe make a difference. Third, we differ on whether aphasia exists in communication deficits that fly different colors. Is the language of the demented patient, the one with a right hemisphere lesion, or the schizophrenic patient aphasic? If not totally, how about partially?

Does it really matter what you call it? We believe it does, because our failure to settle on the best available definition of aphasia and on the most clinically useful classification of people with the disorder is affecting our clinical practice (Rosenbek, 1983). This chapter is about what to call aphasia. We have attempted to temper ebullience for one position or another. Our review is synoptic, but it seeks an ostensive definition of aphasia, a useful system for classifying it, a determination of whether it exists in other neurogenic communication disorders, and the implications of labels and definition. Finally, we end with a definition for this book.

APHASIA IS...!
DIVERGENCE IN DEFINITION

Words have meanings, and faulty assumptions about meaning can precipitate unexpected results. Phineas T. Barnum moved crowds quickly through his New York museum by posting signs announcing "This Way to the Egress." Expecting one of Barnum's fabulous beasts, viewers flocked eagerly to the door through which the Egress could be seen and found themselves outside the museum. Egress turned out to be the exit. Similarly, students and clinicians flock eagerly to the door marked "aphasia," but, depending on their experience with its meaning, they may find themselves where they did not intend to be. Several have attempted to offer direction through definition, but, as we shall see, the directions differ.

Who would have thought, at this late date, we would continue the debate between Broca and Trousseau (Wepman, 1951) held in the 1860s. But, we do. Benson (1979a) observed, "Rather than discussed, viewpoints have often been argued. Much of the controversy can be traced directly to the definition of aphasia" (p. 1). His own definition includes little to argue about.

Aphasia is the loss or impairment of language caused by brain damage. (Benson, 1979, p. 5)

So, we quarrel with it on the basis of what it does not say. Benson's definition is inadequate, for it fails to distinguish aphasia from other acquired disorders of language (Rosenbek, 1982), or, for that matter, from coma or death.

Ryan (1982) stated, "There are probably as many definitions of aphasia as there are scientists and clinicians attempting to define

it" (p. 3). His definition seeks to avoid controversy.

Aphasia is defined as the loss of, or reduction in, the ability to process language as a result of brain injury. It may manifest itself in difficulty with (1) understanding spoken and/or written messages; (2) recognizing pictures and objects; and/or (3) communicating by speaking, writing, and/or gesturing. (Ryan, 1982, p. 3)

Ryan's definition is typical. It is also illustrative of the discrepancy that exists among different definitions of aphasia. It is the "and/or" that separates aphasiologists when they define aphasia. For some, it is "and" and only "and" that makes aphasia aphasia. For others, the "or" is permissible.

THE ANDS: A GENERAL LANGUAGE DISORDER

The contemporary spokesman for the "ands" is Darley (1982). For him, aphasia is:

Impairment, as a result of brain damage, of the capacity for interpretation and formulation of language symbols; multimodality loss or reduction in efficiency of the ability to decode and encode conventional meaningful linguistic elements (morphemes and larger syntactic units); disproportionate to impairment of other intellective functions; not attributable to dementia, confusion, sensory loss, or motor dysfunction; and manifested in reduced availability of vocabulary, reduced efficiency in application of syntactic rules, reduced auditory retention span, and impaired efficiency in input and output channel selection. (p. 42)

The only "ors" in Darley's definition qualify severity, "loss or reduction," and tell what aphasia is not, "dementia, confusion, sensory loss, or motor dysfunction." The "ands" combine symptoms and imply all must be present to be aphasia, "decode and encode," "morphemes and larger syntactic units," "and manifested in reduced ... vocabulary, ...

application of syntactic rules, . . . auditory retention span, *and* impaired . . . input *and* output channel selection."

Darley's definition is consistent with Schuell's (Schuell et al., 1964). For her, aphasia is:

A general language deficit that crosses all language modalities and may be complicated by other sequelae of brain damage. (p. 113)

Thus, Schuell's aphasic patient displays deficits in auditory comprehension, reading, oral expressive use of language, *and* writing. She does not require equal impairment in each modality, but each must show some deficit. A patient who can do everything but write would not be considered aphasic by Schuell or Darley.

THE ORS: ANY OR ALL

A different point of view was offered by Goodglass and Kaplan (1983b). They hold that:

Various components of language may be selectively damaged by aphasia and . . . this selectivity is a clue to (1) the anatomical organization of language in the brain, (2) the localization of the causative lesion and (3) the functional interactions. . .of various parts of the nervous system. (p. 2)

Goodglass and Kaplan arrived at their definition of aphasia by beginning with a definition of normal language.

Normal language may be regarded as depending on a complex interaction between sensory-motor skills, symbolic associations and habituated syntactic patterns, all at the service of the speaker's intent to communicate, and subject to the intellectual capacity that he brings to the task of manipulating them so as to carry out his intent. (p. 5)

Batter the brain of Goodglass and Kaplan's normal language user, and one may observe behavior that represents their definition of aphasia.

Aphasia refers to the disturbance of any or all of the skills, associations and habits of spoken or written language, produced by injury to certain brain areas that are specialized for these functions. (p. 5)

Others (Albert et al., 1981; Benson, 1979a; A. Damasio, 1981) have supported this view. For example, Albert and colleagues (1981) said that:

The assessment of language function must deal with this aspect of dysphasia—its possible selectivity for particular modalities of input or output and—in some instances—for specific input-output combinations. (p. 12)

Similarly, A. Damasio (1981) holds that:

Aphasia is a disturbance of one or more aspects of the complex process of comprehending and formulating verbal messages that result from newly acquired disease of the central nervous system. (p. 51)

Thus, Goodglass and Kaplan's, Albert and colleagues', and A. Damasio's aphasic patient may display deficits in all communicative modalities, or he or she may show selective deficits in one or more modalities. Their patient who can do everything but write would be considered aphasic.

LIGHT ON LANGUAGE, LONG ON IMPAIRED ACCESS

Some (Kreindler & Fradis, 1968; McNeil, 1982) have offered definitions that reduce the importance of language impairment as the salient sign that signifies aphasia. They focus on other issues. For example, McNeil's definition

Aphasia is a multimodality physiological inefficiency with, greater than loss of, verbal symbolic manipulations (e.g., association, storage, retrieval, and rule implementation). In isolated form it is caused by focal damage to cortical and/or subcortical structures of the hemisphere(s) dominant for such symbolic manipulations. It is affected by and affects other physiological information processing and cognitive processes to the degree that they support, interact with, or are supported by the symbolic deficits. (p. 693)

relegates language impairment to almost a secondary status. The primary impairments, he suggested, are "increased fatiguability, increased sensory thresholds, decreased speed of reaction, fluctuation of attention and effort allocation, and inertia of neurophysiological excitation and inhibition" (p. 701).

This subordinate role of language deficit in aphasia has received support from Kreindler and Fradis (1968). They listed six signs they believe are fundamental and common in all aphasic persons. Some are similar to those identified by McNeil—inertness of excitation and inhibition processes and fatigability—but they added others, for example, "blockage within the functional system of the word" (p. 64). These defects, they believe, explain the aphasic patient's language deficits. Kreindler and Fradis described the aphasic patient's difficulty in differentiating among stimuli as resulting from inertness of excitation and inhibition.

Thus, those who suggested aphasia results from impaired access of language have deemphasized the "what"—the "and" or the "or"—and have focused on the "why"—impaired access. Their aphasic patient may display deficits in all communicative modalities, or he or she may show selective deficits in one or more modalities, but this is secondary. Primary is why the deficits exist.

APHASIA AS A COGNITIVE DEFICIT

In the 1970s aphasiologists found cognition. It probably was not lost, but it had not been used frequently to explain disrupted language subsequent to left hemisphere brain damage. Today, some discuss "cognitive styles" and "cognitive processes," and they provide us with yet another definition of aphasia.

Martin (1981b) began with the assumption that "language behavior can be described with reference to cognitive processing, that is,

with reference to the internal actions of the individual" (p. 64). He used Neisser's (1966) definition of cognition to refer "to all processes by which sensory information is transformed, reduced, elaborated, stored, recovered, and used" (Martin, 1981b, p. 65). Aphasia for Martin (1981b) "is the reduction, because of brain damage, of the efficiency of the action and interaction of the cognitive processes that support language" (p. 66). This definition differs from others in that aphasia is not viewed as a loss of language or as a primary linguistic impairment. The problem results from reduced efficiency in the use of cognitive processes.

Others (Brown, 1977; Chapey, 1981) have related cognition to aphasia; however, unlike Martin, they did not explain aphasia as solely a cognitive deficit. Brown (1977) suggested:

Every disorder of language also incorporates aspects of a corresponding level in cognition. A change in awareness, an alteration of mood, the presence or absence of delusional or hallucinatory phenomena, these are not additions to the clinical picture but have an inner bond with the aphasia form. (p. 27)

Chapey (1981) defined aphasia as:

An acquired impairment in language and the cognitive processes which underlie language caused by organic damage to the brain. It is characterized by a reduction in and dysfunction of language content or meaning, language form or structure and language use or function and the cognitive processes which underlie language, such as memory and thinking. (p. 31)

Yet others (Lesser, 1978; Rosenbek, 1982) have wondered whether disrupted cognition may not be more apparent in certain types of aphasia, for example, Wernicke's aphasia, than in other types.

If nothing else, the implication of abnormal cognition in aphasia is controversial. Suggest aphasia is a cognitive problem to some, and they will suggest your time will be used more wisely learning the cranial nerves.

For others, any definition of aphasia must include cognition. The latter differ on preponderance and presence; aphasia is a cognitive deficit, or aphasia is a cognitive *and* language deficit, or only some aphasic patients display cognitive as well as language impairment.

SUMMARY

The divergence in definitions of aphasia need not induce ague. Clinicians seeking a definition of aphasia have several choices, and regardless of what they choose, they will not be lonely, nor will they escape controversy. Those who believe aphasia is a general language deficit cannot accept the position that aphasia may be a selective impairment. Those who view aphasia as a processing problem may be more comfortable with those who view aphasia as a cognitive deficit, because both focus on "processes" and "processing." But, both will probably quarrel over what or which "process" or "processes," physiological, mental, or both, are impaired.

Unfortunately, how one defines aphasia will influence how one manages aphasia. Appraisal and diagnosis will differ with different definitions. The general language disorder folks would not call the patient who can do everything but write aphasic. The selective impairment group might. Similarly, treatment will be influenced by definition. The aphasia as a cognitive disorder camp will employ different methods from those who view aphasia as solely a language disorder.

The solution? We suggest taking a position that permits probing. One must have a position, or one cannot practice. However, that position need not be so permanent that it cannot be penetrated by progress and patients. The Russian psychologist Luria (1981), at the end of his career, observed, "We can confidently say that today we are at the very first stage of this very complex course" (p. 246). Those of us influenced primarily by Western thought must remember that the wise men came from the East.

APHASIA WITH AND WITHOUT: THE CONTROVERSY OF CLASSIFICATION

Disagreement does not stop with definition. And, those who divide on definition—general versus specific language impairment—tend to find themselves on opposite sides of the controversy about classifying aphasic patients into various types. The generalists (Darley, 1982; Schuell et al., 1964) eschew fractionating aphasia into types, and those who permit specific impairment (Goodglass & Kaplan, 1983; Kertesz, 1979) divide aphasic patients into groups that can be identified by salient symptoms.

Almost everyone agrees that aphasic patients differ. Some talk a lot; others speak very little; some understand more than others; and so on. But, disagreement begins when one suggests these differences can be used to sort aphasic patients into specific types. Like the rose, some hold that aphasia is aphasia, whereas others specify aphasia may be Broca's aphasia, Wernicke's aphasia, conduction aphasia, etc. Let us examine the arguments for each point of view.

APHASIA WITHOUT ADJECTIVES

Darley (1982) has presented the most recent abstemious view of aphasia. His position is clear: "aphasia is not modality bound" (p. 28). Therefore, using modalities—auditory comprehension, reading, oral expression, writing—to separate patients into different types is superficial and misleading. He suggested:

> Little clinical purpose is served by proliferating adjectives, which are presumed to designate different 'types' of aphasia. These adjectives emerge because they are based on different, at times incomplete or biased, observations; they reflect what people look for and believe in. (p. 42)

Similarly, Wepman's (1951) position was that "aphasic language disorders are considered as affecting all the language modalities and cannot be limited to specific language skills" (p. 18). And Schuell and colleagues (1964) concluded that "there is a dimension of general language deficit in aphasia that is not modality specific" (p. 156).

Support for this view comes from a variety of statistical evidence obtained from factor analysis and cluster analysis of aphasic patients' language performance. For example, Schuell and Jenkins (1959), using a Guttman scale analysis, concluded that the language deficit in aphasia is a unidimensional trait. Similarly, Schuell, Jenkins, and Carroll (1962) performed a factor analysis of patient performance on the Minnesota Test for Differential Diagnosis of Aphasia (MTDDA) (Schuell, 1965a). Their results indicated there is a dimension of general language deficit in aphasia that is not modality specific. Therefore, they argued there is no evidence for a sensory-motor, receptive-expressive, or input-output dichotomy in aphasia. More recently, Powell, Clark, and Bailey (1979), using two types of cluster analysis and a factor analysis of MTDDA performance, observed differences in severity of aphasia among patients but no support to confirm the existence of types of aphasia. Finally, Clark, Crockett, and Klonoff (1979) did a factor analysis of aphasic patient performance on the Porch Index of Communicative Ability (PICA) (Porch, 1967). They concluded that the variance accounted for by a general language factor outweighed the variance accounted for by specific dimensions.

Even those who classify aphasia into types acknowledge the presence of a general language deficit in aphasia. Goodglass and Kaplan (1972), in their factor analysis of the Boston Diagnostic Aphasia Examination (BDAE), observed a factor that included naming, auditory comprehension, reading, and writing. They conceded this could represent a severity or general language factor similar to that found by Schuell and Jenkins (1959). Further, Weisenburg and McBride (1935) used a four-fold classification— predominately expressive, predominately receptive, expressive-receptive, and amnestic,

but they observed that none of the terms is other than descriptive, and none does more than point out the most marked characteristics of the case.

So, Darley (1982) and ilk elect to designate patients as aphasic without adjectives. They believe differences among patients do not represent different types of aphasia but differences in severity, differences in time postonset, or the presence of a coexisting disorder. For example, the global patient is severely aphasic, and the anomic patient is mild, but both, if evaluated thoroughly, will display a general language disorder that crosses all communicative modalities. Similarly, time postonset works its will on classification. Types change over time (Kertesz & McCabe, 1977; Wertz, Kitselman, & Deal, 1981), and this change represents a change in severity. Finally, certain types, for example, Broca's aphasia, do not represent a difference in aphasia but the presence of a coexisting disorder, for example, apraxia of speech. Thus, they view the ability to classify aphasia as adventitious and the practice as infelicitous.

APHASIA WITH ADJECTIVES

The other side of the argument is that the label "aphasia" is inappropriate and should be "the aphasias," because aphasic patients can be sorted into different types of aphasia. For example, Kertesz (1979) suggested:

Most clinicians will agree that although aphasic disability is complex, many patients are clinically similar and will fall into recurring identifiable groups.... There are many classifications, indicating that none is altogether satisfactory, but also that this effort is useful and even necessary to diagnose and treat aphasics or to understand the phenomena. (p. 1)

Goodglass and Kaplan (1983b) expressed essentially the same view.

A century of intensive analysis of aphasic symptoms has produced considerable agreement as to identifiable component deficits. . . . Not only is there wide consensus as to the individual component deficits to be observed, but the common clusters of defects (i. e., the major aphasic syndromes) emerge repeatedly in the interpretive observations of dozens of careful writers, though often under different names based on different theoretic bases. (p. 5)

Thus, systems for classifying the aphasias exist; they have existed for a long time; there are numerous systems from which to choose; and although there is some inconsistency among systems, there is also considerable agreement.

Early systems to classify aphasia resulted from attempts to display brain-behavior relationships. Damage to certain areas of the brain appeared to result in different language deficits from those observed following damage to other areas of the brain. The early attempts, therefore, were prompted by a desire to localize lesions. With time, experience, improved tools for detecting the site of lesions, and interest from a variety of disciplines, the anatomical emphasis was mixed with psychological and linguistic terminology. Today, the popular classification systems utilize anatomic terminology, for example, transcortical motor aphasia; linguistic terminology, for example, anomic aphasia; and labels that identify the contributions of early investigators, for example, Broca's aphasia. All are used to imply the locus of the lesion and a set of behavioral characteristics.

Classification systems vary from binary types such as Weisenburg and McBride's (1935) expressive-receptive, including their synonyms, sensory-motor or input-output, to elaborate typologies suggested by Nielsen (1946) and Luria (1964). For our purposes, we will limit discussion to the currently popular systems; the fluent-nonfluent dichotomy (Goodglass, Quadfasel, & Timberlake, 1964); Goodglass and Kaplan's (1983b) system; and Kertesz's (1979) taxonomy. First, however, we will consider those behaviors used to classify patients into aphasic types.

SALIENT SYMPTOMS

Although all who classify aphasia appraise a patient's auditory comprehension, reading, oral-expressive use of language, and writing, only auditory comprehension and oral-expressive use of language are used to classify. However, the three systems we are considering subdivide oral-expressive language differently.

FLUENCY

All three systems utilize a patient's verbal fluency to classify. In the fluent-nonfluent classification, fluency is the single measure used to classify. Patients who produce longer phrases, five or more connected words, are labeled fluent. Those who produce only single word utterances or short phrases, four or fewer connected words, are labeled nonfluent.

In Goodglass and Kaplan's system (1983b), a patient's fluency is determined by performance on four of the eight characteristics contained in the Boston Diagnostic Aphasia Examination (BDAE) Rating Scale Profile of Speech Characteristics shown in Figure 3-1. The four characteristics that relate to fluency are melodic line, phrase length, articulatory agility, and grammatical form. The most salient of these for determining fluency is phrase length, defined as the longest occasional uninterrupted word runs. However, the other three should show characteristic relationships with phrase length. For example, patients with low ratings, one to four, on melodic line, articulatory agility, and grammatical form should show low ratings, one to four, on phrase length. They would be classified nonfluent. Conversely, fluent patients, those with high ratings, five to seven, on melodic line, articulatory agility, and grammatical form, should show high ratings, five to seven, on phrase length.

Kertesz (1982) employed a descriptive, 0 to 10, rating scale to determine fluency in his Western Aphasia Battery (WAB). Patients rated 5 to 10 are considered fluent, and patients rated zero to four are considered nonfluent.

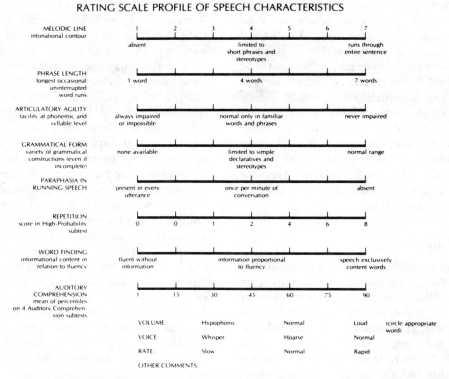

RATING SCALE PROFILE OF SPEECH CHARACTERISTICS

Figure 3-1. Boston Diagnostic Aphasia Examination Rating Scale Profile of Speech Characteristics. From Goodglass, H., & Kaplan, E., (1983a). *The assessment of aphasia and related disorders*. Philadelphia: Lea & Febiger. Reprinted with permission.

Descriptions for each level on the scale incorporate many of the same characteristics—melodic line, articulatory agility, phrase length, and grammatical form—included in the BDAE profile.

Empirical evidence for the use of fluency to classify aphasic patients comes from Goodglass and colleagues' (1964) analysis of patients demonstrating Broca's, Wernicke's, or anomic aphasia. They tested their belief that the significant differences among aphasic patients are revealed in differences in oral-expressive language and not in differences between input and output performance. Comparison of phrase length among the three groups separated the Broca's patients, short phrase length, from the Wernicke's and anomic patients, longer phrase length.

Fluency, therefore, appears to differentiate among types of aphasic patients. Those with global, Broca's, isolation, or transcortical motor aphasia are considered nonfluent, and those with Wernicke's, transcortical sensory, conduction, or anomic aphasia are considered fluent.

AUDITORY COMPREHENSION

How well a patient understands the speech of others is used to classify his or her type of aphasia. Both the BDAE and WAB employ a battery of auditory comprehension subtests, and both use the results similarly to classify. Global, isolation, Wernicke's, and transcortical sensory types display severe to marked or moderate auditory comprehension deficits. Broca's and transcortical motor types display marked to mild auditory comprehension deficits. Conduction and anomic types display moderate to mild auditory comprehension deficits. As observed by Goodglass and colleagues (1964), auditory comprehension is not as precise in separating types of aphasia as is fluency, because severity of auditory comprehension deficit among types overlaps. Thus, auditory comprehension alone will not differentiate among global, isolation, Wernicke's, and transcortical sensory types; among Broca's, transcortical motor, Wernicke's, and transcortical sensory types; or among Broca's, transcortical motor, conduction, and anomic types.

REPETITION

Tests of verbal repetition are included in most aphasia examinations. Patients may display difficulty repeating for one or more reasons. First, they may fail to repeat because their auditory comprehension is impaired, and they do not comprehend the stimulus to be repeated. Second, they may fail to repeat because they lack the verbal ability to produce the stimulus they may have understood correctly. Third, they may fail to repeat because there is a disruption between adequate auditory comprehension and adequate verbal skills. Repetition difficulty is severe to marked in global patients; severe to moderate in Broca's, Wernicke's, and conduction patients; marked to absent in isolation patients; and moderate to absent in transcortical motor, transcortical sensory, and anomic patients. Again, repetition ability may overlap among types and cannot be used as the sole criterion for differentiating among aphasic patients.

NAMING

Difficulty in naming or word-finding appears to be present in all types of aphasia. In fact, it seems to be a hard-core residual deficit even in patients who experience a good deal of improvement in the overall severity of their aphasia. Kertesz and McCabe (1977) and Wertz and colleagues (1981) report that patients who change in their type of aphasia over time tend to migrate toward anomic aphasia.

Both Goodglass and Kaplan (1983a) and Kertesz (1982) included naming subtests in their examinations. However, they rated naming behavior differently. Kertesz employed tests of object naming, word fluency, sentence completion, and responsive speech to evaluate naming behavior. The total correct, 0 to 100, is divided by 10, and the patient's performance is represented by a value from 0 to 10. Goodglass and Kaplan (1983a) also included a variety of naming tests in the BDAE, but they objected to using performance on naming tests as a measure of word-finding difficulty. Total scores, they suggested, do not differentiate the anomic patient from the one who cannot articulate or those with severe restriction of speech. Therefore, Goodglass and Kaplan rated word-finding on the scale shown in Figure 3-1, where informational content is related to fluency. Data for this rating come from the pattern of word-finding displayed in a sample of conversational speech.

Kertesz's approach is easier, and it provides a measure of severity. But, it fails to differentiate among types. For example, naming in the most severe type, global, ranges from zero to six, and naming in the most mild type, anomic, ranges from 0 to 9. Conversely, Goodglass and Kaplan's approach is somewhat less objective and fails to provide a measure of severity. But, it tends to differentiate among, at least, some types.

SUMMARY

The three currently popular methods for classifying aphasic patients—fluent-nonfluent, BDAE types, WAB taxonomy—display similarities and differences in the way patients are classified. The fluent-nonfluent dichotomy uses only the length of utterance to classify. The BDAE and WAB systems use fluency, auditory comprehension, repetition, and naming or word-finding to classify. However, the BDAE rates fluency and word-finding on a scale of speech characteristics and uses subtest performance on repetition and auditory comprehension subtests. The WAB employs a rating scale to determine fluency and uses total performance on subtests of auditory comprehension, repetition, and naming. These different approaches sometimes result in differences in classification, depending upon which system is used.

TYPES OF APHASIA

Now, let us consider the specific types of aphasia and the salient characteristics that represent each type. Included in this discussion will be the differences among the three systems used to classify aphasic patients.

FLUENT-NONFLUENT

Even though Darley (1982) elected not to classify aphasia, he provided an excellent description of the variety of verbal output found in aphasic patients.

> Some patients manage no more than a telegraphic kind of speech, producing primarily substantive words with omission of function words, whereas other patients are relatively unable to produce the substantive words. Still other patients with severe impairment of auditory comprehension may produce a continuous flow of meaningless jargon or fluent speech full of neologisms, seemingly unaware that they are not communicating and even denying that they have a communication difficulty. This copious flow of speech may be largely unintelligible but it resembles the mother tongue by retaining its typical prosodic and some syntactic aspects. (pp. 5–6)

Those who utilize the fluent-nonfluent dichotomy to classify patients recognize the former patients in Darley's description as nonfluent and the latter patients as fluent.

Obtaining a sample to differentiate among patients usually involves engaging a patient in conversation and asking him or her to describe a picture. Deciding whether a patient is fluent or nonfluent may involve the use of Benson's (1967) set of scales, Goodglass and Kaplan's (1983a) determination of phrase length, or Kertesz's (1982) 0 to 10 fluency scale. Regardless of the measure employed, the nonfluent patient

should be characterized by sparse, effortful, sometimes perseverative speech; many pauses; disturbances in prosody; abnormal pronunciation; single word utterances or short phrases; and, sometimes, word substitutions. Conversely, the fluent patient produces a great deal of speech; few pauses; normal prosody; few, if any, perseverations; a lack of abnormal pronunciation; and normal phrase length. As mentioned previously, Goodglass and Kaplan (1983b) suggested the best measure of fluency is phrase length, defined as the longest occasional uninterrupted word runs. Klor and Ratusnik (1980) have reported a significant difference in the mean length of response (MLU) between nonfluent (MLU = 4.96) and fluent patients (MLU = 8.10).

Classifying aphasic patients as fluent or nonfluent gives no indication of a patient's performance in the other language modalities— auditory comprehension, reading, and writing. For example, Poeck, Kerschensteiner, and Hartje (1972) observed no significant differences on the Token Test (DeRenzi & Vignolo, 1962), a measure of auditory comprehension, between groups of fluent and nonfluent patients. This is understandable, because the fluent-nonfluent dichotomy combines a range of auditory comprehension deficits in each group. Nonfluent patients may be Broca's aphasic patients who display moderate to mild auditory comprehension deficits, or they may be global or isolation aphasic patients who display severe auditory comprehension deficits. Similarly, fluent patients may be anomic or conduction aphasic patients with mild auditory comprehension deficits, or they may be Wernicke's or transcortical sensory aphasic patients with severe auditory comprehension deficits.

Orgass and Poeck (1966) suggested that the fluent-nonfluent dichotomy may assist in the general localization of the patient's lesion. Goodglass (1981) listed nonfluent aphasia as resulting from predominantly pre-Rolandic lesions and fluent aphasia as resulting from temporal or temporal-parietal lesions. Generally, therefore, nonfluent patients would have anterior lesions, and fluent patients would have posterior lesions.

Although there is some evidence to support this position (Kertesz, Harlock, & Coates, 1979), the relationship between fluency and the location of a patient's lesion may be influenced by severity, type of aphasia, and time postonset. For example, Broca's patients, nonfluent, tend to have anterior lesions; and anomic and Wernicke's patients, fluent, tend to have posterior lesions. However, global patients, nonfluent, tend to have large lesions that are both anterior and posterior. Further, Kertesz and colleagues (1979) reported three conduction patients, fluent, one with an anterior lesion, one with a posterior lesion, and one with an anterior-posterior lesion. The influence of time postonset on fluency and its relationship with lesion localization is complicated, because some patients migrate from one type of aphasia to another over time. For example, an acute Broca's patient may be nonfluent and display an anterior lesion. However, when this patient becomes chronic, several months postonset, the type of aphasia may have changed from Broca's to anomic. The patient has become fluent, but the lesion has retained its original residence in the anterior region of the left hemisphere. Wertz and colleagues (1981) reported 56 percent of their patients who were nonfluent at 4 weeks postonset were judged fluent at 48 weeks postonset. Conversely, none of their fluent patients became nonfluent as time postonset increased.

Deciding whether a patient is fluent or nonfluent is not too difficult, and clinicians display significant agreement in their decisions. Judge agreement (Wertz et al., 1981) on patients classified fluent or nonfluent at 4, 15, 26, 37, and 48 weeks postonset ranged from 91 percent agreement at 4 weeks to 97 percent agreement at 48 weeks.

Thus, it appears that patients can be classified reliably into fluent and nonfluent types, and the best measure to accomplish the task is a patient's number of words in uninterrupted utterances. We must remember that designating a patient fluent or nonfluent will not necessarily imply severity, the status of language in any modality other than oral expression, or indicate the localization of the lesion.

APHASIC SYNDROMES

We use the heading "aphasic syndromes" to designate specific types of aphasia—global, Broca's, isolation, transcortical motor, Wernicke's, transcortical sensory, conduction, and anomic—and separate these from the more general fluent-nonfluent classification. These specific types have evolved out of a plethora of labels that developed over a century of interest in aphasia. They can, of course, be separated into the fluent-nonfluent dichotomy, but, unlike that classification, the specific types are designed to give information about several aspects of a patient's language behavior—fluency, auditory comprehension, repetition, and naming. They are the types used in most clinics that classify aphasia. They are associated with the Boston school of aphasia, and they are identified, usually, as patterns of performance on two examinations, the BDAE and WAB, designed to detect them.

Table 3-1 shows the signs and symptoms for each aphasic syndrome we are considering. Performance in four language areas—fluency, auditory comprehension, repetition, and naming—is listed as " – ," severe to marked deficit; " – / + ," moderate to mild deficit; or " – " to " – / + ," severe to moderate or mild. Further, the salient sign or signs that typify each syndrome are designated by "S." Although reading and writing show a range of impairment in each syndrome and among syndromes, neither is used to classify a patient on the BDAE or WAB.

Figure 3-2 shows H. Damasio's (1981) major loci of lesions for five of the eight syndromes—Broca's, transcortical motor, Wernicke's, transcortical sensory, and conduction. Localization for global, isolation, and anomic types varies, thus, the loci of lesions resulting in these types cannot be presented with much specificity.

GLOBAL APHASIA. As its name implies, global aphasia is the most severe type of aphasia. Salient signs are severe impairment of all language abilities. Oral expression is nonfluent and reduced to a few words, emotional exclamations, and a few serial utterances. Thus, these patients are nonfluent,

TABLE 3-1.
Salient Signs and Symptoms for Each Aphasic Syndrome.

Aphasic Syndrome	Fluency		Auditory Comprehension		Repetition		Naming	
Global	−	S	−	S	−	S	−	S
Broca's	−	S	−/+		− to −/+		− to −/+	
Isolation	−	S	−	S	−/+	S	−	S
Transcortical motor	−	S	−/+	S	−/+	S	− to −/+	
Wernicke's	−/+	S	−	S	− to −/+		− to −/+	
Transcortical sensory	−/+	S	−	S	−/+	S	− to −/+	
Conduction	−/+		−/+		−	S	− to −/+	
Anomic	−/+		−/+		−/+		− to −/+	S

− = severe to marked deficit; −/+ = moderate to mild deficit; S = salient sign or signs for each syndrome.

and repetition and naming are severely impaired. Auditory comprehension is extremely limited, usually to single words and short phrases. Location of the lesion is variable both in size and location. Damage may involve the entire, left perisylvian region; extend into the underlying white matter; or be represented by two left hemisphere lesions, one anterior and one posterior.

BROCA'S APHASIA. Although patients with Broca's aphasia display some deficits in all language areas, they are identified by their severely impaired fluency. Prosody is abnormal, phrase length is short, articulation is impaired, and grammatical form is characterized by telegraphic utterances that show reduced use of articles, prepositions, auxiliaries, copulas, and inflectional and derivational endings (Goodglass, 1981). Auditory comprehension is less impaired than oral expressive use of language, but if the task is sufficiently difficult, Broca's aphasic patients display moderate to mild problems understanding what they hear. Repetition deficit ranges from severe to mild, depending upon the stimuli to be repeated. Similarly, naming ability shows a range of impairment from severe to mild. Some (Darley, 1982) have suggested that patients classified as having Broca's aphasia show two communicative problems, aphasia coexisting with apraxia of speech. Location of the lesion that causes Broca's aphasia is usually in the left, lower, posterior frontal lobe, Brodmann's area 44. It

can involve the lower portion of the motor strip and territory anterior and superior to area 44.

ISOLATION APHASIA. The syndrome of isolation aphasia is rare. It is characterized by a severe reduction in fluency, auditory comprehension, and naming but only moderate to mild impairment of repetition. Except for the preservation of repetition, these patients would appear globally aphasic. Its name comes from the nature of the lesions that cause it. Essentially, the localization of the damage isolates the speech area from other cortical areas. The disorder was described by Goldstein (1948), and Geschwind, Quadfasel, and Segarra (1968) reported a patient who could sing along with the radio, complete sentences, and repeat sentences, but displayed essentially no auditory comprehension or spontaneous speech. The lesions in this case resulted from carbon monoxide poisoning and surrounded but did not involve the perisylvian speech area. Isolation aphasia is included in Kertesz's (1982) taxonomy, but it is not one of Goodglass and Kaplan's (1983b) types.

TRANSCORTICAL MOTOR APHASIA. "Remarkably well preserved repetition is the hallmark of transcortical motor aphasia" (Goodglass, 1981, p. 10). These patients repeat better than one would expect based on their nonfluent, severely impaired spontaneous speech. Auditory comprehension is moderately to mildly impaired and similar to that seen in

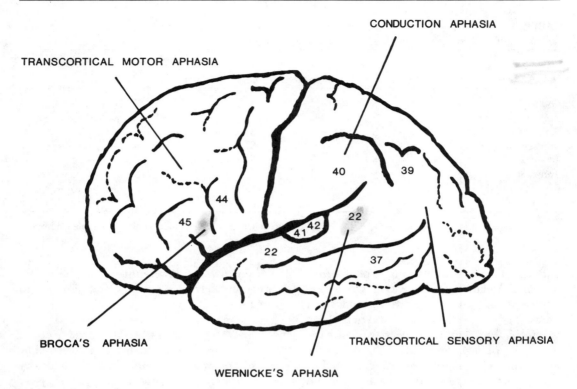

Figure 3-2. The major loci of lesions in five types of aphasia. Broadmann's areas 44 and 45 correspond to Broca's area, area 22 to Wernicke's area, areas 41 and 42 to the primary auditory cortex, area 40 to the supramarginal gyrus, area 39 to the angular gyrus, and area 37 to the posterior part of the second temporal gyrus. Adapted from H. Damasio (1981, p. 29).

Broca's aphasia. Although naming is usually superior to spontaneous speech, it may show a range of impairment from severe to mild. The patient's lesion may be superior to, anterior to, or deep within the classical Broca's area, Brodmann's area 44.

WERNICKE'S APHASIA. Fluent speech and impaired auditory comprehension identify the Wernicke's aphasic patient. Although speech is fluent—good articulation, longer phrase length, evidence of grammatical form, and normal prosody—it is not correct. Paraphasias, both semantic and literal, abound. In severe cases, conversational speech includes neologisms and jargon. Naming shows a range of impairment, severe to mild, as does repetition ability. Auditory comprehension is always impaired, usually severely. The lesion resides in the posterior region of the left superior temporal gyrus, but it may extend into the second temporal gyrus and adjacent parietal region, especially the angular gyrus.

TRANSCORTICAL SENSORY APHASIA. The syndrome of transcortical sensory aphasia is the fluent counterpart of nonfluent, transcortical motor aphasia. Conversation in transcortical sensory aphasia resembles conversation by the Wernicke's aphasic patient—good articulation, decent phrase length, some syntax, and adequate prosody—but it typically abounds with paraphasias and is extremely lacking in nouns. Naming is severely to moderately involved. The salient sign is preserved ability to repeat. Auditory comprehension is impaired, similar to performance seen in Wernicke's aphasia. This type of aphasia results from an extensive lesion in the posterior portion of the middle temporal gyrus that extends into visual and auditory association cortex and, occasionally, into the angular gyrus.

CONDUCTION APHASIA. Unlike the transcortical aphasias, conduction aphasic patients display extremely poor repetition ability. This "selective deficit in repetition is the distinguishing feature of conduction aphasia" (Goodglass, 1981, p. 13). Conversation is fluent—decent articulation, phrase length, syntax, and prosody. Naming deficit ranges from severe to mild. Auditory comprehension deficit ranges from moderate to mild. Thus, extremely poor ability to repeat is highlighted by moderate to mild impairment in other areas. The lesion that causes conduction aphasia is in the supramarginal gyrus, Brodmann's area 40, and the superior temporal lobe.

ANOMIC APHASIA. Some (A. Damasio, 1981) have suggested that pure anomic aphasia is rare. Others (Kertesz, 1979) have reported that it is the most common type encountered, especially in chronic patients. Spontaneous speech is fluent, characterized by good articulation, phrase length, syntax, and prosody. Auditory comprehension and repetition are only moderately to mildly involved. But, these patients have specific difficulty in naming. When anomic aphasia results from a focal lesion, the damage is usually in the angular gyrus or second temporal gyrus.

MIXED NONFLUENT APHASIA. Goodglass and Kaplan (1983b) used this label to describe patients who reside somewhere between global aphasia and Broca's aphasia. It is not included in Kertesz's (1982) taxonomy. The patient displays the nonfluent, sparse verbal output of the Broca's aphasic patient, but auditory comprehension is more impaired than that seen in Broca's aphasia. Naming and repetition abilities are also similar to those seen in Broca's aphasia. These patients are those who were initially globally aphasic and have experienced some improvement over an extended period (Goodglass, 1981). The lesion usually involves the lower posterior frontal lobe and precentral

gyrus, as seen in Broca's aphasia, but it is deeper and extends more posteriorly.

ALEXIA WITH AGRAPHIA. The condition of alexia with agraphia implies impaired reading (alexia) and impaired writing (agraphia) with no oral expressive or auditory comprehension deficits. Should it be considered an aphasic syndrome? Goodglass and Kaplan (1983b) included it in their list; Kertesz (1982) did not. The range of impaired reading and writing is from severe to mild. If there is any speech deficit at all, it resembles mild anomic aphasia. The lesion causing this syndrome is reported to reside in the angular gyrus.

ATYPICAL OR "PURE" APHASIAS

Those who classify the aphasias do not stop with identifying the aphasic syndromes listed previously. They also identify atypical or "pure" aphasias. These are conceded to be quite rare. Identification is by a common feature: impaired performance in a single input or output modality with essentially intact performance in all other modalities.

APHEMIA. Broca (1861) used *aphemia* to describe his patient, Leborgne. Darley (1982) suggested the disorder be called *apraxia of speech* and that it is not aphasia but a motor speech disorder. Goodglass and Kaplan (1983b) described aphemia as "an isolated disorder of articulation in which auditory comprehension, and writing are intact" (p. 98). Initially, the patient may be unable to produce any speech sounds spontaneously or by imitation. An apraxia for oral, nonverbal movements may be present. As the patient improves, articulation is slow and awkward, but syntax is intact, and there is no word-finding deficit. Goodglass (1981) reported that aphemia results from a small, subcortical lesion in the frontal operculum or in the lower end of the precentral gyrus.

ALEXIA WITHOUT AGRAPHIA. The syndrome of alexia without agraphia is also called *pure alexia* (Goodglass & Kaplan, 1983b), and those who display it are rare. As the label implies, the patient cannot read, but he or she can write. Oral expression, auditory comprehension, and repetition are intact. Dejerine (1892) was the first to describe the condition, and Benson and Geschwind (1969) listed a specific set of symptoms. The patient displays a right homonymous hemianopia, inability to identify colors, a calculation disorder, occasional difficulty naming objects, severely impaired reading, and relatively intact writing. The lesion is usually located in the occipital lobe; however, Benson and Geschwind (1969) reported involvement of the splenium of the corpus callosum in 9 of 15 patients. Geschwind (1965) suggested alexia without agraphia results from separation of two cortical areas and the inability to transfer visually perceived stimuli to the angular gyrus where it can be interpreted.

PURE WORD DEAFNESS. Patients with pure word deafness produce error-free spontaneous speech, and naming, reading, and writing are within normal limits. Auditory comprehension is totally absent, but the patient may be able to speech-read. Similarly, repetition is severely impaired except for stimuli that can be speech-read. The patients complain that they cannot "hear"; however, audiometric results, except for speech audiometry, show no conductive or sensorineural hearing loss. Pure word deafness results from bilateral temporal lesions or from a subcortical temporal lesion that spares, but isolates, Wernicke's area in the left hemisphere (Goodglass, 1981).

PURE AGRAPHIA. If a patient can do everything but write, he or she may be classified as displaying pure agraphia. Again, these patients are rare. Oral expression, including spontaneous speech, repetition, and naming, is unaffected. Auditory comprehension is normal. Reading may be mildly involved, or it may be completely intact. The salient sign is a severe writing disorder. Location of the lesion causing pure agraphia is in the angular gyrus. However, Exner (1881) reported a lesion in the foot of the second frontal convolution may result in pure agraphia.

SUBCORTICAL APHASIAS

Traditionally, aphasia has been considered to result from a cortical lesion. Although speech and language deficits have been reported subsequent to thalamic lesions (Fisher, 1959), few have considered these aphasic. With the advent of CT scanning and its ability to identify subcortical lesions that were previously undetected, some (Alexander & LoVerme, 1980; Naeser et al., 1982) have begun to identify subcortical aphasias.

Goodglass and Kaplan (1983b) summarized the belief that left, purely subcortical lesions can result in aphasia. These may result from vascular occlusion or intracerebral hemorrhage. The specified areas of damage are the internal capsule, putamen, or thalamus. The lesions vary in size and extent, anterior and posterior, and both influence the types of speech and language deficits present and their severity.

Speech and language behavior in patients who have suffered left, anterior subcortical lesions that involve the anterior limb of the internal capsule and the putamen is characterized by severely impaired, dysarthric articulation; adequate phrase length, four to six words; mild word repetition deficit; moderate to mild naming problems; mild auditory comprehension deficit; moderate to mild reading problems; and severe to marked writing deficit. Naeser and colleagues' (1982) patients resembled Broca's aphasia in their marked articulation problems and minimal auditory comprehension deficits, but they differed from Broca's aphasia in their preserved syntax and longer phrase length. These patients suffered persisting right hemiplegia.

Patients with left, posterior capsular/putaminal lesions show fluent speech—adequate phrase length, intact syntax, and mild or no articulatory problems. Auditory comprehension and picture naming are severely impaired. Repetition errors are few for single words but present in sentence repetition. Those that occur are verbal paraphasias. Reading and writing are moderately impaired. Naeser and colleagues' (1982) patients resembled the profile seen in Wernicke's aphasia. However, unlike most Wernicke's aphasic patients, they displayed persisting right hemiplegia.

When the left, subcortical lesion is both anterior and posterior, involving the anterior capsule, putamen, and extending into the thalamus, the patient is globally aphasic. Spontaneous speech is limited to stereotyped monosyllables, phrase length does not exceed one word, articulatory agility is severely impaired, and there is no evidence of syntax. Similarly, auditory comprehension, repetition, naming, reading, and writing are severely impaired. These patients suffer persisting right hemiplegia.

Because few patients with subcortical aphasia have been reported, specific speech and language symptomatology is not clearly established. Further, reports indicate anterior and anterior-posterior lesions result in both aphasia and dysarthria. So, these patients suffer coexisting disorders that confound evaluation of the severity and nature of either single disorder.

CROSSED APHASIA

We expect aphasia to result from a unilateral, left hemisphere lesion; however, some patients violate our expectations. Bramwell (1899) introduced the term *crossed aphasia* to describe either right hemiplegia and aphasia in a left-handed person who suffered a left hemisphere lesion or left hemiplegia and aphasia in a right-handed person who suffered a right hemisphere lesion. Today (Hecaen & Albert, 1978), crossed aphasia is used to describe aphasia in right-handed patients who have suffered right hemisphere damage.

These patients are rare. Incidence ranges from less than one percent of aphasic patients (Benson & Geschwind, 1976) to two percent (Zangwill, 1967). Further, the etiologies that result in crossed aphasia differ, in incidence, from the typical, uncrossed aphasia. Boller (1973) estimated that only 23 percent of crossed aphasic patients have a vascular etiology. The majority of cases reported suffered tumor or trauma. This contrasts with traditional aphasic patients, right-handed with a left hemisphere lesion, who show a high incidence of vascular etiology.

Zangwill (1967) and Hecaen (1972) reported that it is difficult to classify the language symptoms in crossed aphasia into one of the traditional syndromes. Agrammatism and writing disturbance seem to be present in most cases, regardless of the site of lesion, and auditory comprehension and naming appear to be minimally affected. However, Wertz (1982a) reported a right-handed patient who suffered a right frontal CVA and displayed the classic signs of Broca's aphasia. In addition, this patient responded to treatment and improved in essentially the same manner and to the same extent as Broca's aphasic patients who suffer a left hemisphere frontal lesion.

SUMMARY

Although neither side of the controversy on whether to classify aphasia has turned the debate into a jihad, a strong difference of opinion exists. Those who classify do so because many aphasic patients tend to cluster in different groups, each of which can be characterized by a salient set of symptoms. These symptoms frequently indicate where in the brain a patient has suffered damage, and classification using salient symptoms aids treatment planning. Conversely, those who avoid modifying aphasia with an adjective do so because all aphasic patients, to be aphasic, must display a general language deficit that impairs, to some degree, all communicative modalities—auditory comprehension, reading, oral expressive use of language, and writing. They hold that differences among patients are explained either by severity or the presence of a coexisting disorder. Classification, for them, is like putting your faith in seed catalogues. That thing with the double-barreled name always turns out to be radishes. Which position is correct? Probably both.

We believe classification of aphasia, for that matter, aphasia's nosology, can be made less eristic by incorporating parts of both positions into one's clinical code. We agree with Darley (1982) and Schuell and colleagues

(1964) that aphasia is a general language disorder characterized by deficits in all communicative modalities. Each modality need not be equally impaired, but if one looks long enough and hard enough, for example, the patient who appears to understand everything will show that he or she does not if the comprehension task is sufficiently difficult. On the other hand, we do not see why this position should prevent one from differentiating among aphasic patients and separating those who understand not everything, but a lot, from those who understand very little or those whose lack of understanding is emphasized when it is compared with their relatively good ability to talk.

Controversy results from exclusion, overemphasis, and inference. For example, we are troubled by texts titled *Aphasia, Alexia, and Agraphia* (Benson, 1979a). One could infer that aphasia involves listening and speaking but not reading and writing. Benson ignored this distinction in his description of aphasia. Similarly, we worry about A. Damasio's (1981) selectivity when he stated, "Aphasia relates exclusively to a disturbance in verbal language as opposed to other forms of language, for example, the language of gestures or of facial expressions" (p. 52). Our clinical experience does not support this view. Conversely, we agree with A. Damasio's (1981) suggestion that it is a mistake to ignore marked differences between modalities that are minimally impaired and those that are markedly impaired.

The "pure" or atypical aphasias require some discussion. We suspect the source of controversy with these stems from overemphasis. For example, we are yet to meet a patient who can do everything but read. Our experience is that the "pure" aphasias simply highlight a salient symptom. We have seen cases of word deafness (Burger, Wertz, & Woods, 1983) and alexia without agraphia (Wertz, Flynn, Green, Rosenbek, & Collins, 1979). The former patient displayed the classic symptoms of word deafness. He also displayed mild residual aphasia persisting from his first left hemisphere CVA. The latter patient displayed a severe reading deficit coexisting with fairly intact ability to write. He also displayed the remnants of aphasia that we had seen a year earlier subsequent to his left, occipital bleed.

A variety of subcortical aphasias are being described (Benson, 1979a), and Ojemann (1975) has demonstrated the contribution of subcortical structures to normal speech and language. Our experience with patients who suffer internal capsule, putamen, and thalamic lesions is that many are dysarthric, and many display aphasic-like language deficits. We suspect that time and attention to these patients will indicate many suffer coexisting disorders, dysarthria and aphasia.

Poeck (1983), we believe, has taken a rational approach in describing aphasic syndromes. He suggested they are identified, primarily, by their expressive aspects. Although language comprehension varies among types of aphasia, it is compromised, to some degree, in all syndromes. Further, he observed that all clinicians construct a profile of aphasic patients' behavior in the different language modalities. If these profiles yield subgroups, Poeck suggested failure to classify the subgroups is an "ideological and not a rational behavior" (p. 88).

So, we are comfortable with the view that aphasia is a diaspora. Probe each patient's language with appropriate measures and you will find aphasic persons are homogeneous. All display some deficit in each communicative modality. However, examine the type of deficit in each modality and compare performance across modalities, and many patients will cluster into groups that may be identified and labeled with an appropriate adjective. We realize that all, perhaps most, patients cannot be classified with confidence. But, as Rosenbek (1983) suggested, the danger in treating aphasia without adjectives is that we may be tempted to treat aphasic patients without regard for their differences. The use of adjectives to describe aphasia is as likely to highlight differences as to conceal them.

ASSOCIATED DISORDERS: WHEN IS "APHASIA" NOT APHASIA?

Nosologic controversy does not stop within the disorder of aphasia, it also exists among disorders that resemble aphasia. These include the language of confusion, dementia, communication deficit subsequent to a right hemisphere lesion, schizophrenia, environmental influence on the language of the normal aged, apraxia of speech, and dysarthria.

Some discuss the presence of aphasia in language and speech disorders that speech-language pathologists consider nonaphasic. For example, Albert and colleagues (1981) and Appell, Kertesz, and Fisman (1982) have discussed aphasia in dementia. Others (Darley, 1982; Wertz, 1982b) have suggested the language deficits of demented patients should not be considered aphasic. Goodglass and Kaplan (1983b) warned:

> Disturbances of language usage that are due to paralysis or incoordination of the musculature of speech or writing or to poor vision or hearing or to severe intellectual impairment are not, of themselves, aphasic. Such disorders may accompany an aphasia, however, and thus complicate the clinical manifestations of the language defect proper. (p. 5)

The disagreement probably stems from differences between general descriptions and attempts to be precise for purposes of patient management. On the one hand, language deficits in associated disorders are sufficiently similar to those seen in aphasia for them to be called aphasia in a quick description of a patient's communicative behavior. On the other hand, clinicians charged with managing these language deficits specify that the treatments and the prognosis for different disorders differ. Although it is not important to fight to the finish these differences in nosology on the beaches of neurology rounds, we should consider some of the differences among disorders that may make a difference.

THE LANGUAGE OF CONFUSION

Darley (1969, 1982) has popularized the label *the language of confusion*. He has used it to describe patients who display reduced recognition and understanding of their environment, faulty memory, unclear thinking, and disorientation in time and space. Their syntax, word finding, auditory comprehension, and ability to repeat are frequently within normal limits. However, responses to open-ended questions will include irrelevance and confabulation. The language of confusion follows bilateral, frequently traumatic, brain damage. It is typified not by impaired language but by irrelevant and confabulatory language. These are the patients who describe their adventures in Salt Lake City during the past weekend when their medical record relates they spent a quiet Saturday and Sunday on the ward. We expect confused language to be transient. If it persists beyond a few weeks, we look for another label. The patient's relatively good language differentiates him or her from the aphasic patient. There are no salient symptoms that signify one of the specific aphasic syndromes.

DEMENTIA

"Dementia is a condition of chronic progressive deterioration of intellect, memory, and communicative function resulting from organic brain disease" (Bayles, 1984, p. 209). Darley (1982) described the demented patient's communicative deficit as "the language of generalized intellectual impairment." Performance initially slips on more difficult language tasks, especially those requiring retention, close attention, abstraction, and generalization. The patient's language deficits are similar in severity to those on other intellectual tasks. Common causes of dementia include Alzheimer's disease; multiple, bilateral infarctions; and idiopathic Parkinson's disease. Although Appell and colleagues (1982) reported demented patients can be classified into the aphasic syndromes, language symptoms appear to represent differences in severity more than differences in type. Bayles, Tomoeda, and Caffrey (1982) have demonstrated gradual, increasing deficits in fluency, phonology, syntax, and semantics as demented patients advance from mild to severe. Certainly, the prognosis and available treatments for dementia differ from those for aphasia.

RIGHT HEMISPHERE IMPAIRMENT

We exclude from this discussion the crossed aphasia patients and focus on those who have left hemisphere language dominance but have suffered right hemisphere brain damage. Myers (1984) reported these patients display few overt language deficits, but they have difficulty communicating. The sources of their problem appear to be lower-order perceptual problems, including left-sided neglect and various visual-spatial deficits; problems with affect and prosody; linguistic disorders; and higher-order perceptual deficits that result in communicative inefficiency. Even the linguistic deficits do not resemble those seen in aphasia. Myers (1984) suggested, "Right hemisphere communication disorders clearly fall outside the continuum of aphasic-like behaviors" (p. 191).

SCHIZOPHRENIA

Some (Chapman, 1966) have suggested that aphasia exists in schizophrenia. Others (Benson, 1973) have not. In fact, debate occurs on whether the schizophrenic patient really has a language disorder at all. Benson (1975) reported that most demonstrate a sizeable vocabulary and correct syntax. He concluded that schizophrenia is characterized by disrupted thinking, not disrupted language. They may dwell on certain themes and perseverate in their ideas, they may be disoriented, and they may confabulate. But, their language differs from that seen in aphasic patients.

ENVIRONMENTAL INFLUENCE ON LANGUAGE

Normal older people placed in what Lubinski (1981) described as a communication-impaired environment may display language deficits that could be mistaken for aphasia. Elderly patients with no evidence of left hemisphere brain damage who find themselves in institutional settings—nursing homes, convalescent hospitals—where few listen or speak, may stop using strategies that normal older persons in noninstitutional environments employ—syntax to cue naming and content to improve comprehension. Deterioration of language abilities in the former is gradual, unlike the sudden onset of deficits seen in aphasia, and it is reversible; change the environment and language improves.

APRAXIA OF SPEECH

A disorder that frequently coexists with aphasia is apraxia of speech. Not all agree it differs from aphasia (Benson, 1979a) or even exists at all (Martin, 1974), but many (Darley, 1982; Wertz, LaPointe, & Rosenbek, 1984) differentiate apraxia of speech, a motor speech disorder, from aphasia, a language disorder. Kent and Rosenbek (1983) define apraxia of speech as:

A sensorimotor speech disorder resulting from brain damage. Symptoms are impaired volitional production of normal articulation and prosody. The articulation and prosodic disturbances do not result from muscle weakness or slowness. Rather they result from inhibition or impairment of CNS programming of skilled oral movements. (p. 231)

Those who immerse apraxia of speech in aphasia do identify its symptoms as disrupted melodic line and impaired articulatory agility. The argument, for the most part, is theoretical and nosologic. And, it is probably not important if the symptoms are managed appropriately.

DYSARTHRIA

Another motor speech disorder that may coexist with aphasia is dysarthria. Wertz (1978) presented Darley's (1969) definition of this disorder.

A group of speech disorders resulting from disturbances of muscular control—weakness, slowness, or incoordination—of the speech mechanism due to damage to the central or peripheral nervous system or both. The term encompasses coexisting neurogenic disorders of several or all the basic processes of speech: respiration, phonation, resonance, articulation, and prosody. (Wertz, 1978, p. 2)

Dysarthria, therefore, is considered to be a motor speech disorder and not a language disorder. It may coexist with aphasia, and it is frequently present in what are now being described as subcortical aphasias.

SUMMARY

We offer several cautions to speech-language pathologists who seek a precise definition of what aphasia is and what it is not. First, many of the labels used above are speech and language diagnoses, not medical diagnoses. For example, the language of generalized intellectual impairment is the speech-language pathologist's term to describe language deficit in what neurologists and psychologists call dementia.

Second, several of the previous disorders may coexist with aphasia. For example, we expect the patient who displays apraxia of speech to also display aphasia. The apraxic signs reside in the patient's prosody and articulation, and the indicants of aphasia reside in syntax, naming, auditory comprehension, reading, and writing. Further, the demented patient who got that way from multiple vascular episodes may have been labeled aphasic following his or her first left hemisphere CVA, and the initial signs of aphasia gradually became submerged in the language of generalized intellectual impairment following additional, bilateral CVAs. And, there is no rule that forbids the patient who suffers the bilateral cortical atrophy of Alzheimer's disease from suffering a focal, left hemisphere CVA and subsequent signs of aphasia.

Third, the speech-language pathologist should avoid professional petulance in his or her insistence on what is aphasia and what is not. One discipline's passion may be another's minimal interest. There is no need to turn off colleagues for the wrong reasons.

Finally, determining what is and what is not aphasia may be important for patient management—appraisal, prognosis, and treatment. Different disorders might dictate different management. But, we remind ourselves that we manage patients and not vocabulary.

A DEFINITION FOR THIS BOOK

We have arrived at the point where we need to give aphasia our definition. Clinicians need some rules to live by. One of these rules dictates that disorders be defined. Definitions should incorporate what we think we know now, but they should be sufficiently flexible to permit modification with what we may soon find out. Definitions, like decisions, can be changed. So, we suggest:

Aphasia is an impairment, due to acquired and recent damage of the central nervous system, of the ability to comprehend and formulate language. It is a multimodality disorder represented by a variety of impairments in auditory comprehension, reading, oral-expressive language, and writing. The disrupted language may be influenced by physiological inefficiency or impaired cognition, but it cannot be explained by dementia, sensory loss, or motor dysfunction.

Let us consider some of the implications in this definition. First, we believe aphasia in adults does not creep, it erupts. The most frequent causes are a variety of CVAs, trauma, infection, and tumor. The latter, of course, may be slow to show its influence. Nevertheless, we include "recent" and "acquired" to differentiate aphasia from the gradual cortical atrophy that signifies dementia or the genetic, congenital, and environmental influences that may affect a child's language development. Our aphasic patients had some competence with language before they became aphasic.

Second, we expect aphasic patients to display a general language disorder that is evident in all communicative modalities—auditory comprehension, reading, oral-expressive language, writing—if we probe each modality with tasks of sufficient difficulty for the patient. But, we believe there is sufficient variety in the severity and symptoms displayed by aphasic patients to classify many, not all, into aphasic syndromes. We caution that the methods one uses to do this may result in a patient receiving a different classification with different methods.

Third, the damage that results in aphasia has occurred in the central nervous system. Typically, it is focal damage in the left hemisphere; however, a rare aphasic patient may have suffered right hemisphere brain damage. When aphasia appears to be present subsequent to bilateral or subcortical damage, one may find a coexisting disorder, perhaps dysarthria, and the patient's speech and language will differ, somewhat, from those patients who have suffered unilateral, left hemisphere, cortical damage.

Fourth, aphasic patients may display physiological inefficiency and cognitive impairment, but neither are sufficient to explain the severity and symptoms that constitute the language deficit. Moreover, both may vary depending upon the location, size, and duration of the patient's lesion.

Fifth, aphasia may coexist with dementia, sensory loss, and motor impairment. But, although diminished intelligence, hearing loss, visual acuity and field defects, paralysis or paresis of the speaking musculature or the upper extremities may be present, and interfere with language use, they do not cause or explain the aphasic language deficits.

Our definition attempts to include and to reconcile different points of view. We do not aim to please anyone. For, to be a mediator great, one must learn to obfuscate. We present, as clearly as we can, what we think our patients have tried to teach us. Thus, our definition represents how aphasia seems to us, right now.

4

APPRAISAL, DIAGNOSIS, AND PROGNOSIS

J. P. astounded us with words that were not only beyond his linguistic experience, or beyond ours, but were beyond anyone's. His brain was starved of oxygen. Dehydration had defoliated his arterial tree. It is difficult to capture this man on paper, because words do not move, and what he said never stood still. His words were shadowless things, and we had been asked to use them to get THERE—to evaluate him, determine what he had, to predict his future, and to decide whether treatment might help. The adding up to get THERE held its own wonder.

The road to getting there usually begins with a request for consultation from a physician, "64-year-old white male s/p CVA in 4/85. Please evaluate and determine need for speech therapy." The speech-language pathologist's journey leads him or her through appraisal, diagnosis, and prognosis to treatment, if treatment is appropriate. We believe it is important to get your train on the right track, because if you do not, every station you come to will be the wrong station. This chapter provides a map and an itinerary for getting THERE.

APPRAISAL

Lore runs both ways between patient and clinician, and, generally, the patient's is more useful than the clinician's, having come straight from life instead of from printed pages. The patient's lore is his or her history, biographical and medical, and his or her performance on the speech and language tasks the clinician administers. The clinician's lore is what he or she elects to administer, how it is administered, and what is done with the results. Clinicians should not confuse their lore with the patient's, and they should be careful not to change what patients have to tell them by the way they seek information. At their very best, clinicians are sentient beings; capable of perceiving and feeling. In appraisal, they must remember they are a part of the audience and not a part of the cast.

Appraisal is the looking. It is the systematic seeking of something one can name if he or she finds it. The naming is diagnosis. And, appraisal can swallow clinician and patient up without a sound. Its purpose is to make a diagnosis, state a prognosis, and, if appropriate, focus treatment without being digested. Moreover, the seeking needs to be sympathetic as well as scientific. Cousins's (1982) advice is sage. Patients need and look for qualities in clinicians beyond pure competence. They want to be reassured. They want to be looked after and not just looked over. They want to be listened to. They want to feel that it makes a very big difference to the clinician whether they improve or not. Most of all, they want to feel they are in the clinician's thoughts. So, clinicians must remember, during appraisal's probing and prodding, that there is a person on the other end of the stimulus.

We begin appraising aphasic patients the same way we appraise all brain damaged patients, because, initially, we do not know they are aphasic. As the evidence mounts to indicate the patient is more likely aphasic than something else, we follow paths that differ from those we would follow if the evidence implied probable dementia, or dysarthria, or something else. We have three sources of data: the patient's biography, his or her medical history and neurological examination results, and his or her performance on our appraisal measures. Comparing each source with the others and sifting all through a sieve constructed of what we know about neuropathologies of speech and language has a high probability of achieving appraisal's purposes—making a diagnosis, stating a prognosis, and, if appropriate, focusing treatment.

BIOGRAPHICAL DATA

We seek who the patient is, what he or she was prior to becoming brain damaged, and what has occurred in his or her life between becoming brain damaged and the time we meet. This information includes: the patient's name and what he or she likes to be called, address, place of birth, date of birth, education, date of onset of brain damage, premorbid and present handedness, racial/ethnic group, previous and present marital status, occupational status at onset and at present, highest occupational level attained, estimate of premorbid communicativeness, estimate of premorbid intelligence, premorbid languages used and an estimate of their usage, present environment, number and kinds of people in the present environment, past and present interests and hobbies, and how the patient currently spends his or her day.

Biographical information does more than simply fill the blank spaces on our forms. Some of it is social; for example, knowing the patient is called "Spark," even though it is not a diminutive for Clarence, is useful and increases the probability of our obtaining his attention. Some is diagnostic; for example,

knowing the patient completed only "three winters" of schooling may indicate all of his or her reading or writing deficits are not explained by brain damage, or knowing that he or she spoke more Spanish than English premorbidly may explain some of the language deficits and that articulatory and prosodic "errors" do not necessarily indicate a coexisting apraxia of speech. Some is prognostic; for example, time postonset, age, education, premorbid handedness, highest occupational level achieved, occupational status at onset, and premorbid intelligence have surfaced in the prognostic literature as possible predictors of improvement. And, if the patient will be treated, some biographical information may influence treatment's goals, organization, and stimuli. For example, premorbidly taciturn talkers do not become verbose after suffering a left hemisphere stroke; therefore, frequency, amount, and content of communication in one patient may more closely approximate premorbid communicative ability than it does in another. Further, knowing where a patient resides and who resides with him or her will indicate whether he or she is within treatment's reach and whether there is someone present to assist with and monitor homework if it is assigned. And, knowing the patient's passions, interests, and hobbies expand the selection of treatment stimuli beyond "cat," "apple," and nonsense syllables.

Most of all, knowledge of a patient's biography permits us to relate to him or her as a person and not only as a patient. We can achieve some of Cousins's criteria—knowing a patient's past assists in providing realistic reassurance about his or her future, permits filling in some of the gaps in his or her communication when we listen, and indicates we are interested in more than his or her ability to demonstrate as completely as possible what he or she does with a toothbrush. We have never harmed a patient by knowing too much about him or her. Some have not received our best, because we did not know enough about them.

Finally, collection of biographical information does not end on the first day of appraisal. We continue to monitor facts that may change; for example, handedness, marital status, living environment, occupational status, etc. And, we probe information that appears inaccurate and seek what is missing. Gradually, we attempt to change the role of historian from family member or friend to the patient. Always, we make the patient a part of the act—seek his or her confirmation or rejection of biographical information regardless of who provides it—because it is his or her play we are doing.

MEDICAL DATA

Although we are interested in a patient's present—how a left hemisphere cerebrovascular accident has disrupted his or her language—and future—how much language deficits will change and how we might influence the change that may occur—we cannot forget the patient has a past—a medical history that began at birth. One of us has said, "History is everything," and he was correct. Appraisal measures may make dissimilar disorders look similar, but history differentiates. It tells us who's who and who's not. Similarly, we should not forget that our patients are not our patients. They originate with the primary care physician—neurologist, physiatrist, internist, surgeon, general practitioner. Thus, "our" patients are loaned to us from the referring physician: He or she provides the patient's recent history in the results of a current neurological evaluation. Some of the information we seek is listed in Table 4-1.

Pieces of a patient's medical history and current neurological examination help complete the pattern that will eventually provide a diagnosis. For example, knowledge of previous central nervous system involvement may explain why a patient who suffered a recent left hemisphere thromboembolic infarct has a significant hypokinetic dysarthria accompanying his aphasia. History may tell us he should, because Parkinson's disease was diagnosed four years prior to the recent CVA.

TABLE 4-1.
Medical Data Collected to Assist in Managing Patients Suspected of Suffering Aphasia.

Variable	Measures
Vision	Acuity, corrected and uncorrected; field abnormalities
Hearing	Acuity, aided and unaided; discrimination; ear pathologies
Limb involvement	Upper and lower; spasticity, weakness, coordination
Brain stem signs	Facial weakness, facial sensory loss; nystagmus, extraocular movement (EOM) and/or gaze impairment; dysphagia; other bulbar signs
Etiology	Type (CVA, trauma, infection, etc.); date of onset
Previous CNS involvement	Type; date of onset
Localization of brain damage	Hemisphere and lobe or lobes for current episode and any previous episode; source (clinical, CT, PETT, MRI, etc.)
Specific, complete diagnosis	For example, thrombosis of left middle cerebral artery, with right hemiparesis, hemisensory defect, hemianopsia, and expressive aphasia
Other major medical diagnoses	For example, diabetes, chronic cardiac arrhythmia
Medications	Number, types, and side effects

Or, one can explain a patient's poor visual matching ability by finding evidence of an old right hemisphere infarct that preceded the recent left hemisphere infarct that brought the patient to our attention. Moreover, knowing premorbid and present visual and auditory acuity may indicate that all of a patient's auditory comprehension and reading deficits are not linguistic. Additional examples could be enumerated, but it should suffice that there is no substitute for a complete medical history.

Information from the current neurological examination can support or confirm the speech and language diagnosis suggested by behavioral data. For example, the absence of hemiplegia and computerized tomographic (CT) or magnetic resonance imaging (MRI) evidence isolating a left hemisphere infarct to the temporal lobe makes one more confident in the speech and language data that suggest a diagnosis of Wernicke's aphasia. Conversely, dense right hemiplegia and CT or MRI evidence indicating damage in the left hemisphere's third frontal convolution and surrounding area bolster our suspicion of Broca's aphasia with coexisting apraxia of speech. And, of course, a history of multiple strokes confirmed by neuroradiological evidence of diffuse and disseminated bilateral brain damage prompt confidence in our speech, language, and cognitive data that indicate the patient is not aphasic and displays multi-infarct dementia.

Medical history and the results of the neurological examination also assist in formulating a prognosis. For example, a negative history of central nervous system involvement, no major coexisting medical problems, and a lesion confined to the left hemisphere third frontal convolution would not only support speech and language data that indicate mild aphasia coexisting with apraxia of speech, but also predict a good prognosis for improvement. Conversely, very sick patients with multiple systems medical problems who have suffered multiple bilateral CVAs would have a poor prognosis for improving their severe deficits in all communicative modalities. Thus, prognosis, an exercise in augury, has a higher probability of being precise when three sources

of data—medical history, neurological evaluation, speech and language behavior—are employed than when one has access to only one.

So, we urge speech-language pathologists to cull each patient's medical history and neurological examination report for information that confirms or challenges what is collected in speech and language appraisal. This requires us to expand our professional parochial boundaries and learn, for example, what a paracentral scotoma is or what lateral gaze impairment signifies. We believe we need to know all there is to know, and we know there are ways of finding out. Again, knowing too much about a patient has never hindered our management of that patient. Knowing too little has.

BEHAVIORAL DATA

Behavioral data on brain damaged patients flow from a variety of sources—neurologist, physiatrist, psychiatrist, neuropsychologist, nurse, occupational therapist, physical therapist, speech-language pathologist, and the patient's family. The list of those who contribute is expanded or abridged depending on what the patient has or the diagnostic dilemma he or she poses. How many of these sources contribute to the reservoir of behavioral data on a brain damaged patient also depends on who is available. Some patients meet only one or two of those who could provide appraisal data. Others are seen by several disciplines but at different times over an extended period of time. And, some are marched or wheeled through the offices of every professional listed during a week or more of intensive evaluation in a major medical center.

Neurologists access brain damaged patients' behavior as a part of or during the clinical neurological examination. Behavioral neurologists, typically, collect more behavioral data on aphasic patients than neurologists, whose primary interest is in muscle disease or neurochemistry. These data include a mental status examination—orientation to time, place, and condition; calculation and attention; registration, measured as the ability to repeat the names of three objects, etc.; an estimate of the patient's language abilities; and, frequently, classification of the type of aphasia. Psychiatrists see aphasic patients whose depression exceeds what is typically seen and expected, and they are called in to render judgments of legal competence. Hemiplegic patients are referred to physiatrists and, eventually, physical therapists to appraise hands, arms, and legs; to determine range of motion; and to detect the presence of limb and dressing apraxias. Occupational therapists contribute information on the patient's ability to perform activities of daily living and how motor deficits may be influenced by visual-perceptual deficits. Neuropsychologists test intelligence, memory, visual perception, and visuospatial abilities. Some, for example, Goodglass and Kaplan (1983b), have provided detailed evaluation of a patient's language. Nurses have close and protracted contact with aphasic people and document their observations of behavior in medical record nursing notes. Family members also have extensive exposure to an aphasic patient's behavior, and they have knowledge of premorbid performance for comparison. Speech-language pathologists administer formal and informal measures of communicative ability to determine the presence, nature, and severity of speech and language deficits and to speculate how these may be managed.

Behavioral data from other disciplines may question, support, explain, or amplify the speech and language data collected by speech-language pathologists. One seeks available data from other disciplines, requests what is missing and necessary, and compares what is obtained with the speech and language data to meet appraisal's purposes—make a diagnosis, state a prognosis, and, if appropriate, focus treatment. Again, Cousins's (1982) caution that the patient wants to be looked after and not just looked over must be remembered. The multidisciplinary Cuisinart approach to appraisal must be shunned. Processing the patient avoids having him or her quartered or diced.

The purposes of this section are to list and discuss the measures speech-language pathologists may employ to appraise aphasic patients, acknowledge recent trends in analysis that differ from more traditional appraisal, present a possible battery of appraisal measures, and demonstrate the battery's use with a patient to meet appraisal's purposes. First, however, we will digress briefly to discuss two properties in the measures we employ—validity and reliability.

PSYCHOMETRICS IN APPRAISING APHASIA

No one ever accused a behaviorist of being imaginative, but most are precise. The quantitative denomination of this ilk recite a litany of psychometric principles when they gather to worship at the altar of appraisal. Cronbach (1970) listed the essential principles, Porch (1967) emphasized their application in aphasia tests, and Lyon (1986) provided a recent review. Here, we consider two principles, validity and reliability.

If a measure does what it is designed to do, it is *valid*. Fine, but measures may be designed to do one or more of several things. For example, a measure of aphasia may be designed to detect the presence of aphasia, determine the severity of aphasia if it is present, differentiate aphasia from other neurogenic communication disorders, predict future performance, or indicate appropriate treatment. We know of no test for aphasia that does all of these things validly. Moreover, one's definition of aphasia may influence whether a measure is valid. For example, if aphasia is defined as a general language deficit in *all* communicative modalities, a measure that can only detect deficits in some but not all modalities is not a valid test for aphasia. However, if aphasia is defined as a language deficit in *one or more* communicative modalities, the same measure would be valid if it detects a deficit in at least one modality. Similarly, if the measure is designed to differentiate aphasia from other neurogenic communication disorders, it would not be valid if demented patients are classified as aphasic on the measure. However, if one believes language deficits in dementia are aphasia, then the measure would be considered to be valid.

Lyon (1986) discussed different types of validity in aphasia tests—content, construct, and criterion-related—and suggested means for determining each. However, he concluded essentially what we do. Different points of view about and definitions of aphasia will result in different decisions about the validity of the measures we employ. Although we do not have a solution, we certainly admire the problem, and we live with it. Perhaps, one should develop internal consistency and employ measures that are valid for one's point of view about and definition of aphasia, acknowledge that there are other measures that are valid for different points of view and definitions, and rejoice in the fact that controversy does not demean us, it ennobles us.

Most, regardless of point of view or definition or judgment about validity, require their measures to be *reliable*. Any change in results should indicate something important— the patient has improved, the patient has suffered another CVA, etc. A change in results should not be traceable to the measure's inconsistency, the clinician's variability, or differences between or among clinicians.

A patient's performance on a measure administered this morning should be essentially the same, within specified tolerance limits, as it would be if the measure were administered this afternoon. Thus, test-retest reliability should be acceptable. This is particularly important if we are using the measure to determine severity, for example, to focus treatment, or if we are seeking to determine improvement that may have resulted from treatment. Without test-retest reliability, assumed severity may vary, and treatment is inappropriately focused, or we cannot assume improvement was evoked by an efficacious treatment. Similarly, if the measure is designed to classify the type of aphasia, test-retest reliability must be sufficient to guarantee a patient who is classified as demonstrating Broca's aphasia today would be classified as demonstrating Broca's aphasia tomorrow. Aphasic patients do change for a variety of reasons—spontaneous recovery, effects of treatment, another neurological episode, depression, fatigue, etc. We must be certain that change reflects a change in the patient and not a lack of stability or inconsistency in the measures we employ to measure change.

We also expect stability and consistency within a clinician who administers measures. The extent to which test-retest scores provided by the same clinician agree indicate intrajudge reliability. If the test is reliable and if nothing has intervened to create change in the patient's performance, a clinician should provide essentially the same scores on repeated administrations of a measure. The extent to which a measure is standardized will influence intrajudge reliability. More rigidly standardized measures typically yield better intrajudge reliability. Further, clinician bias may influence intrajudge reliability. For example, if we have administered 50 hours of treatment to an aphasic patient, our posttreatment appraisal bias may be somewhat different from what it was when we appraised the patient pretreatment. Again, change on appraisal measures should reflect change in the patient. It should not reflect our desire that he or she has improved as a result of our treatment or change in us from having had 50 hours of contact with the patient.

Finally, we expect stability and consistency between and among clinicians. The extent to which test scores agree between or among two or more clinicians indicates interjudge reliability. As always, we want this to be high. If it is not, appraisal of the same patient by different clinicians may imply we are dealing with two patients. Highly standardized measures promote interjudge reliability. Poorly standardized measures reduce it. Without acceptable interjudge reliability, we cannot utilize another clinician's results. And, if we cannot utilize another clinician's results, we lose an effective control for clinician bias— using another clinician to measure change in a patient we have treated.

What constitutes acceptable reliability is difficult to state, and the way reliability is determined may be misleading. Variability between test and retest, intraclinician, and interclinician must be sufficiently below whatever is considered to be a "significant" clinical difference. For example, if we agreed that a 10 percentile change in an aphasic patient's Overall PICA percentile is a significant clinical change, none of this change should be attributable to test-retest, intraclinician, or interclinician variability. We need to know the range of reliability for each, say, plus or minus three percentile units. Then, when a patient changes by 15 percentile units, we can assume, with some confidence, that the magnitude is clinically important and does not result from instability or inconsistency in the test, the clinician, or different clinicians.

Beware the use of correlation coefficients to demonstrate reliability. Two events may be significantly correlated but significantly different. Wertz, Shubitowski, Dronkers, Lemme, & Deal (1985) reported test-retest word fluency measure performance in nonimpaired subjects and three groups of brain damaged adults. Test and retest scores were positively and significantly correlated, above +.95 in all groups, but there was a significant difference (p < .05) between test and retest scores in all groups. Thus, reliability is a question about difference not relationship. And, whatever the statistic used to report reliability, it is more useful clinically if confidence limits are presented.

Most formal, standardized tests for aphasia—the ones we can purchase—give some attention to validity and reliability. But, there are times in appraisal when we need to know things about a patient that the formal, standardized measures do not tell us. For example, for the mildly aphasic patients, most tests lack sufficient "top." The patient performs within the "normal" range. Conversely, for very severe patients, most standardized tests' attempts to command success for the chronically unsuccessful do not work. Thus, there are times when the tests are not testing, and when they are not, those are the times to modify them or seek something else. The something else, typically, is an informal measure the clinician devises to answer questions tests do not.

Modifying a test or employing a nonstandardized measure creates an interesting enigma in validity. We modify or look elsewhere when the test is not testing; essentially, when it is no longer valid for the patient or what we want to know about the patient. However, modifying a standardized test dilutes its validity, and the informal measures we devise do not contain prepackaged validity. Moreover, reliability has not been established for "modified" tests or for our informal measures. Typically, we do not suffer a lot of angst over this, but we do remind ourselves of what we are doing. And, if we elect to use our modifications or informal measures to detect change in our patients, we ensure they are valid and reliable before employing them.

Adherence to psychometric principles in test design can create a means-end reversal where we emphasize how we are appraising aphasic patients and ignore what we are appraising. Validity and reliability are important. Both should be acknowledged and sought, but not worshiped. Some, not all, of the measures that will be discussed here have demonstrated validity and reliability, some are valid depending on your point of view about and definition of aphasia, and some await demonstration that they are valid and reliable.

SPEECH AND LANGUAGE DATA

Appraising potentially aphasic people began with informal documentation of symptoms in the early case reports of Broca (1861) and Wernicke (1874), evolved through the early batteries developed by Head (1926), Weisenburg and McBride (1935), Chesher (1937), and Eisenson (1946, 1954); and culminated in the standardized tests of the 1960s, 1970s, and 1980s by Wepman and Jones (1961), Schuell (1965a), Porch (1967), Spreen and Benton (1969), Goodglass and Kaplan (1972), and Kertesz (1982). Benton (1967) and Tikofsky (1984) provided extensive historical reviews of aphasia testing and acknowledged many whose shoulders we stand on that are not listed here.

More recently, Lyon (1986) and Simmons (1986) presented reviews that make Darley's (1979) list and discussion of 14 tests for aphasia current. Here, we will provide a brief review of selected measures designed to appraise general language ability, performance in specific modalities, motor speech, nonverbal intelligence, and functional communication. We conclude with some of the more recent analyses—language samples, phonological process, semantic, grammatical, pragmatic, discourse, cohesion—that some are exploring to extend what is provided by the more traditional measures. Unfortunately, any list lacks, and this one is no exception. Our purpose is to provide examples and not exhaust what is available to achieve appraisal's purposes.

GENERAL LANGUAGE MEASURES

Most of the general language measures for aphasia share common purposes: to sample behavior in auditory comprehension, reading, oral expressive language, and writing; to permit a diagnosis of aphasia; to indicate severity; and to guide focusing treatment. These include: the Appraisal of Language Disturbance (Emerick, 1971), the Bilingual Aphasia Test (Paradis, 1987), the Boston Diagnostic Aphasia Examination (Goodglass & Kaplan, 1983a), Examining for Aphasia (Eisenson, 1954), the Language Modalities Test for Aphasia (Wepman & Jones, 1961), the Minnesota Test for Differential Diagnosis of Aphasia (Schuell, 1965a), the Neurosensory Center Comprehensive Examination for Aphasia (Spreen & Benton, 1969), the Porch Index of Communicative Ability (Porch, 1967), the Sklar Aphasia Scale (Sklar, 1966), and the Western Aphasia Battery (Kertesz, 1982). Some of these have additional purposes that make them differ from the others. For example, the Bilingual Aphasia Test permits testing an aphasic patient in each of the languages he or she speaks, the Boston Diagnostic Aphasia Examination and the Western Aphasia Battery are designed to classify the patient into one of the specific aphasia types, the Minnesota Test for Differential Diagnosis of Aphasia allows classification of the patient into a prognostic group, and the Porch Index of Communicative Ability includes a profile of the patient's performance to determine which neurogenic communication disorder he or she displays. Four of the

general language measures will be discussed here, two designed to classify the type of aphasia and two that avoid classification.

MEASURES DESIGNED TO CLASSIFY APHASIA

Two popular aphasia tests, the Boston Diagnostic Aphasia Examination (BDAE) (Goodglass & Kaplan, 1983a) and the Western Aphasia Battery (WAB) (Kertesz, 1982), include among their purposes the classification of patients into one of the aphasias—global, Broca's, Wernicke's, etc. The former was developed by neuropsychologists, and the latter was developed by a neurologist. Both tests are quite similar in tasks and stimuli; however, they differ markedly in scoring and methods for classification.

Duffy (1979) provided a comprehensive review of the first edition of the BDAE (Goodglass & Kaplan, 1972). It has been revised (Goodglass & Kaplan, 1983a), but its purposes—diagnose the presence and type of aphasic syndrome and permit inferences about cerebral localization, measure initial severity and detect change over time, and provide a comprehensive assessment of assets and deficits as a guide for treatment—remain essentially unchanged. Tasks include assessment of conversational and expository speech through conversation and picture description; auditory comprehension, ranging from word discrimination to complex ideational material; oral expression, including oral agility, repetition, oral reading, and naming; understanding written language, ranging from symbol and word discrimination through reading sentences and paragraphs; and writing, ranging from the mechanics of writing through written picture description. Supplementary language and nonlanguage tests are available to extend the basic battery. A variety of scores are provided, including a zero to five point Aphasia Severity Rating Scale, a Rating Scale Profile of Speech Characteristics to classify the type of aphasia, and percentiles for each of the subtests. The Rating Scale Profile of Speech Characteristics, shown in Figure 4-1, is used to classify a patient, when possible, in one of several types

Patient's Name __C. F.__   Date of rating __3/15/88__

Rated by __RTW__

APHASIA SEVERITY RATING SCALE

0. No usable speech or auditory comprehension.

1. All communication is through fragmentary expression; great need for inference, questioning, and guessing by the listener. The range of information that can be exchanged is limited, and the listener carries the burden of communication.

2. Conversation about familiar subjects is possible with help from the listener. There are frequent failures to convey the idea, but patient shares the burden of communication with the examiner.

3. The patient can discuss almost all everyday problems with little or no assistance. Reduction of speech and/or comprehension, however, makes conversation about certain material difficult or impossible.

4. Some obvious loss of fluency in speech or facility of comprehension, without significant limitation on ideas expressed or form of expression.

5. Minimal discernible speech handicaps; patient may have subjective difficulties that are not apparent to listener.

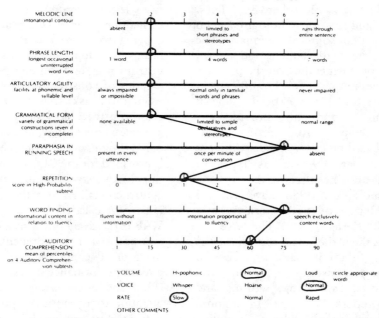

RATING SCALE PROFILE OF SPEECH CHARACTERISTICS

Figure 4-1. BDAE Rating Scale Profile of Speech Characteristics for a 61-year-old man who suffered a left hemisphere thromboembolic infarct in the frontal-parietal area. His profile places him within the range of ratings on each characteristic that is compatible with Broca's aphasia. From Goodglass, H., & Kaplan, E. (1983). *The Assessment of Aphasia and Related Disorders.* Philadelphia: Lea & Febiger. Reprinted with permission.

of aphasia. Goodglass and Kaplan (1983b) provided the rating scale profile range for Broca's, Wernicke's, anomic, conduction, and transcortical sensory aphasia. They described typical profiles for transcortical motor, global, mixed nonfluent, and subcortical aphasias. Classification involves using the patient's subtest summary profile to determine the appropriate rating on each of the eight characteristics in the rating scale. All tests for aphasia have strengths and weaknesses. Listing the latter is influenced by one's point of view about aphasia, experience with the test, and preference. We believe the BDAE is comprehensive in its appraisal of a wide range of abilities within each communicative modality; attempts to standardize profiles for different types of aphasia; provides measures of the qualitative aspects of speech through tallying the number of neologisms, literal and verbal paraphasias, and extended jargon; and assists in communicating with other disciplines, neurologists and neuropsychologists, who adhere to its philosophical rationale. The BDAE can require lengthy administration time, one to four hours depending on the patient's severity; it does not classify 40 to 60 percent of the patients tested into a specific type of aphasia; and it does not provide any empirically based prognostic information. Its validation is based on factor and discriminant analyses; however, the various types of reliability have not been reported.

Risser and Spreen (1985) have provided an extensive review of the Western Aphasia Battery (WAB) (Kertesz, 1982). The WAB was designed to evaluate the "main clinical aspects of language function: content, fluency, auditory comprehension, repetition, and naming, as well as reading, writing, and calculation" (Kertesz, 1982, p. 1). In addition, appraisal of nonverbal abilities, including drawing, block design, praxis, and nonverbal visual thinking as measured by the Coloured Progressive Matrices (Raven, 1962), are included in the battery. Particular emphasis has been placed on using the WAB's subscores to classify patients according to a taxonomic table (Kertesz, 1979) comprising eight types of aphasia: global, Broca's, isolation, transcor-

tical motor, Wernicke's, transcortical sensory, conduction, and anomic. In addition to classification, the WAB provides two major scores, an Aphasia Quotient (AQ) and a Cortical Quotient (CQ). Both range from zero to 100. AQ subtests include spontaneous speech, divided into information content and fluency, and measured by conversation and picture description; auditory verbal comprehension, including "yes-no" questions, auditory word recognition, and sequential commands; repetition of words and sentences; and naming, including object naming, word fluency, sentence completion, and responsive speech. An arbitrary cutoff AQ of 93.8 is used to separate normal from aphasic performance. Performance in four areas—fluency, comprehension, repetition, and naming—is used to enter the taxonomic table and determine the patient's type of aphasia. The CQ includes all AQ subtests plus tests for reading, ranging from letter discrimination to reading comprehension of sentences; writing, ranging from copying to written paragraph description; praxis, including upper limb, buccofacial, instrumental, and complex performance; and a series of constructional, visuospatial, and calculation tasks that require the patient to draw, construct block designs, perform simple arithmetic operations, and complete the Coloured Progressive Matrices. No normal cutoff is provided for the CQ, and none of the additional CQ tests—reading, writing, praxis, or constructional, visuospatial, and calculation—is used to classify the type of aphasia. The WAB is relatively quick to administer, one to two hours; it is comprehensive in its assessment of all communicative modalities; and patient performance is easy to score. Kertesz (1979) and his colleagues have given admirable attention to psychometric principles. Concurrent validity was established through comparison with the revised Neurosensory Center Comprehensive Examination for Aphasia (NCCEA) (Spreen & Benton, 1977), and adequate test-retest, interjudge, and intrajudge reliability has been demonstrated (Shewan & Kertesz, 1980). Classification of patients into one of the eight types by using cutoff scores in the taxonomic table is, as observed by Risser and Spreen (1985), "deceptively simple." Almost every patient can be classified, and the question is whether they are classified correctly. Although WAB classification is based on cluster analysis (Kertesz & Phipps, 1980), the original results generated 10 clusters for acute and 11 for chronic patients, but the taxonomic table employed with the test provides only eight clusters for all patients (Kertesz, 1979, 1982). Thus, the source of the cutoff scores for classification may be, as Risser and Spreen (1985) suggested, "somewhat vague and arbitrary." Moreover, we have evaluated and classified patients with the WAB whose aphasic type has changed from one day to the next, because performance was at the extreme range of the taxonomic cutoff scores on one administration of the test and exceeded the range on the next.

The WAB and BDAE are remarkably similar in some respects and quite different in others. The purposes of each, their content, and patient performance in the various modalities agree; however, whether and how they classify patients differ. Wertz, Deal, and Robinson (1984) compared BDAE and WAB performance by 45 aphasic patients. Correlations between the two tests for fluency, auditory comprehension, repetition, and naming ranged from +.84 to +.94. All were significant (p < .001). However, overall agreement in classification was only 27 percent. Fifteen of the 45 patients were classified as anomic aphasia on the WAB, and only five patients were classified as anomic on the BDAE. Twenty-eight of the 45 patients were unclassifiable on the BDAE, but only five patients were unclassifiable on the WAB. Thus, we have a dilemma. Two tests that are designed to do the same thing actually do it quite differently.

MEASURES THAT AVOID CLASSIFICATION

Schuell's (1965a) Minnesota Test for Differential Diagnosis of Aphasia (MTDDA) and Porch's (1967) Porch Index of Communicative Ability (PICA) are popular examples of general language measures that avoid any attempt to classify aphasia into the traditional aphasia types. Both were developed by speech-language pathologists, and both adhere to a definition of aphasia as a general reduction in language ability in all communicative modalities—auditory comprehension, reading, oral expressive use of language, and writing. And both, unlike the BDAE or WAB, utilize reading and writing performance to determine the presence and severity of aphasia.

Zubrick and Smith (1979) have provided a comprehensive review of the MTDDA. The battery was developed over 17 years and published in 1965 (Schuell, 1965a). Its purposes are to determine the level at which language performance breaks down in each language modality and to provide information about the nature of the deficits observed. Forty-seven subtests are used to appraise performance in five areas—auditory disturbances, visual and reading disturbances, speech and language disturbances, visuomotor and writing disturbances, and disturbances of numerical relations and arithmetic process. Scoring, for the most part, is by plus (+) or minus (−), and totals are obtained for each subtest. In addition, a Clinical Rating is completed using a 0, no observable impairment, to 6, most impaired, scale for understanding what is said, speech, reading, writing, and dysarthria. And a Diagnostic Scale, using 0, no impairment, to 4, no performance, is employed to rate 12 specific auditory, visual, speech, and writing behaviors. Although Schuell did not classify aphasia into the traditional types, she did provide five major and two minor descriptive and predictive diagnostic groups (Schuell, 1965b) based, primarily, on severity and the presence or absence of associated nonlanguage deficits, for example, Group 2: Aphasia with Visual Involvement. Each was assigned a general prognosis for ultimate outcome. The groups were modified later (Schuell & Sefer, 1973) into seven. Certainly, the MTDDA provides an extremely comprehensive sampling of behavior, but one pays a price. Testing time can range from two to six hours. Validity was demonstrated through factor analyses (Schuell, Jenkins, & Carroll, 1962). However, the various types of reliability have not been demonstrated. The MTDDA remains a testimonial to a master clinician's patience, care, and creativity in consolidating almost 20 years of knee-to-knee observation of aphasic patients into a measure for appraising the disorder.

Another example of general language tests for aphasia that was not designed to classify patients into traditional aphasic types is the Porch Index of Communicative Ability (PICA) (Porch, 1967). It has received a comprehensive review by McNeil (1979). The PICA's primary purposes are to provide an accurate and reliable measure of patient performance and a stable estimate of change in performance over time. Eighteen subtests, 17 of which use the same 10 homogeneous stimuli, appraise auditory comprehension, reading, oral expressive use of language, pantomime, visual matching, writing, and copying. These can be administered in one to two hours with most patients. A 16-point

multidimensional scale that describes each response along the dimensions of accuracy, completeness, responsiveness, promptness, and efficiency yields quantified measures for overall, gestural, verbal, and graphic performance. And, in the most recent revision of the PICA (Porch, 1981), scores can be computed for writing, copying, reading, pantomime, auditory comprehension, and visual matching. Percentiles are derived from raw scores for left hemisphere brain damaged patients and bilaterally brain damaged patients. Patient performance is graphed, as shown in Figure 4-2, as a Modality Response Summary—gestural, verbal, and graphic, or as a Ranked Response Summary—tests arranged in the order of difficulty based on performance by a large sample of patients. Three methods for obtaining a prognosis—High-Overall Prediction (HOAP), High-Overall Prediction Slopes (HOAP Slopes), and Intrasubtest Variability—are provided. Validity has been demonstrated through

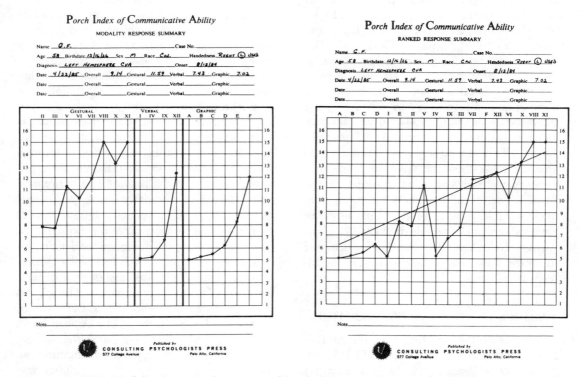

Figure 4-2. PICA Modality Response Summary and Ranked Response Summary for an aphasic patient with coexisting apraxia of speech. Reprinted with permission from Consulting Psychologists Press, Inc., 577 College Avenue, Palo Alto, CA 94306.

factorial and multiple regression analyses, and test-retest, interjudge, and intrajudge reliability is quite acceptable. The PICA's strengths are its description of patient performance, quantification of performance, reliability, indications for treatment planning, opportunity for inter- and intrasubtest comparison, and differentiation among several neuropathologies of speech and language. Its limitations are a somewhat limited sample of communicative tasks, a lack of measures to detect mild aphasia in some modalities, the need for intensive training to ensure validity and reliability, and the necessity to present more difficult tasks prior to easier ones. Certainly, the PICA will not provide all that one needs to meet appraisal's purposes. But, much of what it does provide cannot be obtained with any other measure.

"SCREENING" TESTS FOR APHASIA

The length of some general language measures, one to six hours, has prompted development of several shorter, or screening, measures. Some, the Halstead-Wepman Aphasia Screening Test (Halstead & Wepman, 1949) and the short examination for aphasia (Schuell, 1957), were designed to assist neurologists in assessing aphasic deficits as part of the neurological evaluation. Others, the Aphasia Language Performance Scales (ALPS) (Keenan & Brassell, 1975), Sklar Aphasia Scale (SAS) (Sklar, 1966), Aphasia Screening Test (Whurr, 1974), and Bedside Evaluation and Screening Test of Aphasia (BEST) (Fitch-West & Sands, 1987), were designed to provide a rapid appraisal in most, typically bedside, settings.

Two efforts to devise shorter tests utilized parts of longer batteries. Schuell's (1957) short examination was derived from her longer MTDDA, which was, at that time, in experimental form. DiSimoni, Keith, Holt, and Darley (1975) and DiSimoni, Keith, and Darley (1980) proposed two shortened versions of the PICA, one using four subtests and another using 2 of the 10 PICA objects in 17 subtests.

One wonders, What is the purpose of a screening test for aphasia? If all of the longer batteries contain limitations, what can be accomplished by a brief screening test? Fitch-West and Sands (1987) provided the BEST answer. Shorter length of hospitalization, the variety of patient environments, and rapidly evolving behavior in acutely aphasic patients, they suggested, require a measure that can be administered rapidly and economically in a variety of settings. They observed, however, that the need for convenience carries cautions. Screening tests were not designed to replace longer, more comprehensive measures. Schuell (1966) voiced similar reservations in her reevaluation of the short examination for aphasia. She suggested screening tests are clinical tools for specific purposes, but they do not replace comprehensive evaluations, because they may fail to sample behavior in all communicative modalities, not provide a sufficient sample in the modalities sampled, and obtain insufficient information to make a differential diagnosis. Her alternative to a screening test was to screen with a comprehensive battery by establishing baseline and ceiling performance within each language modality through brief, systematic sampling. This avoids arbitrary selection of a few screening tests that may not be appropriate for the patient, and it permits focusing on tests that are appropriate.

SPECIFIC MODALITY TESTS

General language measures, typically, sample behavior in all communicative modalities, but they may be limited in their range of appraisal in one or more modalities. Thus, some patients may show no deficits in some modalities, and we must look further. Other patients may display deficits within a modality that suggest the need for treatment, and we look for where and how that treatment should be focused. In both situations, we employ tests designed to explore a specific communicative modality—auditory comprehension, reading, oral expressive language, writing, and gesturing—more thoroughly. Simmons (1986) has suggested an appropriate rationale for modality specific tests. The purpose should be clear, and the expected return must justify the cost of patient and clinician time, energy, and funds.

AUDITORY COMPREHENSION

Kearns and Hubbard (1977) observed that severely aphasic patients performed essentially the same as mildly impaired patients on the two PICA subtests that appraise auditory comprehension. For the former, we seek measures that assist in focusing treatment for auditory comprehension deficits, and for the latter, we seek measures that probe auditory comprehension to determine whether sufficient deficits are present to justify treatment. Measures exist to provide the information needed.

DeRenzi and Vignolo (1962) introduced the Token Test as a means to detect minimal aphasia. It employs 20 tokens that vary in three dimensions—color, shape, and size. Four sets of minimally redundant stimuli are used to increase the length of the auditory stimulus systematically, and a fifth set manipulates the grammatical complexity. Since its introduction, the Token Test has undergone a number of modifications (Boller & Vignolo, 1966; DeRenzi & Faglioni, 1978; Spreen & Benton, 1969). This evolution has been reviewed by Wertz (1979). McNeil and Prescott (1978) introduced the Revised Token Test (RTT) as a standardized elaboration of the earlier efforts and included a series of subtests that systematically manipulate syntactic variables and permitted scoring with a multidimensional scale. The RTT can take 15 to 75 minutes to administer. It provides the virtue of the earlier versions of the Token Test, detection of mild auditory comprehension deficits, and it is precise in determining how much and what kinds of deficits are present as a guide for focusing treatment.

Shewan (1979) developed the Auditory Comprehension Test for Sentences (ACTS) to specify different kinds of deficits, determine where auditory comprehension breaks down, and focus treatment. Sentences that vary systematically in length, vocabulary, and syntactic complexity are read aloud by the examiner, and the patient responds by selecting a picture from a matrix of four choices.

The ACTS takes approximately 15 minutes to administer, and performance can be compared with normative data or analyzed quantitatively by the types of errors made.

The Functional Auditory Comprehension Task (FACT), developed by LaPointe and Horner (1978), was designed to determine how aphasic people comprehend what they hear when they are not being tested. Patient responses are gestural, following a variety of instructions that gradually increase in difficulty. Common objects and aspects of the environment are used as stimuli, and these are manipulated, systematically, by introducing variables, for example, length and complexity, known to influence auditory comprehension. LaPointe, Holtzapple, and Graham's (1985) comparison of FACT performance with performance on the Token Test and the Communicative Abilities in Daily Living (CADL) (Holland, 1980a) support its use as a measure of "functional" auditory comprehension. Subsequent reports have examined potential error patterns in FACT three-part commands (LaPointe, Holtzapple, & Graham, 1986) and the influence of contextual relevance on auditory comprehension (Graham, Holtzapple, & LaPointe, 1987).

READING

Beyond the reading subtests in the standard language measures, little has been available to push and probe reading deficits in aphasic adults. Some have employed reading tests developed for children; for example, the Gates-MacGinitie Reading Tests (1965). Unfortunately, the tasks and, especially, the stimuli in these measures are not appropriate for older people who have spent a lifetime perusing print. LaPointe and Horner (1979) offered the first reading modality measure to contain appropriate tasks and content for aphasic adults when they introduced the Reading Comprehension Battery for Aphasia (RCBA).

The RCBA contains 10 subtests that appraise reading comprehension of words, sentences, and paragraphs. Word reading subtests explore the influence of visual, auditory, and semantic similarity in the stimuli. Subtests for paragraph comprehension compare comprehension of factual material with comprehension of material that must be inferred. Additional subtests examine functional reading, synonyms, and morphosyntax. Scoring is plus (+) or minus (−) and the entire battery takes, on the average, 30 minutes to administer. The RCBA provides excellent information for focusing treatment, and it can be used as a change measure to evaluate the effects of treatment.

ORAL EXPRESSIVE LANGUAGE

A variety of measures have been developed to expand appraisal of aphasic patients' oral expressive language abilities. These include the Reporter's Test (DeRenzi & Ferrari, 1978), the Boston Naming Test (Kaplan, Goodglass, & Weintraub, 1983), and a variety of word fluency measures. Each probes specific oral expressive performance to determine deficits that may not be detected on other measures and, if deficits are found, assists in focusing treatment. In addition, each provides a means for detecting change in performance that may not be observable in reevaluation with general language measures.

DeRenzi and Ferrari (1978) utilized the format and stimuli in the 36 item shortened Token Test designed to measure auditory comprehension (DeRenzi & Faglioni, 1978) to obtain a measure of oral expressive language. The Reporter's Test requires the patient to state the examiner's manipulations of the tokens so they could be understood by a hypothetical third person. The patient's reports are scored plus (+) or minus (−) or can be calculated as a weighted score that gives credit for each correct word used to report the examiner's action. As in the auditory comprehension Token Test, length is gradually increased and, eventually, syntax is manipulated. Cutoff scores have been established to separate aphasic from nonaphasic performance. The test appears especially useful in differentiating mildly aphasic from normal performance (Wener & Duffy, 1983).

Problems with naming are found in all types of aphasia and in a variety of other neurogenic communication deficits. Kaplan, Goodglass, and Weintraub (1983) developed the Boston Naming Test to explore naming ability beyond the limits of its sampling on the general language measures. Sixty drawings that represent picturable nouns are presented from easy (bed), to difficult (abacus). The patient is requested to name each, and if he or she fails because of visual misperception of the picture, a stimulus cue, for example, "No—it's something to eat" is given. For other failures, a phonemic cue, the first sound of the target word, is given. Scoring includes the number of correct responses, the number of stimulus cues given and the number correct following the cue, and the number of phonemic cues given, and the number correct following the cue. In addition, the latency for each response is recorded. Norms, based on performance by small samples of children, nonaphasic adults, and aphasic adults are available. The Boston Naming Test may be particularly useful in detecting mild word-finding problems or differentiating among aphasic and nonaphasic naming disorders.

Word fluency measures are controlled association tasks that require the production of as many words as possible beginning with a specified letter of the alphabet or representatives of a specified category (animals, fruit, supermarket items) in a specified period of time (Wertz, 1979). The BDAE and WAB include word fluency for animals as a subtest, and the NCCEA includes a word fluency subtest for letters—F, A, and S. Borkowski, Benton, and Spreen (1967) introduced the measure as a sensitive means to detect the presence of brain damage. It has been used by Chapey (1981) to assess divergent language production, and Adamovich and Henderson (1984) and Collins McNeil, Lentz, Shubitowski, & Rosenbek (1984) have explored its use in differentiating among different neuropathologies of communication and types of aphasia. Typically, the patient's score is the number of words produced in one minute for the specified category or letter. The contribution of word fluency measures to understanding and managing aphasia is not too clear. Its potential for measuring change in patient performance is seriously challenged by its lack of test-retest reliability (Wertz et al., 1985).

WRITING

We know of no specific measures designed to explore writing beyond the way it is sampled in the general language measures. Milner (1964) has employed a written word fluency measure to differentiate intra- and interhemispheric lesions. And, written picture description can be analyzed using the methods employed to assess oral expressive communicative efficiency, grammar, discourse, and cohesion. These will be discussed later.

Recent reports by Hansen and McNeil (1986) and Hansen, McNeil, and Vetter (1987) have indicated assessment and analysis of aphasic writing should proceed with caution. Using a battery of copying, writing to dictation, automatic writing, and written picture description tasks, they explored dominant and nondominant handwriting in a group of neurologically normal individuals. Perceptual and computer-assisted measurements indicated several differences between dominant and nondominant hand production. Moreover, the writing of these normal individuals was not error free. Thus, appraisal of aphasic writing must consider hemiplegia's influence on dictating the use of a nonpreferred hand to write and the probable presence of errors in the patient's premorbid writing. All deficits cannot be explained by brain damage, and Hansen and her colleagues' results indicate we should use normative, not normal, as our comparison. Dentistry reminds us that normal is teeth without cavities, and normative is what most of us have; teeth with cavities. Similarly, when we explore the holes in aphasic persons' performance, our best comparison is with what is normative.

GESTURE

Treatment for severe aphasia often encourages the patient to use pantomime and gesture to convey what cannot be said or written. Similarly, we counsel family, friends, and hospital personnel to accompany their words to patients with appropriate gestures to facilitate comprehension. Some general language measures appraise the patient's ability to pantomime, for example, the PICA, and others include gesture and pantomime subtests to detect the presence and severity of limb apraxia, for example, the WAB. None, however, assesses the patient's ability to understand pantomime. The New England Pantomime Tests (Duffy & Duffy, 1984) do.

Three measures, the Pantomime Recognition Test, the Pantomime Expression Test, and the Pantomime Referential Abilities Test compose the battery. To test recognition, the examiner pantomimes an action, and the patient selects an appropriate picture from a matrix of four pictures. Expression is tested by showing the patient a picture of an object and having him or her demonstrate its use. Both tasks are scored with the PICA multidimensional scoring system. The Pantomime Referential Abilities Test assesses the patient's ability to communicate with pantomime. A third party is enlisted to receive and interpret the patient's pantomimic messages. Success is measured by the third party's ability to select an object associated with the patient's pantomime. Normative data are provided for the Recognition and Expression tests. Duffy and Duffy have provided a means for appraising, focusing treatment, and evaluating progress in the gestural modality.

FUNCTIONAL COMMUNICATION TESTS

Some have criticized standardized, traditional tests for aphasia as being poor measures of a patient's functional communication. They suggest the metalinguistic nature of traditional tests does not permit the patient's functional communicative ability to shine through. If there are places on the aphasic patient's body where this is a possibility, he or she is not communicating—he or she is leaking. Nevertheless, efforts to assess aphasic patients, abilities to communicate in natural environments have culminated in the Functional Communication Profile (FCP) (Sarno, 1969) and the Communicative Abilities in

Daily Living (CADL) (Holland, 1980a). Both provide information that is not provided by the more metalinguistic, traditional measures, but their comparison with the general language measures indicates differences among tests may be more apparent than real. For example, Holland's (1980a) validation studies with the CADL demonstrated patient CADL performance correlated significantly with performance on the PICA (+.93), FCP (+.87), and the BDAE (+.84). Thus, although functional tests and metalinguistic tests may not be totally fungible, they are quite familiar.

Sarno's (1969) FCP uses informal interaction and interviews with the patient to rate 45 behaviors on a nine-point scale. Five areas—movement, speaking, understanding, reading, and other—are assessed. Each samples a variety of functional communication abilities, for example: movement, ability to indicate "yes" and "no"; speaking, saying greetings; understanding, awareness of gross environmental sounds; reading, reading newspaper headlines; and other, time orientation. Adjectives—poor, fair, good, normal—correspond to the nine-point rating scale. Scores in each area are totaled, and a percentage score for each is derived from a table. In addition, each area score is weighted, and an overall percentage score can be obtained by totaling the weighted scores. Scoring of some items may need to be inferred from the interview, the patient's report, or reports from family members. Nevertheless, interrater reliability is quite acceptable. Validity is based on comparisons with the MTDDA, clinicians' ratings of communicative adequacy, and other clinical measures.

The CADL (Holland, 1980a) was designed to assess how aphasic people communicate in everyday encounters. It does not replace traditional aphasia tests, but it does supplement them by providing information that they do not. A three-point scale is used to score 68 items that seek information in 10 categories: reading, writing, and using numbers to estimate, calculate, and judge time; speech acts; utilizing verbal and nonverbal context; role playing; sequenced and relationship-dependent communicative

behavior; social conventions; divergencies; nonverbal symbolic communication; deixis, movement-related or movement-dependent communicative behavior; and humor, absurdity, and metaphor. The CADL's content includes a number of items that differ from those in traditional tests, and the examiner plays roles—doctor, receptionist, store clerk—to elicit some responses. Cutoff scores are provided to separate normal from aphasic performance, and the influence of living environment, institutionalized versus noninstitutionalized, is considered. Holland's validation studies show CADL performance correlates positively and significantly with performance on the PICA, FCP, and BDAE. More importantly, CADL performance correlates positively and significantly with a validation measure that included observation of patients communicating in their everyday environments and information from interviews with patient family members or other caregivers. Thus, the CADL appears to do exactly what it was designed to do, appraise communicative abilities in daily living.

MOTOR SPEECH EVALUATION

Two motor speech disorders, apraxia of speech and dysarthria, may coexist with aphasia. It is necessary to determine whether either is present, and if present, to rate the severity. Certainly, the presence of dysarthria or apraxia of speech may be detected in the patient's oral expressive performance on the general language measures. And, some measures, for example the MTDDA, contain subtests that are particularly sensitive to the presence of dysarthria or apraxia of speech. Additional, supplementary tests to probe motor speech disorders are available, and one may elect to administer these when in doubt or to seek additional information.

Dabul (1979) developed the Apraxia Battery for Adults (ABA) to detect the presence of apraxia of speech and to provide an estimate of its severity. Six subtests—diadochokinetic rate, increasing word length, limb apraxia and oral apraxia, latency and utterance time for polysyllabic words, repeated trials, and inventory of articulation characteristics of apraxia—are scored with a variety of methods. Scores are used to complete a checklist of apraxic features and rate impaired performance on each subtest as either mild to moderate or severe to profound.

Wertz, LaPointe, and Rosenbek (1984) collected stimuli and tasks from a variety of sources, including Darley, Aronson, and Brown (1975) and Johns and Darley (1970), and combined them in a Motor Speech Evaluation. The tasks include: conversation, vowel prolongation, rapid alternating movements, repetition of multisyllabic words, repeated production of the same word, repetition of words that increase in length, repetition of monosyllabic words that begin and end with the same phoneme, repetition of sentences, counting forward and backward, picture description, and oral reading. Scoring can be done by a variety of methods—type of error (aphasic, apraxic, dysarthric), PICA multidimensional scoring, or transcription. Severity is rated on a one, (mild) to seven, (severe) scale. The purpose of this evaluation is to detect the presence of apraxia of speech or dysarthria and if either is present, to rate its severity. In addition, the sample often provides sufficient information to classify dysarthria into a perceptual type or types (Darley et al., 1975).

Two standardized measures for assessing dysarthria are available. One, the Frenchay Dysarthria Assessment (Enderby, 1983), rates 29 behaviors with a nine-point scale and provides a profile for classifying the dysarthria into a specific type; for example, upper motor neuron lesion, mixed upper and lower motor neuron, etc. The other, Assessment of Intelligibility of Dysarthric Speech (Yorkston & Beukelman, 1981), is appropriate for patients who can read words and sentences. For those who cannot, repetition can be used, but sampling and scoring is a bit more cumbersome. Several measures can be derived, including intelligibility for single words, intelligibility for sentences, speaking rate, rate of intelligible speech, rate of unintelligible speech, and a communication efficiency ratio. In addition, a sufficient sample is collected to permit classification into a perceptual type of dysarthria.

NONVERBAL INTELLIGENCE MEASURES

Intelligence, verbal and nonverbal, is extremely difficult to assess in aphasic patients (Lebrun & Hoops, 1974; Wertz, 1985). Nevertheless, many of us attempt to, and when we do, we are never quite sure what the results mean or what we can do with them. Simmons (1986) provided as good a rationale for this effort as we have heard. She suggested nonverbal measures may assist in selecting a treatment; for example, visual action therapy (Helm-Estabrooks, Fitzpatrick, & Barresi, 1982), or indicate a channel for nonverbal communication, for example, drawing or graphics (Lyon, 1984). The increased participation of neuropsychologists in assessing aphasic patients permits us to rely on them and their tools to appraise intelligence. But, we know about and have used some of the measures that are discussed here.

The most popular nonverbal intelligence measure employed by speech-language pathologists is probably the Coloured Progressive Matrices (CPM) (Raven, 1962). It is reported to be a test of nonverbal visual thinking, and it is included as one of the WAB subtests that provide the Cortical Quotient. Thirty-six items, divided into three sets of 12, require the patient to select one of six alternatives to complete a visual pattern. The number of correct responses can be compared with sparse normative data for different ages. We find no strong relationship between CPM performance and severity of language impairment. There is some evidence (Wertz, 1966) that frontal lesions impair CPM performance more than posterior lesions, regardless of the side of the lesion or the severity of the patient's language impairment. When we see a high CPM score in a severely aphasic patient, we may make an extra effort to locate a lane that will let his or her intellect flow. But, we are not overwhelmed by our success.

Some (Tikofsky & Reynolds, 1962, 1963; Wertz, 1967) have used Grant's (1954) Wisconsin Card Sorting Task to evaluate intellectual ability in aphasic adults. The task requires the patient to sort cards that vary along three dimensions—color, form, and number. After each response, the patient is informed whether the response was right or wrong and he or she can use the information to make the next response. The task is constructed so that the correct category is changed without informing the patient after every tenth consecutive correct response. The patient is expected to use the knowledge of results provided by the examiner to detect a shift has occurred and to modify the next response. Tikofsky and Reynolds (1962, 1963) found aphasic patients made significantly more errors than nonaphasic people in their sorting behavior. Wertz (1967) reported similar results; however, he noted that frontal lesions resulted in poorer performance than posterior lesions regardless of the side of the lesion, and he found no significant relationship between card sorting performance and severity of language impairment. What does the Wisconsin Card Sorting Task tell us about nonverbal intelligence in aphasia? Essentially, it is a nonverbal, trial-and-error learning task. The patient must search, systematically, for the correct solution. When it is found, he or she must continue to use it until there is a change in the problem. When this occurs, the patient must return to search behavior. Thus, optimum performance requires formulating a plan to reduce active uncertainty, recognizing that the plan has worked, and utilizing it until it is no longer appropriate. Perhaps the same procedure is appropriate in communication, but there appears to be no relationship between a patient's ability to use it in a nonverbal problem solving task and his or her severity of aphasia.

. Smith (1973) adapted the Symbol Digit Modalities Test from the Digit Symbol subtest of the Wechsler Adult Intelligence Scale (WAIS) (Wechsler, 1955). Smith's version requires the patient to substitute numbers for symbols by using a key that pairs a number with a nonsense symbol. The number of correct number for symbol substitutions in a specified time is the patient's score. Smith permits two forms of the test, written or spoken. This type of task is extremely sensitive to the presence of brain damage, but it is of little use in predicting the laterality of a lesion (Lezak, 1983). Tissot, Lhermitte, and Ducarne (1963)

reported that WAIS Digit Symbol scores by aphasic patients are low, but this results from exceedingly slow performance that is essentially error-free.

The Test of Nonverbal Intelligence (TONI) (Brown, Sherbenou, & Johnson, 1984) is reported to be appropriate for testing aphasic people. To our knowledge, anyone who has used it to do this has not reported the results. Nevertheless, the TONI is offered as a language-free measure of cognitive ability. It is similar to the CPM. Fifty items require the patient to search four to six alternatives and find the one that completes a pattern. Five rules govern relationships among the stimuli: simple matching, analogies, classification, intersections, and progressions. Two equivalent forms are available. Raw scores are converted to TONI Quotients and percentiles, based on normal performance, in a variety of ages from 5 to 85 years. The TONI appears to be a somewhat longer and more difficult black and white alternative to the more colorful CPM.

TRENDS IN APPRAISING APHASIA

We observed earlier that when tests are not testing, they should be modified. Another approach is to employ something else. Many are doing the latter. These efforts include assessment of communicative efficiency; phonologic, semantic, syntactic, and pragmatic analyses; and discourse analysis. Simmons (1986) has provided a thorough review of these recent trends in analyzing aphasic language. Only a few will be considered briefly here.

CONTENT AND EFFICIENCY

Yorkston and Beukelman (1977, 1980) developed a means to quantify connected speech samples of moderately to mildly involved aphasic people. A verbal picture description is elicited, and two measures are derived: content units, the amount of information conveyed; and efficiency, the speaking rate in syllables per minute and the number of content units per minute. The measure indicates that the amount of information conveyed, content units, declines as severity of aphasia increases; however, mildly aphasic speakers tend to convey as much information as nonaphasic speakers. The efficiency measures, speaking rate and content units per minute, on the other hand, separate aphasic speakers from nonaphasic speakers. Thus, mildly aphasic patients provide essentially nonaphasic content, but they are inefficient in doing so. The measure is appropriate for appraising mildly aphasic patients who "top" the more traditional measures and, perhaps, for detecting change if we elect to treat their communicative efficiency.

PHONOLOGICAL ANALYSIS

Controversy continues to surround the nature of articulation errors in people with left hemisphere brain damage. Some (Martin, 1974) have objected to the term *apraxia of speech*. Others (Johns & Darley, 1970) have suggested apraxia of speech is a motor speech disorder that differs from the language disorder, aphasia. If the two are different, then the clinician should manage them differently (Wertz et al., 1984). Thus, one of appraisal's tasks is to differentiate between articulatory errors in aphasia and those that may result from apraxia of speech. Kearns (1980) and Bowman, Hodson, and Simpson (1980) suggested phonological process analysis may provide a means for determining which is which.

Ingram (1976), Hodson (1981), and Shriberg and Kwiatkowski (1980) have employed phonological process analysis to establish the dominant patterns of articulation errors in children. Phonological processes describe systematic strategies that reduce or modify the contrastive elements in an utterance. At least 10 basic phonological processes have been described; for example, reduction of syllables, stopping of continuants, and fronting of velars. In addition, miscellaneous phonological processes may be employed in the analysis, for example, postvocalic devoicing, depalatalization, and affrication. The task is to determine the frequency of occurrence for each of the basic and miscellaneous processes.

Simmons (1986) observed the use of phonological process analysis has not been popular in appraising neurogenic communication disorders. One can guess why. Bowman and colleagues (1980) analyzed over 4,800 phoneme productions in 20 patients to determine which of the 10 basic processes were appropriate for each error. Then, errors were classified further into 16 miscellaneous processes. Perhaps the advent of computer programs (Weiner, 1984) will lessen the labor and popularize this pastime.

SEMANTIC ANALYSES

Vocabulary and meaning in aphasic language are typically probed by confrontation naming or tallying content words in spontaneous speech. Crystal (1982) has suggested neither are adequate, because semantics may vary across situations and must be related to both grammar and lexicon. His Profile in Semantics (PRISM) provides an elaborate analysis of semantic deficits and, he has suggested, a means for organizing treatment. The PRISM-L inventories minor and major lexical items in four main sections and in subcategories within each section. The PRISM-G is a system to analyze meaning as it is conveyed by different grammatical elements. Content for both analyses comes from the patient's spontaneous speech samples.

Simmons (1986) observed the procedure is cumbersome. We agree and add extremely time consuming. Nevertheless, this kind of analysis may indicate the consistency or variability of semantic deficits in a variety of contexts. And, it is certainly a sophisticated step beyond limiting appraisal of semantics to confrontation naming. Development of computer programs (Bennett & Alter, 1985) to assist in semantic analysis of speech samples may ease the burden and make this approach more practical.

GRAMMATICAL ANALYSIS

Some traditional measures, BDAE and WAB, detect and classify grammatical deficits and differences in and among aphasic patients. But, none provides elaborate analysis or precise information for focusing treatment. Tonkovich (1979) suggested the use of case grammar to explore the relationships between semantic and syntactic components of aphasic utterances and made a case for its application in focusing treatment for Broca's aphasia. Others (Kearns & Simmons, 1983; Penn, 1983) have employed Crystal's (1982) Language Assessment, Remediation, and Screening Procedure (LARSP) to appraise aphasic patients' grammar.

The LARSP provides a profile based on seven developmental stages of syntax acquisition; however, it is reported to be applicable for both children and adults (Crystal, Fletcher, & Garman, 1976). For a full assessment, approximately 30 minutes of conversation between clinician and patient is obtained and then transcribed for analysis. Information is organized into four main areas: syntactic ability at the sentence, clause, phrase, and word levels; the main stages of grammatical acquisition; the main patterns of grammatical interaction between the two communicative partners, clinician and patient; and quantitative information, including the total number of sentences, mean number of sentences per conversational turn, and the mean sentence length. The results indicate the patient's syntactic deficits and identify what he or she may be doing to compensate for his or her grammatical problems. Both, Simmons (1986) suggested, may assist planning appropriate treatment.

PRAGMATIC ANALYSIS

Holland (1977) observed that aphasic persons often communicate better than they talk. Traditional measures tend to focus on how aphasic people talk, especially in one context, taking an aphasia test. So, there has been a search for a means to evaluate how aphasic people communicate. What some have found is pragmatics; the use of language in context, especially interpersonal, social situations. Application of pragmatic principles to aphasia has been elaborated by Davis (1983), Wilcox (1983), Davis and Wilcox (1981), and Wilcox and Davis (1977).

Pragmatic analysis of aphasic communication has been assessed with the Communication Profile (Gurland, Chwat, & Wollner, 1982) and the Pragmatic Protocol (Prutting & Kirchner, 1983). The former looks at the aphasic patient's interaction with various communication partners. The latter was originally developed with children and has been employed recently (Prutting & Kirchner, 1987) with brain damaged adults. It includes 30 pragmatic aspects of language divided into verbal, paralinguistic, and nonverbal aspects. About 15 minutes of conversation between the patient and a familiar conversational partner is collected. Each of the 30 aspects is rated as "appropriate," "inappropriate," or "no opportunity to observe." A severity score is shunned, because some of the aspects are considered to handicap communication more than others. One can tally the number of instances of each inappropriate pragmatic aspect and calculate the percentage of inappropriate behaviors.

Application of the Pragmatic Protocol with aphasic patients has yielded some interesting results. Binder (1984) compared Pragmatic Protocol performance by aphasic patients with performance on the WAB and CADL. It failed to correlate significantly with either. Prutting and Kirchner (1987) compared Pragmatic Protocol performance by aphasic patients who had suffered a left hemisphere CVA with performance by patients who had suffered a right hemisphere CVA but were not aphasic. Mean percentage of appropriate pragmatic behaviors was similar in the two groups, 82 percent for aphasic patients and 84 percent for right hemisphere patients. However, the kinds of pragmatic deficits differed between groups. Aphasic patients' deficits were primarily in the verbal aspects parameters—specificity and accuracy of expression, pause time in turn taking, quantity and conciseness of the message, fluency, and the variety of speech acts produced. Conversely, right hemisphere patients' inappropriate behaviors were distributed across verbal aspects—turn taking adjacency, contingency, and quantity and conciseness; paralinguistic aspects—prosody; and nonverbal aspects—eye gaze. Roberts, Wertz, Bernstein-Ellis, & Shubitowski (1987) demonstrated that nonfluent aphasic patients display more inappropriate pragmatic behaviors than fluent aphasic patients and that improvement in pragmatic performance differs between the two types of aphasia and from improvement measured by traditional tests or a measure of syntax.

So, appraisal of pragmatic performance appears to yield information not sampled by other measures, WAB and CADL, and it appears to differentiate among left and right hemisphere brain damage and nonfluent and fluent aphasia. Both support its inclusion as part of an aphasia appraisal battery. For the patient, pragmatics may be an attempt to obtain equilibrium. Aphasia has shifted his or her world, and he or she shifts to maintain his or her angle to the world. This shifting, compensation, rebalancing may be viewed in preserved, appropriate, pragmatic performance but go unnoticed on other measures that focus on words that have flown. For the clinician, appraisal of pragmatics may provide equilibrium in the way he or she views the shifted world of aphasia.

DISCOURSE ANALYSIS

Ulatowska and Bond (1983) have traced the interdisciplinary interest in discourse—the naturally occurring unit of language—and the application of discourse grammar (Berko-Gleason et al., 1980; Ulatowska, North, & Macaluso-Haynes, 1981; Ulatowska, Doyle, Freedman-Stern, Macaluso-Haynes, & North, 1983; Ulatowska, Freedman-Stern, Doyle, Macaluso-Haynes, & North, 1983) to analyze aphasic patients' communication. Connected samples of a patient's language are used to examine the relationships among pragmatic, cognitive, and linguistic aspects of communication. Each can be observed in four types of discourse: conversational, speaker and listener take turns in exchanging information; expository, discourse is focused on a specific topic; procedural, focus is on relating how something is done; and narrative, description of something that happened with emphasis on who did what. Each type has its own grammar, and specified units and levels are employed in the analysis. For example, narrative discourse contains three essential components that are established by its grammar: a setting, a complicating action, and a resolution. The setting includes who, when, and where; the complicating action relates the events in the story and their sequence; and the resolution provides how everything turned out.

Analysis of narrative discourse has been popular in aphasia (Ulatowska & Bond, 1983). Typically, the patient is asked to retell a story, describe a story from a sequence of pictures, or tell a story from memory. Discourse analysis of these productions indicates that aphasic patients produce shorter and less complex narratives than nonaphasic subjects, but the aphasic patients retain the essential elements—setting, complicating action, resolution—established by narrative discourse grammar. The errors that occur in aphasic discourse are typically problems in cohesion, the conceptual linkage of propositions. Although there are several linguistic devices that maintain cohesion, aphasic patients appear to have inordinate difficulty with three: reference—establishing who or what is being discussed; sequence of tense—frequency of and appropriateness in shifting verb tense; and connectors—temporal, causal, or locative organization of information across propositions. Lemme, Headberg, and Bottenberg (1984) and Piehler and Holland (1984) have provided specific methods for analyzing cohesion in aphasic speakers' language, and Armstrong (1987) reported that cohesive harmony in aphasic discourse is significantly related with judged coherence.

Ulatowska and Bond (1983) suggested discourse analysis can make important contributions to patient management. In appraisal and treatment, discourse analysis permits evaluating the influence of context—the setting and the knowledge shared between speaker and listener—on performance. Further, it allows assessing information in different modalities—speaking, writing, and gesturing. And, its units of analysis identify salient errors and suggest the most profitable targets for treatment.

SUMMARY

The game of appraising aphasia has been a victim of its own success. Marie (1883) used three papers to appraise aphasia. Today's clinician may choose from an array of standardized and nonstandardized measures that permit a brief screening of behavior; an exhaustive inventory of a range of ability in each communicative modality; classification of aphasia into a taxonomy; elaborate exploration of auditory comprehension, reading, oral expressive language, or gesture; functional communication; and detailed probing of phonology, semantics, syntax, pragmatics, or discourse. We pedal to keep up, and our feet only rarely hit the ground.

Sometimes, we are asked, "What test should I buy?" Usually, we stifle the response this question deserves, "Should you be working with aphasic patients?" No single test will provide anamnesis, and too many will evoke titubation. Moreover, tests and testing constitute only a portion of appraisal. There is no substitute for history—biographical and medical. The measures we administer are dictated by our purposes—diagnosis, prognosis, focusing treatment—and the preferences our experience has established. One has little faith in the potency of measures that one has never personally experienced.

AN APPRAISAL BATTERY

If time and the patient's condition permit, we employ a battery that includes a motor speech evaluation, a measure of general language ability, and a look at orientation and the patient's fund of general information. Evaluating motor speech indicates the presence or absence of coexisting apraxia of speech and/or dysarthria. The general language measure provides an overall impression of severity, strengths, and weaknesses in each modality, and suggestions for further exploration with specific modality measures. Appraising orientation and fund of general information assist in deciding whether what we are seeing is aphasia, confusion, or dementia.

If time does not permit, there is usually a reason that can be paraphrased into a purpose that guides appraisal: the patient is being discharged this afternoon and wonders whether he or she should return for additional appraisal and subsequent treatment as an outpatient; the patient is a diagnostic enigma, and Neurology has requested our assistance in differentiating between aphasia and dementia before grand rounds at noon; the patient has been ill and unresponsive, there is a bed but no speech-language pathology services available in the nursing home where he or she will be placed and is this o.k.; and so on. Each of these purposes is met by abridging what we usually do, cutting and splicing available measures, and employing informal tasks we make up. We do not consider it an apostasy to trim the turgidities of our traditional appraisal when conditions dictate we must.

Our use of modality specific measures is guided by the questions that persist after administering a general language evaluation and the direction we need for focusing treatment and evaluating its efficacy. For example, if our patient has little success on the general language measure's reading subtests, we may administer the RCBA to determine whether reading is preserved on some of its more comprehensive subtests. Conversely, if our patient "tops" the auditory comprehension subtests on the general language measure, we may push him or her further by administering one of the varieties of the Token Test to determine whether longer or more complex auditory stimuli uncover what we have failed to find. Or, if we plan to treat the patient with severe oral expressive deficits by developing gesture as an alternative means of communication, we may administer the New England Pantomime Tests to establish a baseline for intervention and subsequent reference for assessing improvement.

Phonological, semantic, syntactic, pragmatic, and discourse analyses are not a part of our standard appraisal. We may employ one or more of these to guide treatment's focus and evaluate its efficacy. Currently, most of these are too expensive. The cost in time for us to become competent and to collect and analyze the data is beyond our busy, clinical budgets. Nevertheless, we hope those who are competent will ultimately provide clinically practical packages. So, although we do not hope we have read the "last of the cohesions," we do await the condensed edition.

Appraisal need not be the slow boat to China, a long afternoon on the front porch watching the paint dry, a day at the frog races, a drive to Ordway. But, it can seem that way. We do not hesitate to mix appraisal and treatment. Enough appraisal to focus some treatment, if the patient is a treatment candidate, is enough appraisal to initiate treatment. So, we may divide the patient's subsequent visits into some treatment and some continued appraisal to answer persisting questions. Like so many seemingly slow occasions, appraisal should avoid the patient's passing out from ennui. At best, it is a calm reflecting pool of amiability. The following is representative of how we appraise aphasic people.

ONE PATIENT'S APPRAISAL

Parts of P. G. were temporarily overlaid with speechlessness, and, at times, it permeated her. She was 64 years old when we met, right handed, and had used her 16 years of education to teach elementary school. A left hemisphere thromboembolic infarct in the frontal-temporal-parietal area had left her aphasic six months earlier. Our neurologist's reading of a current CT scan revealed an old right hemisphere parietal area infarct. The date of this was unknown, because P. G. could not remember having suffered a previous stroke. Although there was weakness in her right arm and hand, it did not prevent her from writing or gesturing. Visual acuity was corrected adequately by glasses, and auditory acuity was unimpaired. There were no signs of brain stem involvement, and her health was good.

P. G. had retired from teaching prior to her recent left hemisphere infarct. After becoming aphasic, she received one month of treatment at two months postonset. Her clinician told us she displayed "moderately severe aphasia and moderate oral-nonverbal apraxia and apraxia of speech." "Good progress" had

been achieved during the month of treatment. P. G. lived with her daughter and was awaiting placement in the state veterans home.

Time permitted the leisure of a complete appraisal. We administered a motor speech evaluation, the PICA, the WAB, and orientation and fund of general information questions from the Mayo Clinic Procedures for Language Evaluation. Auditory comprehension and reading were probed further with the Spreen and Benton (1977) version of the Token Test and the RCBA. We questioned her classification on the WAB, so we administered sufficient subtests from the BDAE to seek confirmation.

The motor speech evaluation revealed no difficulty in vowel prolongation or rapid alternating movements for /pʌ/, /tʌ/, or /kʌ/. Combined rapid alternating movements for the sequence /pʌ-tʌ-kʌ/ showed a flurry of errors, but the reason for these was undetermined. Repetition of monosyllabic words was pristine. Repetition of multisyllabic words and words that increase in length showed an occasional articulatory error, as did repeated production of the same word. Again, the nature of these occasional errors was not obvious. Repetition of sentences slayed her. But, the reason for her errors could not be easily pinned on motor speech deficits as opposed to language deficits. Conversation, picture description, and oral reading revealed fluent aphasic speech with frequent articulatory errors. We agreed she was not dysarthric, but opinion varied on the presence of apraxia of speech or literal paraphasia.

P. G.'s PICA performance is shown in Figure 4-3. We used the bilateral norms to derive an 83rd Overall percentile. Modality performance was 83rd percentile, Gestural; 42nd percentile, Verbal; and 97th percentile, Graphic. Auditory comprehension was correct but showed a few delayed responses. Reading was also correct but incomplete and, infrequently, delayed. Visual matching was fine except for one delay in picture-object matching, and pantomime ranged from related responses to mostly complete and correct responses. Verbal performance was depressed. Repetition of words included an error and two rejections amidst mostly correct responses. Sentence completion was poor, and naming

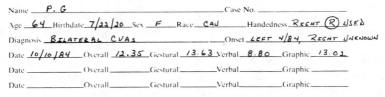

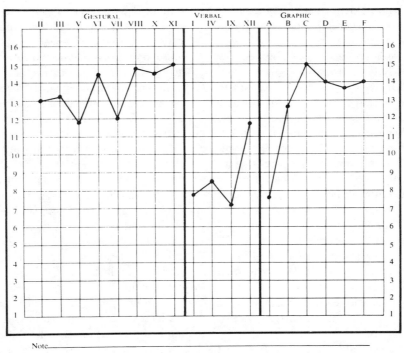

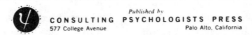

Figure 4-3. PICA Modality Response Summary for P. G., who had suffered bilateral CVAs. Reprinted with permission from Consulting Psychologists Press, Inc., 577 College Avenue, Palo Alto, CA 94306.

and sentence formulation were not much better. Writing sentences was beyond P. G.'s ability, but most responses were reasonable facsimiles of the targets. Writing names was better, and writing to dictation and copying were better yet.

WAB performance showed fluent, aphasic speech; mild auditory comprehension deficits; extremely poor repetition; and severe naming problems. P. G.'s Aphasia Quotient was 54.6.

Cortical Quotient subtests indicated moderate reading and writing problems, no oral-facial or limb apraxia, and no overt constructional deficits. The Coloured Progressive Matrices portion of the Constructional subtests led us to believe P. G. was as smart as she had been premorbidly. Her Cortical Quotient was 66.6. She profiled as conduction aphasia in the WAB taxonomy.

Mayo orientation and fund of general

information subtests were 95 percent correct. The one error was an error and not an irrelevant response or confabulation. Again, her responses included frequent articulatory errors, but their type and nature did not signify clearly apraxia of speech as opposed to literal paraphasia.

Token Test performance was 80 percent correct and revealed more auditory comprehension deficits as the stimuli increased in length and complexity. RCBA performance was 84 percent correct, and functional reading, paragraph-picture comprehension, and morphosyntax subtests accounted for almost all of P. G.'s errors.

We administered sufficient subtests from the BDAE to obtain a rating on the severity scale and a profile of P. G.'s speech characteristics. The results are shown in Figure 4-4. Her severity rating was 2 on the six-point scale, and she seemed to be the patient Goodglass and Kaplan (1983b) had in mind when they constructed the conduction aphasia profile. P. G.'s speech was fluent, and her auditory comprehension was at the 60th percentile. Paraphasias, mostly literal, abounded; repetition was poor; and word-finding problems were obvious. Thus, the BDAE confirmed the WAB's classification of conduction aphasia, but we continued to wonder whether the articulatory errors implied the presence of apraxia of speech.

P. G. had received about five hours of appraisal. We achieved two of appraisal's purposes—provide a prognosis and focus treatment. Debate about her diagnosis created a good deal of late afternoon conversation and, ultimately, continued into her treatment.

DIAGNOSIS

Appraisal provides the data, but the data are not the diagnosis (Rosenbek & LaPointe, 1981). Appraisal usually includes administering tests, but tests do not diagnose; clinicians do (Wertz, 1986b). Appraisal is the looking. Diagnosis is the finding—applying the label, stating what something is as opposed to what it could be. Sometimes, diagnosis is a neat mutation. Sometimes, it is as difficult as putting socks on snakes. Always, diagnosis gives a clinician an opportunity to stretch his or her mind.

This section is about diagnosing aphasia; differentiating it from what it could be but is not. What was done in appraisal, usually, will assist, but not always. To nonclinicians, brain damaged people appear to be trying to talk alike and not succeeding. To clinicians, brain damaged people can be assigned to various groups—aphasia, dementia, language of confusion, apraxia of speech, dysarthria, etc. Some patients are assigned to more than one group, because the location and extent of the lesion or previous episodes leave them with coexisting disorders; for example, aphasia coexisting with apraxia of speech. Other patients speak with shadows on their tongues. The features are there, but they are not seen clearly. Every patient deserves a diagnosis, but not all receive one; at least, not immediately. For these, the best diagnostician is not the speech-language pathologist. It is the patient. If we sit down, shut up, listen, and watch, the patient will eventually tell us his or her diagnosis. The danger is not in having no idea what to call it. It is in having no idea that we have no idea.

By now, it should not be surprising that clinicians do not always agree. Chapter 3 implied that definitions of aphasia differ. The appraisal section in this chapter suggests that different clinicians hunt for a diagnosis with different tests. One's definition and one's tools will influence what one bags. Some, for example, find aphasia in demented patients (Appell et al., 1982). Others (Wertz, 1982b) believe this is not very useful and urge the two disorders be separated. What follows is the way it seems to us, and we do not always agree.

We believe that aphasic people are not flat. Each is a complex landscape with promontories of great wealth and occasional canyons of weakness. Each deserves to be judged as a whole and not diagnosed on the basis of a single feature. The definition we apply in diagnosing aphasia is that the disorder is a general language deficit affecting all

Patient's Name ___P. G.___ Date of rating ___10/15/84___

Rated by ___R. T. W.___

APHASIA SEVERITY RATING SCALE

0. No usable speech or auditory comprehension.

1. All communication is through fragmentary expression; great need for inference, questioning, and guessing by the listener. The range of information that can be exchanged is limited, and the listener carries the burden of communication.

2. Conversation about familiar subjects is possible with help from the listener. There are frequent failures to convey the idea, but patient shares the burden of communication with the examiner.

3. The patient can discuss almost all everyday problems with little or no assistance. Reduction of speech and/or comprehension, however, makes conversation about certain material difficult or impossible.

4. Some obvious loss of fluency in speech or facility of comprehension, without significant limitation on ideas expressed or form of expression.

5. Minimal discernible speech handicaps; patient may have subjective difficulties that are not apparent to listener.

RATING SCALE PROFILE OF SPEECH CHARACTERISTICS

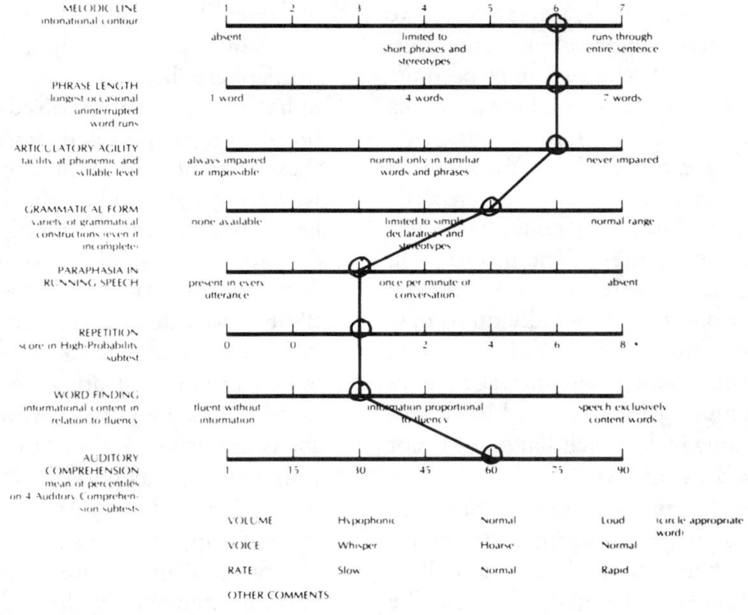

Figure 4-4. BDAE Aphasia Rating Scale and Rating Scale Profile of Speech Characteristics for P. G. The profile is indicative of conduction aphasia. From Goodglass, H., & Kaplan, E. (1983). *The Assessment of Aphasia and Related Disorders*. Philadephia: Lea & Febiger. Reprinted with permission.

communicative modalities—auditory comprehension, reading, oral-expressive language and writing. The deficit does not result from dementia, sensory loss, or paralysis or paresis. Typically, it exists subsequent to left hemisphere brain damage. We have discussed the data we collect—biographical, medical, and behavioral—to make a diagnosis. These data and our definition are employed to place the label, aphasia.

Diagnostic errors in aphasia are two: diagnosing aphasia when the patient's disorder is something else or diagnosing something else when the patient is aphasic. Unfortunately, there is no "gold standard" that everyone agrees defines aphasia. Thus, no single attribute of the disorder provides sufficient specificity or sensitivity for us to say when we observe it, "Ah ha! This is aphasia." So, we collect the patient's attributes and sort them to determine who is who and who is not. Here, we discuss that sorting by comparing those attributes that signify aphasia with those that signify something else—normal language, dementia, confusion, schizophrenia, right hemisphere communication deficit, apraxia of speech, and dysarthria. Always, however, we remind ourselves that disorders may coexist.

APHASIA VERSUS NORMAL LANGUAGE

When aphasia is moderate or severe, we seldom confuse it with normal language. But, when aphasia is mild, the two may be quite similar. Duffy (1981) has discussed the gray area between mild aphasia and normal language. PICA performance by left hemisphere brain damaged patients above the 90th percentile overlaps with performance by nonaphasic subjects (Duffy & Keith, 1980). The problems in differentiating mild aphasia from normal language are two. One, some individuals may appear aphasic, but the explanation for this is not left hemisphere brain damage. Two, some individuals may have suffered left hemisphere brain damage, but their language is not easily identified as aphasia.

Language deficits in those who have not suffered brain damage can be traced to several sources. The behavioral data we collect indicate the presence of language deficits. The explanation is in the person's biography or medical history. Those who show adequate auditory comprehension and oral-expressive language but depressed reading and writing are not aphasic. Their biography indicates a lack of education, and their medical history indicates no evidence of brain damage. They are, essentially, illiterate. Not all talents were meant to be encouraged in school. They do not meet our definition of aphasia, a general language deficit in *all* communicative modalities. Others may display a depression of ability in all modalities and their biography

may indicate 12 or more years of education and an occupational history requiring literacy. But, their medical history gives no indication of brain damage and their decline was gradual. Although we could be viewing dementia, there is another explanation. If the person's biography indicates he or she began to display communication problems after being placed in a nursing home, we might suspect the influence of what Lubinski (1981) called a communication-impaired environment. She has documented the effects an abnormal environment can have on the normal aged's communicative ability. The coping strategies employed by the normal aged to communicate (Obler & Albert, 1981) are eroded by an atmosphere where there are rules against talking and no one listens. The result may masquerade as aphasia, but it is not.

Some who are aphasic following left hemisphere brain damage never were very aphasic or they have evolved to that level. The problem in diagnosis is determining whether these patients are aphasic or no longer that way. Biography and medical history are little help. Both show a rapid onset of brain damage. The answer must be sought in the patient's behavior. Raymer and LaPointe (1986) have listed the signs of mild aphasia and discussed standardized and nonstandardized means of demonstrating their presence. Ultimately, it is the patient who decides if he or she is aphasic. We do not hesitate to ask, "Is your language as good as it was before your stroke?" Moss's (1972) account of his own aphasia supports the sanity of this approach.

So, to differentiate between aphasia and normal language, we look for the reasons— education, environment—that make the person appear aphasic when he or she is not, and for the mildly aphasic patient, we push performance beyond the limits of traditional measures, including asking the patient, to determine whether the aphasia that was once there still remains.

APHASIA VERSUS DEMENTIA

If one believes the language deficits in dementia are aphasic, one does not differentiate aphasia from dementia. However, we believe there are sufficient differences in the language behavior, the prognosis, and the management between the two disorders to differentiate one from the other. The recent interest in slowly progressive aphasia, however, complicates the task for those who would separate aphasia from dementia.

Biography and medical history contain powerful information to separate aphasia from dementia. Deal, Wertz, and Spring (1981) compared aphasic patients with demented patients. Their results indicate that aphasia erupts (100 percent of the aphasic patients had a rapid onset, under 10 days), and dementia creeps (87 percent of the demented patients had a slow onset, over 10 days). All aphasic patients brain damage was confined to the left hemisphere. Ninety-three percent of the demented patients had bilateral brain damage. All aphasic patients had focal lesions. Ninety-three percent of the demented patients had diffuse and disseminated brain damage. Thus, rapidity of onset; localization of brain damage; and the extent of brain damage, focal or diffuse and disseminated, assist in differentiating aphasia from dementia.

Bayles (1984) and Bayles and Kaszniak (1987) have listed several behavioral differences between dementia and aphasia. These, along with some of our observations, are summarized in Table 4-2. Deterioration of language in dementia is quite orderly. It proceeds from semantic deficits through syntactic disruption to phonological problems as the disorder progresses. Conversely, all three— semantics, syntax, and phonology—may be disrupted in aphasia, depending on the patient's type of aphasia, at any time postonset and at all levels of overall severity. Similarly, aphasic patients may be divided into fluent and nonfluent groups at any time postonset and at all levels of overall severity; however, demented patients are fluent until they become quite severe, and even at this level, fluency may be retained. Organization and relevance are apparent in aphasic patients unless auditory comprehension deficits prevent understanding. Demented patients are irrelevant and disorganized, and both deteriorate further as the disorder progresses. Memory and cognition are usually intact in aphasia, and this can

be demonstrated if one can establish a clear channel to deliver requests and an intact performance modality. Memory and cognition are disrupted in dementia at all levels of severity. Aphasic patients may be depressed and sometimes frustrated, but their mood and behavior are usually appropriate. Demented patients are labile and withdrawn, and some can become inappropriately agitated.

Although we believe aphasia and dementia differ, we do not deny that the two can coexist. For example, an aphasic patient who suffered a focal left hemisphere infarct may, over the years, develop bilateral cortical atrophy indicative of probable Alzheimer's dementia. Similarly, the patient with probable Alzheimer's dementia may suddenly appear aphasic, because he or she has sustained a left hemisphere CVA. Multi-infarct dementia is more problematic. It may begin with aphasia subsequent to a left hemisphere infarct and progress to coexisting dementia and aphasia as the patient suffers additional bilateral infarcts. Or the patient may be demented as a result of multiple, small, bilateral infarcts and not take on the additional burden of aphasia until he or she sustains a major left hemisphere infarct.

Mesulam's (1982) report of slowly progressive aphasia without generalized dementia challenges the contention that aphasia erupts and dementia creeps. Language deficits as the first sign of a dementing disease are not novel. Several reports (Wechsler, 1977; Holland, Swindell, & Forbes, 1985) have documented this is not uncommon in Pick's disease. And, Pogacar and Williams (1984) discussed a case of Alzheimer's disease whose major symptom was aphasia during the first two years. The question is whether the language deficits in these patients represent aphasia or linguistic decline in dementia. Administering an aphasia test will not tell us. Appell, Kertesz, and Fisman (1982) demonstrated demented patients can be classified as aphasic on the WAB. Some (Wertz, 1982b) do not accept this as evidence to demonstrate demented patients are aphasic. Duffy (1987) provided a careful review of slowly progressive aphasia and concluded it "probably does exist" (p. 354). If it does, we need to, as Duffy

TABLE 4-2.
Differences between Aphasia and Dementia.

Variable	Aphasia	Dementia
Onset and course	Rapid onset, symptoms improve	Slow onset, progressive deterioration
Semantics	Word-finding problems, semantic and literal paraphasias	Ranges from mild word-finding problems through visual misrecognition to marked reduction in vocabulary
Syntax	Can be divided into a fluent and nonfluent dichotomy	Intact in mild patients, reduced complexity in moderate and severe patients
Phonology	Impaired in nonfluent patients and may be present as literal paraphasias in some fluent patients	Preserved in mild and moderate patients, sometimes disrupted in severe patients
Verbal repetition	Impaired to some degree in most patients	Intact in mild and moderate patients and in most severe patients
Fluency	Patients can be divided into fluent and nonfluent	Mild and moderate patients are fluent, some severe patients may be nonfluent
Pragmatics	Socially appropriate	Mild to severe inappropriate pragmatic behavior depending on overall level of severity
Organization and relevance	Generally unimpaired, severe auditory comprehension deficits may result in irrelevance due to misunderstanding	Mild to severe irrelevance and disorganization depending on overall level of severity
Memory	Generally intact	Poor to global failure depending on overall level of severity
Cognition	Generally intact	Ranges from subtle deficits to global failure
Mood and behavior	Generally appropriate, may be depressed or frustrated	Labile, withdrawn, sometimes agitated

Adapted from Bayles (1984).

suggested, reconsider some of our definitions for aphasia, consider the prognosis for slowly progressive aphasia, and determine whether it can be managed efficaciously.

Most dementing illness, we believe, can be differentiated from aphasia. The rapidity of onset, location and type of brain damage, and behavioral symptoms differ between the two disorders. More importantly, the prognosis and methods of management differ. Because they do, we believe it is clinically essential to determine whether a patient is aphasic or demented.

APHASIA VERSUS LANGUAGE OF CONFUSION

Darley (1982) described the language of confusion as an impairment of language that is often traumatically induced. It is characterized by reduced understanding and recognition of the environment; faulty memory;

unclear thinking; and disorientation in time, place, and condition. Language may be normal in semantics, syntax, and phonology; however, the content may be highly irrelevant and confabulated. Darley suggested this is not aphasia. We agree.

Traumatic brain injury (TBI) can result in confusion, and we have seen confused patients who suffered anoxia (Wertz, 1985). Chedru and Geschwind (1972) discussed several patients with confusion resulting from metabolic and toxic disorders. All agree the onset is rapid, the brain damage is diffuse and not well localized, and the salient signs are irrelevance and confabulation. Rapidity of onset does not differentiate confusion from aphasia, but localization and the language symptoms do. Aphasia results, typically, from a focal left hemisphere lesion. Confusion results from diffuse bilateral brain damage. Aphasic patients, if they understand the request and have an intact performance modality, respond appropriately. Confused patients are irrelevant and confabulate. When asked the capitol of the United States, an aphasic patient does not reply, "Banda Oriental was the former name for Uruguay." A confused patient might. When asked how many years he or she went to school, an aphasic patient will tell you or indicate he or she can't say it. We know a confused patient who had a master's degree in education who answered the question with a 10-minute monologue about having three degrees, including a combined doctorate in theology and dentistry that required him to write a dissertation on the "metaphysics of basic tooth structure." Confused patients are irrelevant and confabulate. Aphasic patients are not and do not.

Confusion frequently follows TBI, and so does dysarthria and, sometimes, aphasia. What is present depends on which parts of the brain have been traumatized. If the trauma has placed a focal lesion in the left hemisphere, we are not surprised to find aphasia coexisting with confusion, cognitive deficits, and the other sequelae of TBI. However, many TBI patients have suffered diffuse and disseminated bilateral brain damage with no focal left hemisphere lesion. Their communicative deficits are not aphasic, but different measures will classify these patients differently. Bernstein-Ellis, Wertz, Dronkers, & Milton (1985) reported that WAB performance by 15 TBI patients classified 14 as aphasic. Conversely, discriminant function analysis of PICA performance by the same 15 patients classified only one as aphasic. Sarno (1980) observed, "The boundaries which usually help to identify and classify patients with linguistic deficits after brain damage do not seem to hold to the same degree for the head trauma patients as they do in the stroke population" (p. 692). She (Sarno, 1980, 1984) divided TBI patients into three groups: aphasia, dysarthria with subclinical aphasia, and subclinical aphasia. Holland (1982), on the other hand, suggested most TBI patients are not aphasic.

The TBI patients we see, typically, are not aphasic. The language of confusion is the best of available labels, but it is not completely adequate. We rely on the set of symptoms shown in Table 4-3 to differentiate TBI patients from aphasic patients. Those who have suffered diffuse, bilateral brain damage and have no focal lesion in the left hemisphere tend to confabulate and are irrelevant. They show cognitive and memory deficits. Their language is better than their ability to communicate. And, most display a personality that differs substantially from their premorbid personality. Conversely, aphasic patients do not confabulate, and they are relevant. Cognition and

TABLE 4-3.
A Comparison of Patients with Aphasia Subsequent to Left Hemisphere Brain Damage and Behavior in Patients Who Have Suffered Bilateral Traumatic Brain Injury.

Behavior	Aphasia	Traumatic brain injury
Confabulation	−	+
Irrelevance	−	+
Cognitive deficits	−	+
Memory deficits	−	+
Language worse than communication	+	−
Personality change	−	+

+ = symptom is present, − = symptom is not present.

memory are intact if one can find a means to demonstrate both. Their language is worse than their ability to communicate. And, we see little difference between their reported pre- and postmorbid personalities. TBI patients who have suffered a focal left hemisphere lesion do not surprise us with their aphasic symptoms that reside within the signs of bilateral TBI. Further, we are not amazed by their dysarthria resulting from cerebellar, brain stem, or bilateral upper motor neuron damage.

APHASIA VERSUS SCHIZOPHRENIA

Jaffe (1981) asked whether the sudden onset of Wernicke's aphasia in a schizophrenic patient would be noticed. Some (Benson, 1973; DiSimoni, Darley, & Aronson, 1977) would notice, because they differentiate between language disturbance in aphasia and schizophrenia. Others (Chapman, 1966; Farber & Reichstein, 1981) would not, because they believe schizophrenic language is aphasic or, at least, a subgroup of schizophrenic patients display a language disorder that could be called "schizophasia."

We agree with Benson's (1973) position that schizophrenia is a thought disorder that may be observed as a language disturbance in the patient's speech. And, we agree with DiSimoni and colleagues (1977) that schizophrenic speech and language performance is different from the speech and language performance seen in aphasia. In addition, biographical and medical histories differ between the two disorders.

Aphasia, typically, erupts. Schizophrenia creeps, and it is usually seen first as a psychiatric disturbance in late adolescence or early adulthood. The sudden onset of schizophrenia in an adult would be considered a psychiatric anomaly. Conversely, the sudden onset of aphasia in an adult is not uncommon. Medical history for the schizophrenic patient should indicate a history of psychiatric disturbance, and a current neurological evaluation would show no evidence of left hemisphere brain damage. The typical aphasic patient presents with the opposite, no history of psychiatric disturbance and evidence of left hemisphere brain damage. Behavioral data show schizophrenic patients' language is typified by irrelevance and confabulation and an absence of specific language deficits in auditory comprehension, reading, oral-expressive language, and writing. Aphasic patients display no confabulation and little irrelevance. Their language deficits are present in all communicative modalities.

Therefore, history of psychiatric disturbance, slow onset, absence of observable brain damage, and no general language impairment differentiate the schizophrenic patient from the aphasic patient. Those who suffer schizophrenia may sustain brain damage and display aphasia. However, this results in the coexistence of two disorders, schizophrenia and aphasia, and behavior differs from the presence of either alone.

APHASIA VERSUS RIGHT HEMISPHERE COMMUNICATION DEFICITS

Right hemisphere brain damage results in communicative deficits (Myers, 1984), but these differ, except in a few, rare patients, from the general language deficit seen in aphasia. Most house language in the left hemisphere. A few who are right handed and have right hemisphere language dominance display crossed aphasia after suffering right hemisphere brain damage (Hecaen & Albert, 1978). Estimates of incidence range from 0.4 percent (Hecaen, Mazurs, & Ramier, 1971) to 10 percent (Branch, Milner, & Rasmussen, 1964). These patients display a general language deficit and are appropriately diagnosed as aphasic. They differ from patients who have left hemisphere language dominance and sustain a right hemisphere lesion.

Beyond the location of the lesion, the general sign that separates the right hemisphere brain damaged patient from the left hemisphere aphasic patient is the former's relatively good language ability and generally poor communication compared with the latter's poor language ability and relatively good communication. Myers (1979, 1984) listed several signs that constitute right hemisphere communication deficit: failure to integrate information on a perceptual level, tendency to itemize rather than interpret information, irrelevance, lack of affect, and abnormal sense of humor. Kent and Rosenbek (1982) added the frequent occurrence of dysarthria following right hemisphere brain damage and significant aprosody. In addition, Prutting and Kirchner (1987) have listed inappropriate pragmatic behaviors following right hemisphere brain injury—disrupted turn taking, prosody, and eye contact.

Even though some (Archibald & Wepman, 1968) have reported "aphasic-like" behavior in right hemisphere brain damaged patients, and Deal, Deal, Wertz, Kitselman, & Dwyer (1979) found 62 percent of their right hemisphere sample was classified as aphasic based on a discriminant function analysis of PICA performance, we have little difficulty in differentiating aphasia from right hemisphere communication deficits. When we find a case of crossed aphasia (Dronkers, 1987; Wertz, 1982a) we acknowledge it and treat it with the rarity it deserves.

APHASIA VERSUS APRAXIA OF SPEECH

Some (Martin, 1974) have no difficulty in differentiating aphasia from apraxia of speech, because they deny the latter exists. Those who do acknowledge the existence of apraxia of speech (Wertz, LaPointe, & Rosenbek, 1984) must seek its presence among the signs that signify aphasia, because the two disorders typically coexist. The search is guided by the location of the lesion, but the identification relies on the presence of specific motor speech deficits that constitute apraxia of speech.

Mohr (1973, 1980) and Mohr and colleagues (1978) reported apraxia of speech is common following damage in the left hemisphere's third frontal convolution, Broca's area. We agree, but we add, so is aphasia. Further, we have seen apraxia of speech result from damage in other areas of the brain. So, we use location of the lesion as one piece of evidence

to confirm the presence of apraxia of speech, but we rely on the presence of a set of salient symptoms to make the diagnosis.

We have defined aphasia as a general language disorder crossing all communicative modalities. Our definition of apraxia of speech is:

A sensorimotor speech disorder resulting from brain damage. Symptoms are impaired volitional production of articulation and prosody. These symptoms do not result from abnormal strength, tone, or timing; or from aphasia, confusion, generalized intellectual impairment, or hearing loss. Rather, they result from inhibition or impairment of neural programming of skilled movements (Wertz, LaPointe, & Rosenbek, 1984, p.4).

Four clinical characteristics indicate apraxia of speech is present (Wertz, LaPointe, & Rosenbek, 1984, p. 81):

1. Effortful, trial and error, groping articulatory movements and attempts at self-correction.

2. Dysprosody unrelieved by extended periods of normal rhythm, stress, and intonation.

3. Articulatory inconsistency on repeated productions of the same utterance.

4. Obvious difficulty initiating utterances.

All signify the presence of this motor speech disorder, and all differ from the general language disorder we call aphasia.

Confusion in differentiating apraxia of speech from aphasia flows from three sources. First, the severely aphasic patient may not produce sufficient speech to permit identifying the four signs listed here. Many of these patients eventually develop sufficient verbal output to confirm our early suspicion that they suffer a severe apraxia of speech coexisting with severe aphasia. But, early postonset the paucity of verbalization does not permit diagnosis of apraxia of speech. Rosenbek (1985) suggested there is no need to worry, because one typically elects to treat these patients' aphasia. Later, when the patient is talking more, there is sufficient information to decide whether he or she is apraxic.

Second, by definition, apraxia of speech coexists with Broca's aphasia. Goodglass and Kaplan's (1983b) rating scale of speech characteristics shows Broca's aphasic patients have disrupted melodic line and articulatory agility. We consider these signify disturbed prosody and the effortful, groping articulatory movements, articulatory inconsistency, and difficulty initiating utterances that constitute apraxia of speech. The short phrase length, disrupted grammatical form, tendency to produce primarily content words, word-finding problems, and mild auditory comprehension deficits represent Broca's aphasia. Thus, two disorders, apraxia of speech and Broca's aphasia, coexist. Some have difficulty in accepting the coexistence of disorders and elect to combine all symptoms into one disorder, Broca's aphasia.

Third, some patients who suffer apraxia of speech have sufficient phrase length and grammatical form to classify them as displaying fluent aphasia. However, their prosodic abnormality and poor articulatory agility makes them different from the typical fluent aphasias—Wernicke's, transcortical sensory, conduction, and anomic. Thus, they are unclassifiable on the BDAE. Moreover, the apraxic errors are sometimes similar to the literal paraphasic errors one sees in some of the fluent aphasias, especially conduction aphasia. We employ the characteristics listed in Table 4-4 to differentiate apraxia of speech

coexisting with fluent aphasia from conduction aphasia. And, we remind ourselves that apraxia of speech is a symptom complex, and literal paraphasia is a symptom.

APHASIA VERSUS DYSARTHRIA

Differentiating aphasia from dysarthria also requires separating a language disorder from a motor speech disorder. And, although the two disorders may coexist, we do not usually see significant dysarthria resulting from left hemisphere cortical lesions. Damage that includes the facial and oral areas of the left hemisphere motor strip may result in a lower right facial involvement and some restriction of lip and tongue mobility. But, the presence of dysarthria in these patients is almost subclinical, especially when compared with their obvious aphasia. The recent attention being given to subcortical aphasia reminds us that aphasia and dysarthria can coexist. For example, Goodglass and Kaplan (1983b) pointed out that anterior subcortical aphasias that involve the anterior limb of the internal capsule and the putamen are characterized by sparse verbal production but no notable agrammatism. In addition, severely impaired articulation and hypophonic voice indicate the presence of a significant, coexisting dysarthria.

Darley and colleagues (1975) described dysarthria as a group of speech disorders that result from disturbance in muscular control—weakness, slowness, or incoordination—of the speech mechanism due to central and/or

TABLE 4-4.
Signs That Differentiate Apraxia of Speech from Conduction Aphasia.

Apraxia of Speech	Conduction Aphasia
Lower proportion of sequencing errors	Higher proportion of sequencing errors
Predictable substitutions	Unpredictable substitutions
Abnormal prosody	Normal prosody
Initiation difficulty	No initiation difficulty
Usually anterior brain damage	Usually posterior brain damage
Frequently right hemiplegic	Usually not hemiplegic

peripheral nervous system damage. Any or all of the basic processes of speech—respiration, phonation, resonance, articulation, and prosody—may be impaired. The salient signs include disrupted speech intelligibility, abnormal voice quality, changes in rate, hypernasality, abnormal stress, etc., depending on the location of damage. All differ markedly from the general language disturbance that characterizes aphasia. It is common to see dysarthric patients with no signs of aphasia and aphasic patients with no significant dysarthria. Coexisting aphasia and dysarthria, however, does not surprise us. For example, the patient who displays aphasia subsequent to a left hemisphere lesion may, after suffering a second CVA in the right hemisphere, display spastic, or pseudobulbar, dysarthria resulting from the bilateral upper motor neuron damage caused by the two strokes.

SUMMARY

Diagnosis, putting a label on the problem, has two primary purposes: providing a prognosis and indicating appropriate management. What we call it is influenced by our definition of it and how we have looked for it in appraisal. And, sometimes, even the most concise definition and the most precise appraisal do not permit a confident diagnosis. This occasional amazement is enough to keep us addicted to diagnosis. It is one of the speech-language pathologist's abilities that elevates him or her above being only a therapist.

Why is diagnosis, at times, difficult? Well, patients' brains differ, and so do their social, educational, and medical histories. In addition, all conditions are not static. Some evolve. Plus, the boundaries between and among disorders are somewhat arbitrary. We have established specific labels, but we may be flawed in our use of them. Those who think labeling is always possible are abusing the labels. Sometimes, we just don't know. Labels are hypotheses to which clinicians assign probabilities. They give structure to what would otherwise be structureless. And, they brighten what is otherwise a very dull activity.

It is good to know glasses are to drink from. The bad thing is not knowing what thirst indicates.

New ways of seeing have disclosed new things. The radio telescope revealed quasars and pulsars. The scanning electron microscope showed the whiskers of the dust mite. Similarly, the CT and MRI disclose lesions we and our patients did not know existed. PET and SPECT now make it necessary to distinguish between the structural lesions established by CT and MRI and the functional lesions implicated by these measures of cerebral blood flow. Idling brain differs from activated brain. And, as some suggest, the gain in brain is mainly in the stain.

Certainly, new ways of seeing have generated new ways of thinking. The comfortable contention that aphasia is a disorder of cortex has been challenged by the advent of subcortical aphasias. Traditional belief that aphasia erupts must deal with reports of slowly progressive aphasia. Static diagnostic security must cope with the current dynamics in diagnosis. It is an exciting time to be a clinical aphasiologist, and it is no time to let your brain get so full of things that you have no room to think.

ONE PATIENT'S DIAGNOSIS

E. D. is a lesson in how some of what we know is not so. He also provided the comfort of confirming that some of what we know is so. Evolution of his symptoms is listed in Table 4-5. The infinite darkness of every clinician's ignorance can be illuminated by the right patient. E. D. turned on a few lights for us.

A left hemisphere thromboembolic infarct brought him to our attention. Evaluation of his motor speech and language revealed a mild Broca's aphasia and mild coexisting apraxia of speech. Neuroradiology confirmed the recent left hemisphere CVA involved the frontal and parietal areas. In addition, an "old" right hemisphere parietal infarct was detected. This was news to E. D., who had no knowledge of suffering a previous stroke. Additional evaluation indicated he had significant stenosis of both the right and left carotid arteries. A right

TABLE 4-5.
Evolution of Speech, Language, and Voice Symptoms in E. D.

Events	Date	Diagnosis
Right hemisphere CVA	Unknown	Asymptomatic
Left hemisphere CVA	September 15, 1985	Mild aphasia
		Mild apraxia of speech
Right carotid endarterectomy	September 30, 1985	Mild aphasia
		Mild apraxia of speech
		Dysphonia
Right hemisphere CVA	October 1, 1985	Mild aphasia
		Mild apraxia of speech
		Dysphonia
		Spastic dysarthria

carotid endarterectomy was performed approximately two weeks after he suffered the left hemisphere CVA. We visited E. D. on the evening of his surgery. His aphasia and apraxia persisted, and we detected a breathy voice quality that was not present prior to surgery. Otolaryngology was consulted and found paralysis of his right vocal fold, apparently resulting from the endarterectomy. That night he suffered a right hemisphere infarct that was subsequently localized in the right frontal-parietal area. Our evaluation the next day indicated he had added a significant dysarthria to his list of disorders.

E. D. taught us brain damage can exist without anyone's knowledge. His first right hemisphere infarct was asymptomatic and introduced itself during a CT scan following his left hemisphere infarct. We wonder how many other patients who are believed to have a first, single left hemisphere infarct may also have one of these "silent" lesions. E. D. also permitted us to employ our textbook knowledge and clinical experience as we followed him through the evolution of his symptoms. The left hemisphere frontal-parietal infarct involved the left hemisphere motor strip and surrounding territory, including the third frontal convolution. His Broca's aphasia and apraxia of speech were consistent with this localization. The right carotid endarterectomy apparently nicked or compressed the vagus nerve as it courses vertically down the neck in the carotid sheath. This would explain the presence of right vocal fold paralysis and our perception of breathy voice quality. Finally, the second right hemisphere frontal-parietal infarct involved the right motor strip and surrounding territory. Combined with his previous left hemisphere infarct, E. D.'s bilateral upper motor neuron involvement supports our perception of spastic, or pseudobulbar, dysarthria.

E. D. did not write the book, but he confirms it. His evolution of symptoms demonstrates how medical data can be combined to support what we see and hear. With him, we had no need to vacillate in our diagnoses, and that is the question—isn't it?

PROGNOSIS

Any aphasic patient who keeps up a running quarrel with his language deficits leaves a history like a dog's track on the beach. You can tell by the meanderings and sorties and retreats where the enormous wave almost engulfed him, and where the dead crab stank beneath the heaped Sargassa, where the rubber boot enticed for other purposes behind the dune. If you follow far enough, you can learn where the expedition ended—at the surf's edge in the obliterating sea or on a cliff surveying where he had been. Prognosis for the aphasic patient is an attempt to predict the future and, most importantly, where the expedition postonset will end.

Prognosis consists of several outcomes and the probability of each following a symptom, sign, or disease (Longstreth, Koepsell, & van Belle, 1987). In the best of worlds, we would know the complete natural history from the time of onset of a condition to its end. Unfortunately, in aphasia, we do not. What we know is sparse and influenced by our interventions. What we know we use to manage patients and answer their questions about what management will accomplish.

Aphasic patients can live through a day, if they can live through a moment. What creates despair is their imagining a future filled with millions of moments and thousands of days. This may drain them so they cannot live the moment at hand. Prognosis provides information about what the future will be. It ranges from near normality to persisting, severe language impairment. We say near normality, because return to normal from aphasia does not occur in the patients we see. In those that it does, it occurs in a matter of hours, and these patients seldom become our patients. We also acknowledge that prognosis for some patients is persisting, severe language deficits, because we have worked with some who ended that way despite their best efforts and ours. Most are in between. To forecast their future we cull prognostic variables, ponder behavioral profiles, employ statistical prediction, and, for some, we employ brief bouts of prognostic treatment.

PROGNOSTIC VARIABLES

Aphasic people have different social, education, and medical histories. Over the years, clinicians have observed how these differences may influence improvement in aphasia or the lack of it. Typically, a trait, or variable, is considered as a positive or a negative prognostic sign. For example, some have used age at onset as a predictor of improvement. Until recently, it was believed that young aphasic patients have a better prognosis for improvement than older aphasic patients. These prognostic variables have received considerable review (Darley, 1972, 1975, 1982; Wertz, 1983, 1985). We discuss here biographical,

medical, and behavioral variables that may assist in predicting the aphasic patient's future.

BIOGRAPHICAL VARIABLES

Age, gender, premorbid intelligence, and occupational history have surfaced as possible prognostic variables in aphasia. Evidence on the potency of each conflicts.

Most reports no longer support the notion that age influences prognosis. The observations that younger patients improve more than older patients (Eisenson, 1949; Marquardson, 1969; Marshal & Phillips, 1983; Sands, Sarno, & Shankweiler, 1969; Vignolo, 1964; Wepman, 1951) conflict with other reports (Basso, Capitani, & Vignolo, 1979; Culton, 1969; Deal & Deal, 1978; Hartman, 1981; Heinemann, Roth, & Chichowski, 1987; Keenan & Brassell, 1974; Kertesz & McCabe, 1977; Porch, Collins, Wertz, & Friden, 1980; Sarno & Levita, 1971) that show age has no effect on improvement in aphasia. Recently, however, Holland, Greenhouse, Fromm, & Swindell (in press) have reopened the question by demonstrating age, favoring younger patients, was significantly associated with language improvement early postonset.

The influence of gender on recovery is also debatable. McGlone's (1977) report that male patients are more likely to become aphasic after a left hemisphere CVA was not supported by DeRenzi, Motti, & Nichelli (1980), Kertesz and Sheppard (1981), or Obler, Albert, Caplass, Mohr, & Geer (1980). Moreover, Kertesz and McCabe's (1977) and Heinemann and colleagues' (1987) observations of no difference in improvement between male and female patients contrasts with Edwards, Ellams, and Thompson's (1976) report that persisting aphasia is more severe in male than in female patients. Holland et al. (in press) found gender, favoring male patients, was only moderately related to improvement. And, Basso, Capitani, and Moraschini's (1982) results are enigmatic. Their female aphasic patients improved significantly more in oral expression than male aphasic patients, but there were no differences in auditory verbal comprehension.

Similar conflicting answers are given regarding the influence of premorbid intelligence on improvement in aphasic patients. Eisenson (1949) suggested above average premorbid intelligence is a negative prognostic sign. These patients become depressed when they realize how far they have fallen. However, Wepman (1951) and Messerli, Tissot, & Rodriguez (1976) reported patients with higher premorbid intelligence make more improvement after becoming aphasic than those with lower premorbid intelligence.

Occupational history, the kind of work a patient did and whether he or she was working at the onset of aphasia, has been explored for its prognostic significance. Sarno, Silverman, & Sands (1970) and Keenan and Brassell (1974) agreed that how a patient earned his or her living has no influence on improvement after he or she becomes aphasic. However, Sarno and Levita (1971) observed that patients who were working at the onset of aphasia improved more than those who were not working at onset. Conversely, Marshall, Tompkins, and Phillips (1982) found employment at onset had no influence on improvement.

Additional biographic variables—education, handedness, etc.—have been examined, and all show similar conflicting results. Thus, we are not able to state with any confidence that, for example, a young, intelligent, female lawyer who was practicing law at the time she became aphasic has a better prognosis than an old, male, retired custodian of average intelligence. Our experience indicates that no single biographical variable provides much power for predicting prognosis. And, like the medical and behavioral variables we will discuss, we remind ourselves that variables do not simply exist; they coexist. Therefore, even if one indicated a positive prognosis, its coexistence with one or more negative prognostic variables may pilfer its potency.

MEDICAL VARIABLES

Cause of aphasia, location and extent of brain damage, health during recovery, and time postonset are among the medical variables that have been suggested to be prognostic. Although there is agreement on the power of some of these to predict aphasic patients' futures, some conflicting opinions exist.

Aphasia results from a variety of causes, and one cause may carry a more favorable prognosis than another. Several (Alajouanine, Castaigne, Lhermitte, Escourolle, & Ribancourt, 1957; Eisenson, 1964, 1984; Luria, 1963) suggested patients who suffer closed head trauma improve more than patients who are aphasic subsequent to a vascular etiology. Butfield and Zangwill (1946) observed 60 percent of their patients who suffered trauma were much improved compared with only 32 percent of their vascular and tumor patients. Kertesz and McCabe (1977) reported that their traumatic patients improved rapidly, within the first three months postonset, and their vascular patients showed slower improvement, up to three or more years postonset. Gloning, Trappl, Heiss, and Quatember (1976), however, found cause of aphasia, traumatic or vascular, had no specific influence on improvement. Among the vascular causes of aphasia, Glosser, Kaplan, and LoVerme (1982) suggested that aphasia resulting from subcortical hemorrhage improves more slowly than aphasia following vascular accidents in the cortex. And, Eisenson (1964) pointed out that aphasia following a single CVA has a better prognosis than aphasia that follows multiple CVAs.

The location and extent of brain damage influences how much improvement an aphasic patient can expect. These variables receive some support from data. Yarnell and colleagues (1976) observed a large lesion, many small lesions combined with one large lesion, and bilateral lesions have a poor prognosis for improved language. Gloning and colleagues (1976) found that bilateral lesions are associated with less language improvement. Penfield and Roberts (1959) and Eisenson (1964) reported damage in the temporoparietal area results in the most severe and persisting aphasia. Rubens and his colleagues provided data on the relationship between site and size of brain damage and recovery of specific language abilities. Superior temporal-inferior parietal and insula-putamen lesions result in persistent poor naming ability (Knopman, Selnes, Niccum, & Rubens, 1984). Extensive damage in the Rolandic cortical region and underlying white matter result in persisting nonfluent aphasia (Knopman, Selnes, Niccum, & Rubens, 1983). Very extensive left hemisphere lesions slow and restrict improvement in single word comprehension (Selnes, Niccum, Knopman, & Rubens, 1984), and lesions in the posterior superior temporal and infrasylvian supramarginal regions are associated with poor improvement in auditory comprehension (Selnes et al., 1983). Ludlow and colleagues (1986) examined the influence of lesion size and location on improvement of nonfluent aphasia in traumatic brain injured aphasic patients. Larger lesions with greater posterior and deep extension resulted in less improvement than smaller lesions confined to the anterior cortex.

Aphasic patients' general health after onset appears to influence their prognosis for improvement in language. Anderson, Bourestom, and Greenberg (1970) and Eisenson (1949, 1964) agreed that healthier patients with no sensory deficits have a more favorable prognosis for language improvement than those who are ill and suffer sensory deficits. Marshall and Phillips (1983) and Marshall and colleagues (1982) demonstrated general health was a significant predictor of improvement in aphasia. Holland and colleagues (in press) found aphasic patients with a shorter stay in the hospital made more improvement than those with a longer stay. And, Candelise, Landi, Orazio, and Boccardi (1985) observed that reactive hyperglycemia and preexisting diabetes had an adverse effect on the outcome of hemispheric stroke.

Probably the most potent prognostic variable is time postonset. The closer the patient is to onset of aphasia, the more improvement he or she can expect, with or without treatment. Early postonset, the patient receives the benefits of spontaneous recovery. This may continue in CVA patients for two months (Culton, 1969); three months (Lendrem & Lincoln, 1985); or up to six months (Basso et al., 1979; Butfield & Zangwill, 1946; Deal & Deal, 1978; Kertesz & McCabe, 1977; Vignolo, 1964). Wepman (1951) extended spontaneous recovery to a year in traumatic brain injured patients, and Marks, Taylor, and Rusk (1957) observed improvement in some patients after a year postonset. Wertz and colleagues (1981) reported that 65 percent of the total improvement achieved by aphasic patients treated during the first year postonset occurred during the first three months postonset. An additional 18 percent occurred between three and six months, 10 percent between six and nine months, and 7 percent between nine and twelve months.

BEHAVIORAL VARIABLES

Prognostic behavioral variables are linked to prognostic medical variables. For example, the two we will consider here, severity of aphasia and type of aphasia, relate to the size and location of the lesion. Nevertheless, neither severity or type of aphasia surfaces until the patient is massaged with measures. So, we consider these separately.

Initial severity of aphasia is believed to be a powerful predictor of prognosis. Almost everyone agrees that the less severe patient has a better potential for ultimate improvement (Basso et al., 1979; Butfield & Zangwill, 1946; Gloning et al., 1976; Hartman, 1981; Keenan & Brassell, 1974; Kertesz & McCabe, 1977; Messerli et al., 1976; Sands et al., 1969; Sarno & Levita, 1971, 1979; Schuell et al., 1964; Wepman, 1951). But, as Kertesz (1979) has suggested, examination of severity must be separated into amount of improvement and ultimate outcome. For example, patients who are initially very severe may make more overall improvement than patients who are initially mild. However, the severe patient will never achieve the level of performance attained by the mild patient. Shewan and Kertesz (1984) reported that moderately severe patients improved an average of 33 points on the WAB Language Quotient, severely aphasic patients improved 28 points, and mildly aphasic patients improved 20 points. Thus, the severe patients improved more, but they did not reach the level of performance that the mild patients did.

The prognostic value of type of aphasia is controversial. Kertesz and McCabe (1977) and Lomas and Kertesz (1978) advocated using the patient's type of aphasia to predict his or her future. Both report patients who demonstrate conduction or anomic aphasia have a good prognosis for improvement. However, both note that Broca's and Wernicke's aphasia patients also make significant gains. Conversely, Prins, Snow, and Wagenaar (1978) and Lendrem and Lincoln (1985) found type of aphasia was not related to the amount of improvement their patients made. Basso and colleagues (1979) compared improvement in fluent and nonfluent patients and found no significant difference in improvement between the two groups. Shewan and Kertesz (1984) observed 85 percent of their treated Broca's aphasic patients improved, followed by global, 78 percent; Wernicke's, 73 percent; anomic, 40 percent; and conduction, 38 percent.

SUMMARY

Darley's (1979) advice on the use of prognostic variables is sage: "No single negative factor is so uniformly potent as to justify excluding a patient from at least a trial of therapy" (p. 629). Nevertheless, some variables are more predictive than others. For example, patients who are closer to onset will improve more than those who are longer postonset; patients with a single, small lesion that avoids the temporoparietal area have a better prognosis than those who suffer large, multiple, or bilateral lesions involving the left hemisphere temporoparietal area; patients in good health will improve more than patients in poor health; and initially, mildly severe patients will attain higher levels of performance than initially severe patients, although they may not make as much improvement. The influence of etiology is enigmatic. Although patients who suffer closed head trauma may achieve better language proficiency than patients who suffer other etiologies, their persisting cognitive deficits may severely impair communication.

For the other variables—age, premorbid intelligence, occupational history, and type of aphasia—there is sufficient conflicting evidence to make their prognostic prediction effete.

Determining the power of a prognostic variable requires a cohort study, and these have not been done. Because different variables may interact, it is necessary to isolate the variable of interest and hold all other variables constant. Essentially, one must establish and study cohorts who differ only on a single variable. For example, to determine the prognostic power of age, one must establish cohorts that differ only in age—40 to 50 years, 50 to 60 years, 60 to 70 years, etc. All patients in all cohorts must be similar in all other variables—etiology, time postonset, size and location of the lesion, severity, etc. Then, these cohorts are followed and managed in exactly the same way. If one cohort, for example, the 40 to 50 years group, improves more than the other cohorts, then we have evidence that age, favoring younger patients, is prognostic. Of course, since age always coexists with other variables, the process would need to be repeated in cohort studies that manipulate two, and three, and more variables systematically. One can see why we lack data on the prognostic power of specific variables.

BEHAVIORAL PROFILES

Another approach to providing an aphasic patient a prognosis is to use his or her performance on a test that has prognostic validity. This is developed by evaluating patients with a variety of tasks, constructing profiles of their performance, following them over a period of time to determine which patients with which profiles improve and which do not, and then using the results to predict for future patients. Schuell (1965b) pioneered this approach in aphasia, and Porch (1981) used it to predict potential performance on the PICA.

Schuell (1965b) listed five prognostic groups and two minor syndromes based on her retrospective analysis of aphasic patients' improvement on the MTDDA (Schuell,

1965a). Each group and minor syndrome is defined, specific signs are listed, most discriminating tests are identified, and a prognosis is given. Thus, a clinician can administer the MTDDA, compare the patient's performance with that listed for each group or minor syndrome, and obtain a prognosis. For example, patients who meet the definition and signs for Group 1: Simple Aphasia, have a prognosis for "excellent recovery of all language skills. Treatment is usually required for maximal return of language and successful vocational adjustment" (Schuell, 1965b, p. 9). Conversely, prognosis for patients whose MTDDA performance places them in Group 5: Irreversible Aphasic Syndrome, indicates "auditory comprehension may show functional improvement, and reactive responses increase, but language does not become functional or voluntary in any modality" (Schuell, 1965b, p. 14).

Prognosis with the MTDDA is the result of a skilled clinician's careful observation, organization, and patience. It does exactly what it is designed to do: take an aphasic patient's performance early postonset and predict how he or she will perform in the future. Schuell and colleagues (1964) discussed the use of this approach with individual cases. To our knowledge, there has been no report of its precision with a large sample of patients who were given a prognosis, followed over time, and compared with the prognosis given. Sometimes it is difficult to fit a patient's MTDDA performance into one of the five prognostic groups or two minor syndromes, because performance straddles two or more categories. Further, the prognosis is limited to adjectives and brief descriptions. And, Smith (1972) found that although MTDDA performance was correlated with overall improvement, other significant predictors of improvement—nonlanguage ability, somatosensory function, age, and motivation—had to be added to the prognostic equation. Nevertheless, Schuell provided a tool and direction for giving aphasic patients and their families a view of the future.

Porch (1981) developed three methods for predicting an aphasic patient's future performance on the PICA: High-Overall Prediction (HOAP), High-Overall Prediction Slopes (HOAP Slopes), and Intrasubtest Variability. These utilize a patient's present performance as a "best guess" of future performance. Figure 4-5 shows a PICA score sheet that contains all of the information necessary to provide a prognosis with each method.

The HOAP method requires administering a PICA, computing the overall and nine high (mean of the patient's nine best subtests) scores, and using the PICA Manual to predict future performance. There is a computer program, the PICA Pad (Katz & Porch, 1983), that will take a lot of the work out of this effort. N. S., the patient shown in Figure 4-5, performed at the 28th overall percentile at one month postonset. The mean of his nine highs was 13.44. Appendix D in the PICA Manual, High-Low Percentiles for Left Hemisphere Brain-Damaged Patients, indicates that a nine high score of 13.44 corresponds to an overall score of 11.11, which is at the 53rd percentile. Thus, 53rd percentile performance was N. S.'s predicted performance at six months postonset. He was treated three times a week for five months, and he performed at the 63rd percentile at six months postonset. Thus, we underestimated his potential performance by 10 percentile units.

The HOAP Slopes method is used when the patient is more than one month postonset. HOAP Slopes, provided in the PICA Manual, require determining where the patient's current overall percentile and time postonset intersect, and traveling up the slope to find the predicted performance at six months postonset. For example, N. S. performed at the 55th percentile at three months postonset. Using the HOAP method at one month postonset, we had predicted he would be at the 53rd percentile at six months postonset. Because he had already met our six month prediction at three months, we used the HOAP Slope method to revise our six month predicted performance. The appropriate slope in the PICA Manual predicted 73rd percentile performance at six months postonset. As indicated previously, N. S. was at the 63rd percentile at six months postonset. Thus, with this method, we

Porch Index of Communicative Ability

SCORE SHEET

Name _N. S._   Onset _1/6/87_   No. _____

Date _2/9/87_ By _RTW_   Time _9:05_ to _10:06_ Total Time _61 mins._

Test Conditions _STANDARD_

Patient Conditions _Good, COEXISTING APRAXIA OF SPEECH_

Glasses: _No_   Hearing aid: _No_   Dentures: _No_   Hand Used: _LEFT_

ITEM	I	II	III	IV	V	VI	VII	VIII	IX	X	XI	XII	A	B	C	D	E	F
1. Tb	3	12	13	3	5	15	11	15	2	13	15	4	3	⑤	⑤	8	14	14
2. Cg	3	15	12	3	⑤	15	11	15	2	15	15	3	4	⑤	⑤	6	10	14
3. Pn	3	12	12	3	⑤	13	12	15	2	15	15	3	3	⑤	⑤	6	14	14
4. Kf	3	13	13	3	⑤	13	12	15	2	13	15	3	3	⑥	⑤	8	14	14
5. Fk	3	13	15	3	⑤	15	12	15	2	15	15	3	3	⑥	⑤	6	7	12
6. Qt	3	12	12	3	⑤	9	12	15	2	15	15	3	3	⑤	⑤	8	14	11
7. Pl	3	12	12	3	⑥	13	12	15	2	15	15	3	3	⑤	⑤	8	14	10
8. Mt	3	7	12	3	⑤	15	12	15	2	15	15	3	3	⑤	⑤	6	14	11
9. Ky	3	15	15	4	⑤	15	12	15	2	15	15	3	3	⑤	⑥	6	14	14
10. Cb	3	9	15	4	⑤	15	12	15	2	15	15	3	3	⑤	⑥	6	14	14
TIME	9⁰⁷	9¹¹	9¹⁴	9¹⁷	9²⁵	9²⁶	9²⁷	9²⁸	9³⁰	9³¹	9³²	9³⁴	9³⁷	9⁴²	9⁴³	9⁵⁶	9⁵⁹	10¹⁴
MINUTES	2	4	3	3	8	1	1	1	2	1	1	2	3	5	5	13	3	7
MODALITY	VRB	PTM	PTM	VRB	RDG	AUD	RDG	VIS	VRB	AUD	VIS	VRB	WRT	WRT	WRT	WRT	CPY	CPY
MEAN SCORE	3.0	12.0	13.1	3.2	5.0	13.8	11.8	15.0	2.0	14.6	15.0	3.1	3.1	5.0	5.0	6.8	12.9	12.8
%ILE	2/7	80/82	80/81	7	4/12	45	43/44	34/77	0/1	57/62	18/77	4	4	16/28	16/32	46	69	46/48
VARIAB.	0	30	19	8	0	12	2	0	0	4	0	9	9	0	0	12	11	12

	OVERALL	WRITING	COPYING	READING	PANTOMIME	VERBAL	AUDITORY	VISUAL
MPO _1_								
	8.73	4.98	12.85	8.40	12.55	2.83	14.20	15.00
%ile	28	19	63	31	80/81	1	49	35/99
Variab.	128	21	23	2	49	17	16	0
Mean Var.	7.1	5.3	11.5	1.0	24.5	4.3	8.0	0

	Gestural	Verbal	Graphic	9 HI	9 LO	HOAP	Correction	Target
Score	12.54	2.83	7.60	13.44	4.02	11.11	0	
%ile	41	1	43	53	9	53	0	53%

CONSULTING PSYCHOLOGISTS PRESS
577 College Avenue   Palo Alto, California

Figure 4-5. PICA score sheet containing information to provide a prognosis with the HOAP, HOAP Slope, and Intrasubtest Variability methods. Reprinted with permission from Consulting Psychologists Press, Inc., 577 College Avenue, Palo Alto, CA 94306.

overestimated his performance by 10 percentile units.

Intrasubtest variability employs Porch's concept of the Peak Mean Difference (PMD). The assumption is that the patient's best current performance is prognostic of performance at a future date. PMD utilizes the variability of performance among items in each subtest. It is obtained by subtracting the subtest mean from the best score within that subtest. For example, on Subtest II, N. S.'s mean performance was 12.0, and his best performance on any item was 15. Thus, in the "VARIAB" column, the PMD for Subtest II is 30. Decimal points are ignored. Subtest variability is summed to obtain overall variability and variability within each modality. These are listed below the percentiles at the bottom of the score sheet. Porch states, "If the PMD is high (+ 400), the patient is demonstrating a large discrepancy between his potential level of functioning and his actual performance, and therefore he has the capacity for improvement" (Porch, 1981, p. 104). On the other hand, a low PMD, under 200, indicates little variability in performance and poor potential for change. N. S.'s overall variability at one month postonset was 128. Although this indicated little capacity for change, he improved 35 percentile units between one and six months postonset.

Wertz, Deal, and Deal (1980) evaluated the precision of the HOAP and HOAP Slope methods with 85 patients who had suffered a single left hemisphere infarct and had received at least two PICAs within the first six months postonset. Correlations between predicted performance and performance actually obtained were significant (p <0.001) for both methods. However, predicted performance with either method placed no more than 67 percent of the patients within plus or minus 10 percentile units of the PICA score actually obtained.

Aten and Lyon (1978) evaluated the Intrasubtest Variability (PMD) method for providing a prognosis. Seventy-two patients were followed between one and nine months postonset. The results indicated that the amount of variability in performance within a subtest did not predict the amount of improvement their patients made.

Porch and Callaghan (1981) suggested that both tests of PICA predictive methods contain "some methodological and interpretive limitations" (p. 188). They indicated that HOAP methods should yield a normal distribution around the predicted score. Thus, approximately two-thirds of the predictions should fall within 10 percentile units of the performance attained. This interpretation is supported by the data from Wertz and colleagues (1980). Up to 67 percent of the patients in each of their prediction groups achieved scores within plus or minus 10 percentile units of those predicted. And, some patients missed the predicted score by as much as 40 percentile units. Porch and Callaghan explained Aten and Lyon's (1978) negative results using PMD

as a problem in pooling patient data. They suggested that intrasubtest variability will differ in different patients at different points in time. Thus, combining patient performance is not an accurate test of the potency of PMD prediction.

PICA prediction, like Schuell's behavioral profiles, can make a very accurate statement about the future for many patients. For some, however, they are inaccurate, and the patients make substantially more or less change than predicted. Both approaches permit revision in prognosis as patients progress through management. We use both, but we caution ourselves and our patients that we may err in either direction, overprediction or underprediction. Patients are more comfortable with our "best guesses" than we are, and they, fortunately, are more forgiving.

STATISTICAL PREDICTION

The use of statistical procedures—multiple regression, discriminant function analysis, multiple logistic regression—is becoming popular in providing a prognosis for aphasic patients. Multiple regression techniques test the power of a variable or variables to predict change in aphasic performance. Discriminant function analyses identify variables that distinguish between patients who achieve significant improvement and those who make less or minimal improvement. And, multiple logistic linear regression, like multiple regression, assesses the relative importance of predictor variables on improvement.

In multiple regression and multiple logistic linear regression, an equation that employs a priori measures collected during an initial evaluation is used to predict future performance. For example, the patient's age, education, and auditory comprehension, reading, speaking, and writing performance on a language measure at one month postonset may be used to predict language performance at one year postonset. The analysis may include one or more steps. In step one, a prediction is attempted using the predictor (for example, auditory comprehension at one month postonset) that has the highest correlation with the criterion variable (for example, severity of aphasia at one year postonset). An analysis of variance is performed on all other variables to determine whether their inclusion in the equation significantly increases predictive precision. If including an additional variable increases predictive precision, step two is performed by adding the second predictor (for example, speaking ability at one month postonset) to the equation. This stepwise procedure is continued until no additional predictor significantly increases prediction or all a priori predictors have been included in the equation. The test of predictive power is the relationship between the predicted performance and the performance actually obtained. Several have employed this procedure with varying degrees of success.

Porch and colleagues (1980) used the patient's age and PICA modality scores—Gestural, Verbal, and Graphic—collected at one month postonset to predict PICA Overall performance at 3, 6, and 12 months postonset. The predicted scores correlated significantly ($p < 0.001$) with the scores patients actually obtained at the three different points postonset. Marshall and colleagues (1982) used 11 predictors to forecast the amount of improvement made on the PICA between an initial test and a final test. All 11 predictors produced the highest correlation, +0.704, between predicted and obtained improvement, but three variables—number of treatment sessions, months postonset, and age—provided most of the predictive power. VanDemark (1982) employed multiple regression analysis to predict posttreatment performance on the BDAE. For aphasic patients who had suffered vascular lesions, three BDAE subtests—confrontation naming, complex ideational material, and body part identification—yielded a multiple correlation coefficient, R, of .91. Thus, for most of her patients, posttreatment performance on the BDAE was predicted with impressive accuracy. Lendrem and Lincoln (1985) used stepwise multiple regression analyses to predict spontaneous recovery in untreated aphasic patients between 4 and 34 weeks postonset. Age, four-week PICA Gestural, Verbal, and Graphic scores,

and measures of nonverbal ability were entered in the equation. Only the PICA Gestural, Verbal, and Graphic scores at four weeks postonset contributed significantly to predicting the PICA Overall score at 34 weeks postonset. Lendrem and Lincoln concluded that improvement in aphasia by 34 weeks postonset can be predicted by performance at four weeks postonset. Finally, Holland and colleagues (in press) used multiple logistic linear regression to determine the power of eight variables for predicting recovery in aphasia as indicated by a WAB Aphasia Quotient at 93.8 or above. Variables that were significantly associated with recovery included age, favoring younger patients, and length of hospital stay, favoring shorter stays. Gender, favoring male patients; type of stroke, favoring hemorrhage; and side of lesion, favoring the right hemisphere, were moderately associated with recovery. Neither race nor a history of previous stroke were significant predictors of recovery.

Marshall and Phillips (1983) employed a stepwise discriminant function analysis to test the predictive value of 10 prognostic variables for identifying aphasic patients who eventually obtain the ability to communicate verbally. Six variables—initial severity of aphasia, number of months postonset, auditory comprehension ability, age, speech fluency, and general health—identified eventual speaking ability in 86 percent of the patients studied. Occupational status at the onset of aphasia, ability to self-correct errors, progress during the first month of treatment, and the number of treatment sessions did not contribute significantly to identification. Patients who achieved good eventual speaking ability were identified with slightly more precision, 91 percent, than patients who achieved poor eventual speaking ability, 83 percent.

Statistical prediction of improvement in aphasia is more promising than precise. None of the multiple regression formulas is ready for application with individual aphasic patients. For example, Deal and colleagues (1979) utilized the predictive equation developed by Porch and colleagues (1980) to provide a prognosis for 90 aphasic patients. Correlations between predicted PICA performance and the performance the patients obtained were significant ($p < 0.001$). However, less than half of the 90 patients obtained a PICA score that was within plus or minus five percentile units of the score predicted. Nevertheless, in order to get anything right, we are obligated to get a great many things wrong. We wander about looking for techniques and targets. Statistical prediction appears to be an appropriate technique for determining how an aphasic patient will perform in the future. The work to be done is improving statistical prediction's ability to hit the target accurately with individual patients.

PROGNOSTIC TREATMENT

The most precise prognostic methods, we believe, are the most expensive. Prognostic treatment requires patient and clinician to invest several sessions to determine whether treatment will influence the patient's future. We employ the single-subject designs discussed in Chapter 5 to see whether a patient can learn, generalize improvement on treated stimuli to untreated stimuli, and retain what has been accomplished, and whether he or she is willing to practice. If the patient can achieve all four in a few sessions, prognosis is good, and we invest more time and effort in more sessions. If he or she does not learn, generalize, retain, or practice, prognosis is poor, and we assist the patient in making a life rather than making language.

ABILITY TO LEARN

Names abound to identify treatment methods—facilitation, stimulation, reorganization, etc. All require the patient to learn what is being worked on in treatment. If the patient learns, prognosis is good. If he or she does not, prognosis is poor.

From our appraisal data, we select a behavior that may respond to treatment. We place it in a single subject treatment design—examine performance in baseline for a few sessions to determine its stability, intervene with treatment to determine whether the patient learns, and then withdraw to view retention

during a period of no treatment. For chronic patients, those beyond the influence of spontaneous recovery, the A-B-A Withdrawal design is appropriate. For patients who are close to onset, a multiple baseline design will show whether treatment has any power to produce more than is occurring through spontaneous recovery.

Figure 4-6 shows the use of an A-B-A Withdrawal design to test G. O.'s ability to learn. He was eight months postonset when his wife contacted us to inquire whether speech therapy would help. Appraisal indicated 59th Overall performance on the PICA, and the WAB classified him as displaying Broca's aphasia. A motor speech evaluation revealed a moderate coexisting apraxia of speech. Some informal testing during appraisal showed G. O. profited from phonetic priming. When he was given auditory and visual

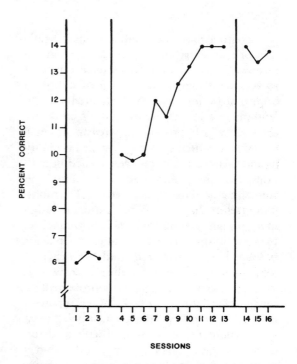

Figure 4-6. A-B-A Withdrawal design used to determine G. O.'s ability to learn confrontation naming. Performance is shown as the mean of 20 productions scored with the PICA multidimensional scoring system.

information about a word's first sound, he was fairly successful in producing it. The A-B-A design shown in Figure 4-6 was used to determine whether he could learn confrontation naming if treated with phonetic primes. Twenty pictures were selected and baselined. His performance, measured on the PICA multidimensional scale, was stable. Ten treatment sessions followed and consisted of giving him a phonetic prime; the sound and articulatory position for the first sound in the name of each picture. Performance was measured after each session by having G. O. name each picture without any priming assistance. In the first three treatment sessions, performance leaped and then stalled, but thereafter it continued to improve. During withdrawal, G. O. sagged, but only a bit. This man learned during prognostic treatment, and that learning prompted us to predict a good prognosis for additional improvement.

GENERALIZATION

Neither patient or clinician has the time to work on every bit and piece of language necessary to communicate. We expect patients to generalize their gains on treated stimuli to improved performance on untreated stimuli. Without generalization, prognosis is bleak. So, one piece of prognostic treatment may examine a patient's ability to strut his ability attained on treated stimuli across their boundaries and show improved performance on something we have not worked on. The multiple baseline single subject treatment design indicates whether this occurs. Performance on two or more sets of stimuli or tasks is baselined, one is treated, and the other or others continue in the baseline condition. If the patient generalizes, we see improvement on the untreated stimuli or tasks. When a patient is close to onset and is receiving a boost from spontaneous recovery, it is difficult to determine whether generalization results from a spread of a treatment effect or from spontaneous recovery. We do not worry about why generalization occurs in these patients, because our question is prognostic. If generalization occurs, the patient is improving on things we

have not treated, and that is what we want to know.

D. G.'s generalization is shown in Figure 4-7. He arrived with very little and did even less with what he had. PICA Overall performance was at the 12th percentile, and the WAB classified him as global aphasia. We suspected he also carried a heavy load of apraxia of speech, but his only utterance was "May," and it did not provide enough information to permit a diagnosis beyond severe aphasia. At 14 months postonset, D. G. didn't convince us he would break any prognostic records. Nevertheless, we wondered whether he could develop some articulatory gestures, realize they had meaning, and produce them volitionally. This is monumental, upstream work. Its results are shown in Figure 4-7. Three vowels—/i/, /a/, and /o/—were baselined. Treatment began on /i/ based on the rationale that it was part of the diphthong in his recurring utterance, "May," and we might get it by laying on some hands. The other two stimuli, /a/ and /o/, were followed in baseline to see

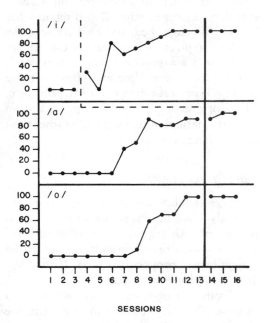

SESSIONS

Figure 4-7. Multiple baseline design used to determine D. G.'s ability to generalize verbal repetition from treated /i/ to untreated /a/ and /o/. Performance is shown as the percent correct for 10 repetitions of each stimulus.

if generalization might occur. We had so far to go with D. G., we needed all of the help we could get. Treatment consisted of strong auditory and visual stimulation, "Watch me and listen to me and say what I say," plus spreading his lips into the appropriate articulatory position. Data points in Figure 4-7 represent 10 productions from repetition only. Baseline for all three stimuli got only "May." This continued through the first two treatment sessions on /i/ with only a hint of what was desired. In the third session, D. G. got hold of /i/ and started to run with it. Both /a/ and /o/ remained in baseline, and both began to move without treatment during the fourth through fifth treatment session on /i/. Did this represent generalization? We think it did. By the end of the tenth treatment session, all three responses were 90 to 100 percent correct in repetition, and all held up during withdrawal. D. G. learned to produce /i/ during treatment, and he generalized his performance to improvement on untreated /a/ and /o/. Although prognosis remained guarded in this severely aphasic man, a flicker of a future was there, and we moved on to other targets.

RETENTION

What patients learn, we hope they will retain. After a brief treatment trial, performance may sag when treatment is withdrawn. If improvement occurred during treatment, the posttreatment drop in performance usually indicates the need for additional treatment. Eventually, however, we want patients to maintain their treatment gains and display minimal sag during withdrawal. The ability to retain, we believe, is prognostic. Those who maintain treatment gains have a better prognosis than those who need additional refurbishing of what was formerly achieved. The withdrawal portion of an A-B-A Withdrawal or multiple baseline single-subject treatment design gives us a look at retention.

J. P. had two passions: football and fishing. When he was not watching one, he was doing the other. And, when schedules or weather did not permit doing either, he liked to read about both. A left hemisphere CVA had not interfered with watching football or going fishing, but the aphasia that followed it had eroded his ability to read much about either. At 10 months postonset, he performed at the 61st Overall percentile on the PICA, and the WAB classified him as displaying anomic aphasia. His reading was just about right for single words if he received a lot of help. RCBA performance was 60 percent correct, and the bulk af his accuracy was on the single word subtests. We set up the multiple baseline design shown in Figure 4-8 to obtain a prognosis for J. P.'s potential to improve his reading. It also gave us a look at how he retained the reading ability he gained. Two sets of stimuli, printed names and pictured mascots or logos for 20 NFL football teams and printed names and pictures of 20 fish, were baselined in three sessions. Treatment was initiated on the football stimuli, and the fish stimuli were followed in extended baseline. J. P.'s task was to match the printed name of each football team with the correct picture of the team's mascot or logo in a response matrix of 10 stimuli. If he failed, additional information was provided auditorily—"It's the team that used to be in Oakland" or "Vince Lombardi used to coach there." The data points in Figure 4-8 represent J. P.'s ability to match each name with each picture without any auditory cues. Performance on football stimuli shot up within five treatment sessions. When he reached our criterion of 90 percent accuracy in three successive sessions, we put football stimuli into withdrawal and began to treat fish stimuli. The treatment remained the same, including appropriate auditory cues—"Some people like to catch this one with a dry fly" or "You told me you caught one of these in the Carquinez Straits, and it weighed 42 pounds." Fish stimuli were a little harder for him to catch than football stimuli, but progress was obvious. More importantly, our look at football stimuli during withdrawal indicated J. P. retained what he had learned during treatment. We read this as a sign that prognosis for improving reading was good. We also learned more about fish than we wanted to know.

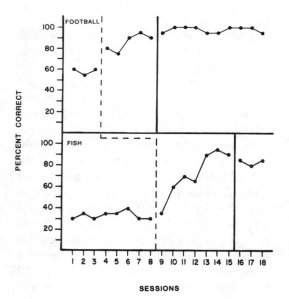

Figure 4-8. Multiple baseline design used to determine J. P.'s ability to retain improvement on treated football stimuli. During sessions four through eight, football stimuli were treated. In sessions nine through 18, football stimuli were followed without treatment. Lack of decline in performance indicates J. P. was able to retain what he learned during treatment. Fish stimuli were followed in baseline during sessions one through eight, treated during sessions 9 through 15, and followed without treatment in sessions 16 through 18. Performance represents the percent correct in matching printed words with appropriate pictures.

WILLINGNESS TO PRACTICE

Aphasia treatment differs from any treatment a patient has received from medicine or surgery during his or her life before becoming aphasic. Typically, physicians and surgeons tell patients there is a lot of that going around, and call me in a week if you are not feeling better; or take three of these each day for 10 days, and they should get it; or we will schedule you for surgery on the 29th and take that thing out. All of these, typically, are effective, but all, from the patient's point of view, are passive. When he or she sees us for aphasia therapy, we tell him or her that improvement is possible with a lot of effort on his or her part over an extended period of time. This requires patients to get active, remain active, and want to be active. Certainly, it differs from their history with hospitals, because it requires them to be willing to practice. We believe those who are willing to have a more favorable prognosis than those who are not. And, when possible, we find a means to identify the willing and add this piece of lore to the prognostic equation. An extended baseline that measures a patient's willingness to practice outside of treatment can provide what we seek.

C. H. lived a sufficient distance from our medical center to preclude more than two visits a week. His 42nd percentile Overall performance on the PICA and WAB classification of severe Broca's aphasia indicated he needed more help than he could get to us to receive. His wife was enlisted to provide some practice for C. H. at home between visits with us. Twenty situation pictures were placed in the Davis and Wilcox (1985) PACE format. C. H. was instructed to convey each picture's content to his wife using all means at his disposal—speech, gesture, writing, or drawing. This was to be done in two thirty-minute sessions each day between treatment visits. When we saw C. H., the first few minutes of each treatment session were used to assess this willingness to practice at home. The extended baseline in Figure 4-9 shows the results. Each data point represents C. H.'s wife's ability to understand his description of the 20 situation pictures. Correct identification rose rapidly during our first six checks on home practice. We believe this represented C. H.'s willingness to practice between our treatment sessions, and prognosis for improvement on additional tasks, practiced in the same format, was good.

SUMMARY

Aphasic patients, like D. H. Lawrence's Mrs. Morel, wait and wait, and what they wait for can never come. It does not help anyone to look forward to the past. After becoming aphasic, one will never be again as he or she had been. But, for many aphasic people, improvement is possible, and for most, it is inevitable. Prognosis is an effort to state the possible and the inevitable.

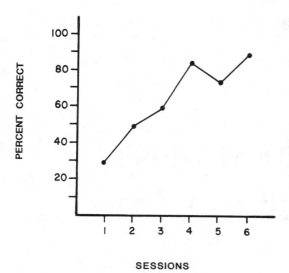

Figure 4-9. Extended baseline used to determine C. H.'s willingness to practice. Each data point represents his wife's ability to understand his description of 20 pictures following practice at home between treatment sessions.

We construct a prognosis by using the patient's biographical, medical, and behavioral variables that may predict improvement or the lack of it. Behavioral profiles on the MTDDA and PICA can be constructed and culled for their contribution. And, prognostic treatment is utilized to determine whether a patient can learn, generalize, and retain, and whether he or she is willing to practice. Statistical prediction, currently, tells us more about prognosis for the aphasic population than it does about prognosis for any individual aphasic patient. Thus, the contributions of variables and behavioral profiles and the results of prognostic treatment are summed to forecast the patient's future. The result is, usually, a descriptive adjective—good, poor, guarded, etc. It should also indicate the cost in time, money, and effort to attain what is predicted. Most of all, it should include answers to the patient's and family's specific questions—"Will he be able to return to work?" or "Will she be able to talk?" "Yes" or "no" are seldom the answers we can provide. Frequently, we counsel patience and suggest that time is the best ally—time for the brain to heal, time for the tongue to untangle, time for treatment to work its will, and time to cope with a devastating disability. When we advise patients to wait, we must be very specific in defining what they are waiting for. It is not normality, but it can be functional communication in specific situations under specific conditions.

A simple, safe prognosis has considerable appeal. But, if it is wrong, it is ultimately neither simple nor safe. Perhaps the world is round to prevent us from seeing too far down the road. However, many of us would be better clinicians if we did not spend so much time watching and waiting for the world to become perfect or predictably precise or flat. The fecundity of our prognostic ability is more fallow than fertile. It is a part of our professional responsibility we need to cultivate, because a crop of "We just don't know" is unacceptable.

5

APHASIA TREATMENT:
ITS EFFICACY

Jacques Lipchitz related he had read somewhere about a papyrus discovered in Egypt having to do with a prayer called the "Song of Vowels," a prayer that was a song composed only of vowels and designed to subdue the forces of nature. Lipchitz's sculpture, *Song of Vowels,* sits in a grassy area in front of the Stanford University Medical Center as a memorial to Dr. Henry Kaplan, the internationally renowned radiologist and cancer research pioneer. Kaplan's efforts resulted in a treatment program that changed Hodgkin's disease from an almost universally fatal cancer to a usually survivable malignancy; truly, a triumph of man over nature.

Clinicians who treat aphasia also sing their song of vowels to combat the havoc nature wreaks on the language of those who suffer left hemisphere brain damage. This chapter considers the power of the song to soothe disrupted semantics and syntax; whether what we do for aphasic patients does any good. The evidence comes from group treatment trials and single-subject designs. The former tell us whether language treatment has any effect on diminishing the severity of the disorder. The latter indicate whether a specified treatment lessened the severity of aphasia in a specific patient. Both approaches have their place in the practice of clinical aphasiology. Results of group studies argue for

or against aphasic patients being treated. Results of single-subject designs indicate whether a patient has been helped by a treatment. Clinicians must know this literature and how to evaluate it. Not all are convinced aphasia treatment helps. A knowledge of the literature and the ability to explain it assists the clinician in convincing those who doubt.

GROUP TREATMENT STUDIES

Writing in the journal *Neuroepidemiology,* Kurtzke (1982) observed that neurologists have two axioms. The first is "Where is the lesion?" and the second is "Be paranoid." Speech-language pathologists who treat aphasic patients have one axiom; "Be paranoid." And, most have discovered that being paranoid does not mean people are not out to get you.

The source of the aphasia clinician's paranoia has been the paucity of acceptable scientific evidence to support the efficacy of language therapy for aphasia. Until recently, research has failed to provide an unassailable answer. Does language treatment for aphasia do any good? Opinion has varied, and so has the evidence generated by studies designed to provide an answer.

Almost 30 aphasia treatment studies have been conducted, and most have produced positive results: treatment for aphasia is efficacious. Few, however, have met the scientific requirements necessary to provide proof that treatment results in significantly more improvement than no treatment. It is not easy to design and conduct an aphasia treatment study. Some (Editorial, *Lancet*, 1977) have suggested it is impossible. The following lists the problems involved in testing whether treatment for aphasia does any good.

COMPLICATIONS IN APHASIA TREATMENT TRIALS

The adequacy of an aphasia treatment study is measured by its ability to cope with four major complications: controlling patient variables that may influence response to treatment, controlling for spontaneous recovery, defining an acceptable no-treatment group, and specifying the treatment administered. Failure to cope with these complications sinks even the most buoyant positive results.

PATIENT VARIABLES

Aphasic patients differ in what made them aphasic, how long they have been that way, how aphasic they are, and so on. These differences are believed (Darley, 1972, 1975; Wertz, 1978; 1983) to influence patients' response to treatment. Therefore, if one wants to test the efficacy of treatment, one must control those variables that may influence the study patients' response to treatment. Mixing patients who have become aphasic as a result of different etiologies, or who vary widely in their duration of aphasia will generate mixed results. And, results should apply to someone. Failure to control variables that may influence response to treatment yields results that apply to no one. Conversely, establishing rigid selection criteria to obtain a homogenous sample limits the number of patients available for study and restricts generalization of the results obtained.

Science demands the latter approach; establishing rigid patient selection criteria. A minimum of these is shown in Table 5-1. Controlling age, education, premorbid literacy in English, etiology, lesion localization, medical status, sensory acuity, time postonset, and severity of aphasia does not eliminate patient variability. It does, however, reduce it. And, for some of the variables that are permitted to vary, for example, aphasic severity, additional control can be obtained through

TABLE 5-1.
Selection Criteria for an Aphasia Group Treatment Trial.

Criterion	Description
Age	75 years or younger
Time postonset	4 weeks at entry
Etiology	First, single, thromboembolic infarct
Localization	Confined to the left hemisphere
Neurologic history	No previous neurologic involvement
Medical and psychological status	No major coexisting medical or psychological disorder
Sensory and Motor Status	
Auditory	Hearing no worse than a 40 dB speech reception threshold, unaided, in the better ear
Vision	Vision no worse than 20/100, corrected in the better eye
Sensory-Motor	Ability in one upper extremity sufficient to gesture and write
Literacy	Premorbid ability to read and write English
Language severity	PICA performance from the 15th through 75th Overall percentile at entry
Informed consent	Patient and patient's representative agree to participate in the study

Adapted from Wertz, Collins et al. (1981)

analysis of covariance in the statistical treatment of the results.

Again, the more rigid the selection criteria, the smaller the sample size. Wertz, Collins et al. (1981) screened over 1,000 patients during a three and one-half year period to find 67 who met the selection criteria listed in Table 5-1. Treatment studies that employ rigid selection criteria tend to obtain samples that are clean but lean.

SPONTANEOUS RECOVERY

Language ability improves in untreated aphasic patients during the first few months postonset. This is called *spontaneous recovery* (Butfield & Zangwill, 1946). Probably, the improvement results from physiological restitution. We know it occurs (Hartman, 1981), but we do not know how much occurs or how long it continues.

Culton (1969), Vignolo (1964), and Lendrem and Lincoln (1985) provided the best evidence. All found no significant change in the language ability of untreated aphasic patients after approximately two months postonset. Others (Eisenson, 1964; Kertesz & McCabe, 1977; Sarno & Levita, 1971) extended this period to three months postonset, and some (Butfield & Zangwill, 1946; Godfrey & Douglass, 1959; Luria, 1963; Marks et al., 1957) suggested spontaneous recovery may continue until six months postonset. These differences in opinion result, probably, from the different patients studied and the different methods used to measure the duration of spontaneous recovery. Nevertheless, spontaneous recovery occurs, and it may continue to evoke improvement in aphasia up to six months postonset.

So, if aphasic patients improve without treatment, those who conduct treatment studies must demonstrate how much of the improvement detected results from the treatment administered and how much results from spontaneous recovery. Two methods for accomplishing this are to study patients in whom spontaneous recovery has run its course or to assign patients to treated and untreated groups. The former approach requires serial testing of patients until significant spontaneous improvement has stopped and then initiating treatment. The latter approach equates the influence of spontaneous recovery by random assignment of patients who meet selection criteria to treatment and no treatment groups. There are scientific objections to waiting, and there are ethical objections to no treatment. Again, conducting an aphasia treatment study is not easy. But, it is essential to control for spontaneous recovery if one intends to demonstrate the efficacy of language treatment for aphasia.

DEFINING A NO-TREATMENT GROUP

Aphasia treatment, like most treatment, has "just growed." Historically, clinicians began treating aphasic patients before they demonstrated that the treatment administered was effective. This leap to treat has created a situation where treatment exists, and because it does, many believe it is unethical to withhold it. But, this is exactly what must be done to demonstrate whether aphasia treatment is efficacious.

The scientifically acceptable test of any treatment is to select patients who are similar in the important characteristics and assign them randomly to treated and untreated groups. If the treated group improves significantly more than the untreated group, then the treatment is considered to be effective. To study treatment for aphasia, random assignment to treated and untreated groups is essential if treatment occurs during the period of spontaneous recovery. If the study patients meet the same selection criteria, random assignment to treated and untreated groups controls for the presence of spontaneous recovery, because it will occur equally in both groups. Thus, if the treated group displays significantly more improvement than the untreated group, one can conclude the difference results from treatment and not spontaneous recovery. This is the scientifically acceptable approach. It is also the approach that is ethically unacceptable.

Only two group treatment studies (Lincoln, et al., 1984; Wertz, Weiss et al.,

1986) have employed random assignment of patients to treatment and no-treatment groups. Lincoln and colleagues avoided the ethical objection of withholding treatment by observing that most of the aphasic patients they studied would not have been treated because treatment was not available (Mulley, 1986). Wertz and colleagues obtained a randomly assigned no-treatment group by deferring treatment for 12 weeks. Patients who met selection criteria were assigned randomly to immediate treatment for 12 weeks or deferred treatment for 12 weeks followed by 12 weeks of treatment. Thus, the deferred group provided a randomly assigned no-treatment group during the first 12 weeks of the study.

Others (Basso, Capitani, & Vignolo, 1979; Hagen, 1973; Shewan & Kertesz, 1984) have employed self-selected or waiting list no-treatment groups for comparison with treated groups. Basso and colleagues' and Shewan and Kertesz's no-treatment groups were composed of patients who lived too far away to receive treatment, rejected treatment, or could not participate in treatment for miscellaneous reasons. Hagen's no-treatment group was composed of patients who were placed on a waiting list. The first 10 patients admitted to the hospital who met selection criteria were assigned to the treatment group, and the next 10 who met selection criteria were assigned to a no-treatment group, because staff were not available to treat them. Both approaches are, probably, more desirable than not having a no-treatment group, but neither is scientifically acceptable. Why patients are not treated may influence the results obtained. For example, Shewan and Kertesz's self-selected no-treatment group was significantly less severe than their treatment group.

SPECIFYING THE TREATMENT

The shortest section in any report of an aphasia treatment trial is the one that describes the treatment. Although it is easy to document how much treatment patients receive—two hours a week for 24 weeks, six to eight hours a week for 48 weeks, etc.—it is almost impossible to specify exactly how the patients were treated. Group treatment trials designed to test the efficacy of aphasia treatment, typically, are not testing *a* treatment or comparing two or more treatments. They are testing the efficacy of treatment in general.

Aphasic patients, including those in group treatment trials, display a variety of overall severity, a variety of severity within the different language modalities, and a variety of responses to different treatment methods. In a single-subject treatment design, one can and must specify how the patient was treated. In a group treatment trial, the 20, or 30, or 40, or more treated patients are, typically, treated differently. Thus, description of the treatment is general; for example, "traditional, individual, stimulus-response type treatment of speech and language deficits in all communicative modalities" (Wertz, Collins et al. 1981, p. 582). Some control over treatment can be exercised by using a treatment protocol that specifies, generally, the types of treatment that will be administered, the language modalities that will be treated, the criteria for selecting treatment tasks, the criterion for success in each task that must be reached before moving on to another task, and so on. But, in a group treatment study, one cannot specify a specific treatment program for all patients, because it may not be appropriate for any patient in the study.

This need for flexibility to meet the individual needs of the patients participating in an aphasia treatment study has been criticized by Howard (1986). He argued it is not sensible to investigate the effects of a set of heterogeneous treatment techniques on a heterogeneous sample of aphasic patients. His solution is to avoid group treatment trials and confine efforts to single case studies that explore the efficacy of a specified treatment for a specific patient. We agree with part of this epistemological position; the need for single-case treatment research. But, we cannot accept eschewing group treatment studies. Results of a single case study will only show whether a treatment was or was not effective for an aphasic patient. Any number of these will never demonstrate whether language treatment is efficacious for aphasia. This question is answered by studying treated and untreated groups of aphasic people to provide the statistical power necessary to demonstrate whether treatment for aphasia does or does not work. One reduces group heterogeneity by establishing rigid selection criteria, but it is essential to permit heterogeneity in the treatment so it will be appropriate for individual patients in the group. This, it seems to us, is somewhat similar to selecting a specific treatment for a specific patient in a single case study.

A HISTORY OF THE EFFICACY OF APHASIA TREATMENT

Historic continuity with the past, Oliver Wendell Holmes, Jr. reminded us, is not a duty, it is only a necessity. Knowing the history of aphasia treatment research is essential for clinicians to defend the efficacy of their efforts. Opinion about whether aphasia treatment helps has bifurcated into two schismatic sects: those who "know" it does and those who "know" it does not. The latter make opprobrious remarks about the worth of the former's efforts and suggest treatment study results are execrable. The clinician who does not know the literature can only make elegiac apologies and consider becoming an anchorite. Even if one knows the literature, it is necessary to know how to interpret it, because the results are not pellucid.

This section reviews the results of remote and recent aphasia treatment trials. We attempt to identify the numerous vigias in the studies and reduce some of the hugger-mugger. What is contained here can be supplemented with reviews by Darley (1972, 1975); David (1983); and Wertz (1987).

EARLY RESEARCH

Broca (1865) advocated aphasic patients be treated, and he implied treatment was effective. However, evidence to support Broca's beliefs was not collected, or it has been submerged in the literature.

Frazier and Ingham (1920) were, apparently, the first to report the results of their efforts. They noted that 16 aphasic patients who had suffered gunshot wounds to the head made marked improvement as a result of treatment. Some of these patients had not changed for several months, and they improved when they were treated.

Weisenburg and McBride (1935) reported the results of treatment with five of their patients. All improved in their language abilities, and all experienced improved attitude and morale.

Butfield and Zangwill (1946) treated 63 patients who varied in their time postonset. Overall, 76 percent the group was either "much improved" or "improved" after treatment. And, those treated before six months postonset made more gains than those treated after six months postonset.

Wepman (1951) reported his results with 68 patients who were aphasic subsequent to traumatic head injury. All were six months or more postonset when treatment began. After treatment, 86 percent of his sample was "much improved" or "improved."

Marks, Taylor, and Rusk (1957) used a four-point rating scale to measure the results of treatment with 324 aphasic patients. Results indicated improvement was excellent in 6.9 percent, good in 22 percent, fair in 21.4 percent, and poor in 49.7 percent.

Vignolo (1964) seems to be the first to compare treated patients with self-selected untreated patients. Pre- and posttreatment comparisons showed no differences between the two groups. However, Vignolo observed patients treated between two and six months postonset and those who received more than six months of treatment made more improvement than patients treated after six months postonset, those who received less than six months of treatment, and those who received no treatment.

Sands, Sarno, and Shankweiler (1969) studied 30 treated patients who were aphasic subsequent to a cerebrovascular accident. The duration of treatment ranged from 2 weeks to 32 months. After treatment, amount of improvement varied, but 27 of the 30 patients showed some improvement. Only three remained the same or became worse.

The second group comparison was conducted by Sarno, Silverman, and Sands (1970). They assigned 31 severely aphasic patients to either traditional treatment, programmed instruction, or no treatment. After 40 hours of treatment, there were no significant differences among the three groups.

These constitute what we call the early research on aphasia treatment's efficacy. The variety of methods among studies make comparison impossible. Only two (Sarno, Silverman, & Sands, 1970; Vignolo, 1964) compared treated and untreated patients, and neither employed random assignment to groups. Cause of aphasia varied both among studies—Frazier and Ingham's (1920) and Wepman's (1951) patients suffered gunshot wounds or traumatic head injury and Sands et al. (1969) and Sarno and colleagues (1970) studied patients who suffered a stroke—and within studies. (Butfield & Zangwill, 1946; Marks et al., 1957). And, apparently, the amount and type of treatment differed within and among studies. Only Sarno and colleagues (1970) specified the amount and type of treatment their patients received.

Darley's (1972) review of these early efforts concluded, "any all-conclusive statement about the efficacy of aphasia therapy would be ill-advised" (p. 7). He suggested, "More data are needed applying to clearly specified samples of the aphasic population subjected to clearly specified regimens of therapy by clinicians, for clearly specified periods" (p. 8). Since this suggestion, at least nine treatment studies have been conducted. Their ability to meet Darley's requirements will be examined below.

RECENT RESULTS

Those of us who follow learn, we hope, from those who preceded. We stand on the shoulders, not the backs, of those who lead. The early efforts have moved what we know from penury to plenty.

Hagen (1973) compared treated and untreated patients who were aphasic subsequent to a single left hemisphere embolic or thrombolic infarct. The first 10 patients who met selection criteria were treated, and the second 10 patients were placed on a waiting list and not treated. All patients were followed for three months. Then the treated group received four hours of individual treatment, eight hours of group treatment, and six hours of independent treatment each week for 12 months. The no-treatment group received all hospital services, (e.g., physical therapy and occupational therapy) except communication treatment for 12 months. Treated patients made significantly more improvement in reading comprehension, language formulation, speech production, spelling, and arithmetic than untreated patients. Hagen's effort was carefully controlled, except for the lack of random assignment to treated and untreated groups, and his results imply that language therapy for aphasia is efficacious.

Deal and Deal (1978) compared five groups of aphasic patients who had suffered a single, left hemisphere cerebrovascular accident: Group I began treatment during the first month postonset; Group II began treatment during the second month postonset; Group III began treatment during the third month postonset; Group IV began treatment during the fourth to seventh months postonset; and in Group V, patients were not treated. The number of patients in each group ranged from 10 to 17, and the amount of treatment in Groups I through IV ranged from 27 to 254 sessions across groups. Treated patients were tested with the Porch Index of Communicative Ability (PICA) (Porch, 1967) when treatment began and again when treatment ended. Group V, the untreated patients, was tested during the first two months postonset and later at 12 months postonset. The results indicated that Group I made significantly more improvement than Groups III to V, Group II made significantly more improvement than Groups IV and V, Group III made significantly more improvement than Group V, and Group IV did not differ significantly from Group V. Deal and Deal acknowledged the limitations of their effort—small sample sizes; patients were not randomly assigned to groups; and failure to control amount, intensity, and duration of treatment. Nevertheless, their results suggested that patients who are treated early postonset, between one and three months, make significantly more improvement than patients who receive no treatment. Further, treatment initiated before one month postonset resulted in more improvement than treatment begun after three months postonset.

Basso, Capitani, and Vignolo (1979) examined the influence of treatment on aphasic patients initiated at three different points postonset—before two months, between two and six months, and after six months. Treated patients received no less than three individual sessions each week for at least six months. Their improvement was compared with that of three groups of self-selected untreated patients examined during the same time periods and reexamined at least six months later. Sample sizes were large; 162 patients in the treated groups and 119 patients in the no-treatment groups. Cause of aphasia was a cerebrovascular accident in 85 percent of the cases, trauma in 11 percent, postsurgical ablation of a benign tumor in 3 percent, and a nonprogressive focal lesion in 1 percent. The results indicated treated patients made significantly more improvement in each of the time postonset groups than untreated patients, and patients treated earlier postonset made significantly more improvement than patients treated later postonset. This is substantial evidence that language treatment for aphasia is efficacious, however it must be filtered through the lack of randomly assigned treatment and no-treatment groups and the mixture of etiologies in both groups.

Holland (1980b) has contributed results from a retrospective, serendipitous treatment study. During her validation of the Communicative Ability in Daily Living (CADL) (Holland, 1980a), she observed 17 of 28 patients tested and retested approximately one year apart showed improved performance on the second test. Efforts to explain this revealed 13 of the 28 had received treatment during the year between the two tests and 15 had not. Comparison of the pre- and posttests showed the 13 patients receiving treatment made significantly more improvement than the 15 untreated patients. Other characteristics—type and severity of aphasia, age, education, and

time postonset—did not differ greatly between groups. Obviously, this effort fails to meet many of the criteria for an aphasia treatment study. Had it been planned, the design would have differed from what was discovered. But, as Holland suggested, "If an efficacy study creeps up on you, PUBLISH" (p. 241).

Wertz, Collins, Weiss, and colleagues (1981) conducted the first Veterans Administration cooperative study on aphasia. This investigation compared individual with group treatment and, indirectly, tested the efficacy of treatment for aphasia. Patients who met the rigid selection criteria listed in Table 5-1 were assigned randomly to either individual treatment by a speech pathologist eight hours a week for 44 weeks or group treatment by a speech pathologist eight hours a week for 44 weeks. In individual treatment, there was direct stimulus-response manipulation of deficits in all language modalities. In group treatment, there was no direct manipulation of speech and language deficits. Treatment consisted of group discussion, group projects, lectures, and recreational activities. A battery of measures was administered at entry, four weeks postonset, and every 11 weeks thereafter, up to 48 weeks postonset. The results indicated that both groups made significant improvement during the 44-week treatment trial and, although group differences were few, those that did occur indicated more improvement in patients who received individual treatment. To test the efficacy of treatment, the authors examined improvement in both groups after six months postonset. They argued that the continued significant improvement observed in both groups implied treatment was efficacious, because significant spontaneous recovery is believed to end by, at most, six months postonset.

Lincoln, McGuirk, Mulley, and colleagues (1984) conducted the first aphasia treatment trial that assigned patients randomly to treated and untreated groups. Treated patients were to receive two one-hour sessions each week for 24 weeks, and untreated patients received no treatment for 24 weeks. Selection criteria excluded acute stroke patients who were unable to cope with testing, patients who had mild aphasia, and patients who were severely dysarthric. Patients with more than one stroke were not excluded, type of stroke was not reported, and lesion localization—left hemisphere, right hemisphere, or bilateral—was not specified. The results indicated patients in both groups improved, and there were no significant differences in language improvement between groups. A review of the treated group indicated that only 26 percent of the patients received 37 to 48 of the 48 hours of treatment specified.

Shewan and Kertesz (1984) compared performance by patients in three randomly assigned treatment groups—language oriented therapy by a speech pathologist, stimulation-facilitation therapy by a speech pathologist, and treatment in unstructured settings by a trained volunteer—with that by patients in a self-selected no-treatment group. All patients had suffered a unilateral first CVA, and all were two to four weeks postonset at entry. Treated patients received three hours of treatment each week for one year. Results indicated that the combined treatment groups improved significantly more than the self-selected no-treatment group, both groups treated by speech pathologists improved significantly more than the self-selected no-treatment group, and improvement in the group treated by volunteers did not differ significantly from that in either group treated by speech pathologists or the self-selected no-treatment group.

The second Veterans Administration cooperative study (Wertz, Weiss et al., 1986) compared treatment in three groups of aphasic patients. Patients who met selection criteria, similar to those listed in Table 5-1, were assigned randomly to clinic treatment by a speech pathologist, 8 to 10 hours each week for 12 weeks, followed by 12 weeks of no treatment; home treatment by a trained volunteer, 8 to 10 hours each week for 12 weeks, followed by 12 weeks of no treatment; or deferred treatment for 12 weeks, followed by 12 weeks of treatment, 8 to 10 hours each week, by a speech pathologist. This design permitted answering the following questions: Is treatment by a speech pathologist efficacious? (comparison of the clinic group with the deferred group who received no treatment until 12 weeks after entry); Is home treatment by trained volunteers efficacious? (comparison of the home treatment group with the deferred treatment group at 12 weeks after entry); and Does deferring treatment for 12 weeks influence ultimate improvement? (comparison of the three groups at 24 weeks after entry, after the deferred group had received 12 weeks of treatment). Results indicated that treatment by a speech pathologist was efficacious. The clinic group displayed significantly more improvement at 12 weeks than the deferred group who had received no treatment. Home treatment was enigmatic. Improvement in home treatment patients did not differ significantly from that in the clinic or deferred groups at 12 weeks. And, delaying treatment had no effect on ultimate improvement. There were no significant differences among groups at 24 weeks after entry.

Poeck, Huber, and Willmes (1986) examined the effects of treatment on aphasic patients with "predominantly vascular etiology." Patients were grouped according to time postonset—early, between one and four months postonset; late, between four and seven months postonset; and chronic, over seven months postonset. All received two hours of treatment each day for six to eight weeks. Performance was measured before and after treatment, and improvement was corrected for "mean spontaneous recovery rates obtained in another study." Ninety-six percent of the early treatment group showed significant improvement, but this was reduced to 79 percent after the correction for spontaneous recovery was applied. Similarly, after correcting for spontaneous recovery, 56 percent of the late and 67 percent of the chronic groups showed significant improvement. The authors concluded that even in the chronic stage, aphasia improves under the influence of intensive speech therapy.

COMPARISON OF TREATMENTS

We have reviewed efforts that employed two types of designs. In one, a group of aphasic patients is selected, treated, and improvement or the lack of it is examined. In the other, at least two groups of patients are compared—treated patients with randomly assigned untreated patients or self-selected untreated patients. A third approach, comparison of one treatment with another, has been used. This was employed in the previously discussed comparison of individual and group treatment (Wertz, Collins et al., 1981) and included in the treatment and no-treatment studies by Shewan and Kertesz (1984) and Wertz, Weiss et al. (1986). Other examples exist.

Three efforts from the United Kingdom (David, Enderby, & Bainton, 1982, Meikle, Wechsler, Tupper, et al., 1979; Quinteros, Williams, White, & Pickering, 1984) conducted similar aphasia treatment trials that compared improvement in patients treated by speech pathologists with improvement in patients treated by volunteers. Amount of training and professional assistance to volunteers varied among the three studies, and patients' characteristics varied within and among studies as did the intensity and duration of treatment. The results, however, were remarkably similar. Patients in all three studies displayed significant improvement, and there were no significant differences between groups treated by speech pathologists and groups treated by volunteers. The lack of group differences, unfortunately, has been interpreted by some to indicate treatment for aphasia is not efficacious, and speech pathologists can be replaced by volunteers. Both assumptions are fallacious. First, a comparison of treatments, e.g., speech pathologists vs. volunteers, is not a test of treatment. The efficacy of treatment is tested by comparing it with no treatment. Patients in both groups in all three studies improved. The lack of a no-treatment group in any study does not permit determining whether either treatment, speech pathologist or volunteer, was efficacious. Second, the results do not support replacing speech pathologists with volunteers. In all studies, speech pathologists performed initial and final evaluations, provided information and some training to volunteers, and monitored the volunteers' activity during the treatment trial. Thus, volunteers worked under the direction of speech pathologists. This,

possibly, suggests an additional role for speech pathologists. For patients who live beyond traditional treatment's reach, who cannot afford frequent and protracted treatment, or who would not be treated by a speech pathologist for other reasons, a speech pathologist may consider serving as a consultant to the patient, family, and a volunteer and provide appraisal, diagnostic, and treatment planning and monitoring services rather than providing traditional face-to-face treatment. Before assuming this role, we would be comforted by evidence that demonstrates treatment for aphasia by trained volunteers is efficacious. The two efforts that have compared volunteer treatment with no treatment (Shewan and Kertesz, 1984; Wertz et al., 1986) have shown no significant differences between treatment by volunteers and no treatment.

Another, recent comparison of treatments investigation was conducted by Hartman and Landau (1987). Aphasic patients who met selection criteria were assigned to either conventional language treatment by a speech pathologist, two visits a week for six months, or patient and family counseling by a speech pathologist, two visits a week for six months. Patients in both groups improved, and there was no significant difference in improvement between groups. Unfortunately, the authors concluded that their results indicate conventional treatment is ineffective. This, of course, is incorrect, because again a comparison of treatments is not a test of treatment. All Hartman and Landau demonstrated was that the two managements do not differ. The absence of a no-treatment group prevents them from declaring whether either management is or is not effective.

CONCLUSIONS

What are we to conclude about the value of language treatment for aphasia from the variety of positive and negative results collected in investigations that studied a variety of patients with a variety of treatments for a variety of durations? Well, we can conclude that the answer to the question of whether therapy works varies. But, we would like something more definitive.

Those who have provided conclusions also vary. Darley (1979), for example, reviewed the evidence and concluded, "We do not depend on sentiment or intuition in declaring that aphasia therapy works. It works so well that every neurologist, physiatrist, and speech-language pathologist responsible for patient management should refuse to accede to a plan that abandons the patient to neglect" (p. 629). Benson (1979b) agreed. David (1983), however, also reviewed the evidence and concluded, "In spite of the volume of research which has been undertaken, our understanding of the effects of treatment on acquired aphasia is still incomplete (p. 23)." And Siegel (1987) contended that the question "Does therapy work?" is not a proper question for research.

So, have we been marching in marmalade; working hard but getting nowhere? Perhaps, especially if one seeks the definitive answer, positive or negative, in a single definitive study. That study has not been and is not likely to be done. Inquiry is more likely to find an answer if we rephrase the question: Whom does aphasia treatment help? This permits examining results of treatment studies, filtering them through controlled and uncontrolled variables, and arriving at specific patient characteristics and treatment conditions that predict a positive or negative outcome. So, what do we know?

The evidence (Basso et al., 1979; Hagen, 1973; Shewan & Kertesz, 1984; Wertz, Collins et al., 1981; 1986) suggests that patients who are aphasic subsequent to a single occlusive infarct, moderately to mildly severe, and less than six months postonset are good treatment candidates. They will benefit from language treatment if it is provided at least three hours a week for at least five months (Basso et al., 1979); three hours a week for 12 months (Shewan & Kertesz, 1984); eight hours a week for 11 months (Wertz, Collins et al., 1981); 8 to 10 hours a week for three months (Wertz et al., 1986); or 18 hours a week for 12 months (Hagen, 1973). Conversely, patients who suffer single or multiple unilateral or bilateral strokes do not benefit from 48 hours of treatment or

less during a 24 week period (Lincoln et al., 1984). Similarly, chronic, severely aphasic patients do not benefit from 7 to 46 hours of treatment during a 4 to 36 week period (Sarno, Silverman, and Sands, 1970).

Listing what we know also identifies what we do not know. Rosenbek (1983) observed that clinical researchers need not fear all of the questions have been answered. Those that remain encompass how much, of what, for whom, and when. The answers will come one slog-step to the next, the only way we have ever known to get a thing done. We wish we were older and wiser guessers, able to come on some angle of insight that would declare: Here, these are the answers. We are not. In the meantime, those of us who treat aphasic patients can utilize the evidence at hand to select appropriate treatment candidates. And, we can see how malleable aphasic behavior is by probing what we do not know with single-subject treatment designs.

SINGLE-SUBJECT DESIGNS

Case reports on aphasic patients have been and continue to be numerous. Broca's (1861) was a pioneer. But, those that mentioned treatment and its influence on improvement were not very precise and confined their empirical evidence to adjectives. Like Broca's (1865), many case reports implied that intensive and protracted treatment would or did effect considerable change in the aphasic patient's condition. Readers admired these authors' efforts and assumed their honesty, but we lacked the comfort data provide to document a verbal description of deeds.

LaPointe's (1977a) Base-10 system, shown in Figure 5-1, was a long first step toward demonstrating and documenting a treatment's influence on an individual aphasic patient's performance. It required specification of the task (e.g., verbal sentence completion from auditory stimuli), setting criterion performance (e.g., 90 percent correct in three consecutive sessions), stating the scoring system (e.g., plus or minus), and describing the treatment method (e.g., the clinician says "Finish the

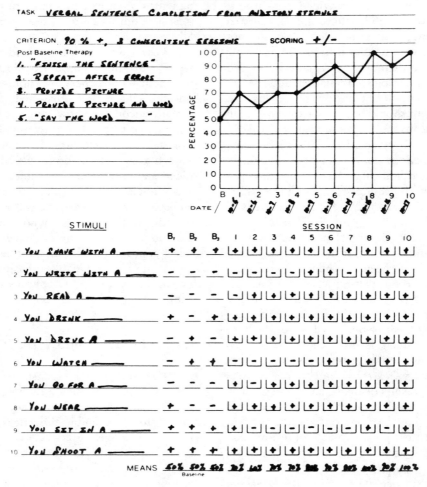

BASE-10 RESPONSE FORM

PROGRAMMED SPEECH-LANGUAGE STIMULATION

TASK _VERBAL SENTENCE COMPLETION FROM AUDITORY STIMULI_

CRITERION _90 % +, 3 CONSECUTIVE SESSIONS_   SCORING _+/-_

Post Baseline Therapy
1. _"FINISH THE SENTENCE"_
2. _REPEAT AFTER ERRORS_
3. _PROVIDE PICTURE_
4. _PROVIDE PICTURE AND WORD_
5. _"SAY THE WORD ____"_

Figure 5-1. Patient performance on a Base-10 treatment task designed to improve verbal sentence completion. From LaPointe, L.L. (1977). Base-10 programmed stimulation: Task specification, scoring and plotting performance in aphasia therapy. *Journal of Speech and Hearing Disorders, 42,* 90–105. Reprinted with permission from PRO-ED.

sentence, You shave with a ____." if the patient makes an error, the stimulus is repeated; if the error persists, the clinician presents a picture of the desired response; if still incorrect, a picture and the printed word are provided, and, finally, if necessary, the clinician has the patient repeat the desired response, "Say razor"). Ten stimuli are selected, and pretreatment performance is collected for a baseline. This is followed by 10 treatment sessions or

until the patient reaches criterion performance. Any error is scored wrong and followed by as many of the treatment steps as necessary to evoke a correct response. Soon, aphasia clinicians began documenting their deeds with data provided by the Base-10 system, and the results of these efforts began appearing in print (Czvik, 1976; Marshall & Holtzapple, 1976).

Introduction of the Base-10 system also opened the world of single-subject experimental designs to many who treated aphasic patients. We began to discover powerful methodologies previously hidden in psychology and related disciplines (Hersen & Barlow, 1976; Sidman, 1960). And eventually McReynolds and Kearns (1983) elaborated the potential of single-subject experimental designs for managing communication disorders. Aphasia clinicians seized this tool and began to document the results of their efforts (Davis, 1978; LaPointe, 1979b; Rosenbek, Green, Flynn, Wertz, & Collins, 1977). Currently, clinicians have and use a variety of single-subject designs to answer a variety of questions about the influence of a specified treatment on a specific patient We applaud this advance, and we urge all aphasia clinicians to employ single-subject designs to find out whether what they are doing does any good.

GROUP VERSUS SINGLE-SUBJECT DESIGNS

Again, neither design for determining the efficacy of aphasia treatment, group or single subject, is better than the other. They are different, and some of these differences are listed in Table 5-2.

How many aphasic patients do you need to treat to find out whether treatment works? The answer for a single subject is easy. You need one, the patient being treated, to determine whether treatment helps him or her. For a group design, the answer is more difficult, and we tend to forget it is. Too often one reads, "Fifteen aphasic patients were compared with 15 nonaphasic adults with no history of brain damage." Why 15? Usually, it is because 15 were available, or there was only time to study 15, or 15 is all the budget would allow. The answer to how many patients one needs in a group treatment study is enough—but not too many. More precision comes if one can specify power and effect size. Power is defined as $1-\beta$, where β is the probability of failing to find the specified difference to be statistically significant. Power is a practical control over the Type II error; for example, failing to declare two groups are different when, in fact, they are (Fleiss, 1981). A power of .80 is, typically, the minimum acceptable (Kirk, 1982). Effect size (Cohen, 1969) involves specifying the difference

TABLE 5-2.
Comparison of Single-Subject and Group Designs for Studying the Efficacy of Treatment for Aphasia.

Single Subject	Group
Minimum number of subjects necessary is one	Minimum number of subjects depends on selected effect size and statistical power
Provides data on the "typical" behavior of a single subject	Provides data on the behavior of a "typical" member of a group
Not necessary to assume subjects respond similarly to an experimental condition	Necessary to assume subjects respond similarly to an experimental condition
Subjects must be run more than once in each experimental condition	Not necessary for subjects to be run more than once in each experimental condition
Can generalize to the "typical" behavior of the subject studied	Can generalize to the "typical" behavior of the mean or median group member studied
Difficult to control for order and sequence effects	Relatively easy to control for order and sequence effects
Statistical procedures for assessing the reliability of results are not well developed	Statistical procedures for assessing the reliability of results are well developed
Can generalize to the population from which the subjects are selected on a logical basis	Can generalize to the population from which the subjects are selected on a statistical basis

Adapted from Silverman (1977); Wertz and Rosenbek (1978).

one wants to detect. For example, clinical experience may tell us a 15 percentile difference on the Porch Index of Communicative Ability (PICA) (Porch, 1967) is a meaningful difference in an aphasic patient's language ability. A patient who is 15 percentile units or more higher on the PICA understands, reads, talks, and writes noticeably better than a patient who is 15 percentile units lower. If the difference is any smaller, we could not differentiate between patients. So, in this example, if we compared treated patients with untreated patients, we would want to see the treated group perform 15 percentile units better on the PICA after treatment to conclude treatment resulted in a meaningful clinical change compared with no treatment. Armed with these two figures, power and effect size, one can utilize formulas (Fleiss, 1981; Kirk, 1982) to determine how many subjects are necessary to achieve a specified power and effect size. Moreover, it becomes clear why there is more single-subject research in aphasia than there is acceptable group research.

A single-subject design tells us about the "typical" behavior of the patient being treated. He or she is observed over several sessions, and his or her typical performance is recorded. It is not necessary to assume that other patients would respond similarly to the treatment, because we are interested in only one patient, the one being treated. Conversely, a group design tells us about the behavior of the "typical" group member being treated. Thus, it is necessary to assume that all patients in the group respond similarly to the treatment. This, of course, is the assumption that is frequently violated and appropriately criticized (Howard, 1986). Because, as noted earlier, aphasic patients differ in a number of characteristics that may influence their response to treatment, it is more likely they will respond differently to the treatment. Group studies can combat this problem in three ways. First, rigid selection criteria are employed to make the group more homogeneous. Second, the treatment protocol can permit tailoring the general treatment to fit each individual member of the group. Third, the statistical analysis of results (e.g., analysis

of covariance) can equate group members on certain variables (e.g., initial severity, time postonset). In addition, measures of variability (e.g., standard deviation, range) indicate how "typical" are the results.

Because one looks for a patient's "typical" behavior in a single-subject design, it is necessary to observe his or her behavior on several occasions. As will be discussed later, single-subject treatment designs employ a "baseline" phase before treatment is initiated, a treatment phase when the patient is being treated, and a withdrawal phase after the treatment has been stopped. Several observations are made in each of these phases to determine what is "typical" for the patient being studied. Group designs do not require these multiple observations. Typically, a group design obtains a pretreatment measure on all patients who will be treated and a posttreatment measure for comparison with pretreatment performance. In longer group treatment studies, several periodic measures may be collected at specific points in time during the treatment trial to determine whether and how much improvement occurred when.

A single-subject design permits one to generalize results to the typical behavior of the patient that was studied. Comparison of performance pre-, during, and posttreatment can be considered typical for the patient within the condition he or she was observed. In a group study, performance by patients is pooled. Thus, one can generalize to the "typical" behavior of the mean or median member of the group.

It is difficult, if not impossible, to control for order or sequence effects in a single-subject treatment design. With one patient, one cannot determine how what came first affected performance on what came second. Thus, all single-subject designs are confounded, somewhat, by order, sequence, and time. Conversely, a group study can control for order and sequence effects by counterbalancing—random assignment of patients in the group to different orders or sequences.

There are few statistical tools to assess the reliability of results in single-subject treatment designs. Kitselman, Deal, and Wertz (1981) have discussed why analysis of variance models and time-series analysis are either inappropriate or too cumbersome. Revusky (1967) has proposed the R_n statistic, but it is only appropriate for analyzing results of a multiple baseline design. Statistical procedures abound for analyzing the results of group treatment studies for example, analysis of variance and analysis of covariance. Again, however, acceptable group treatment studies are those that state effect size and power and include the appropriate number of patients to accomplish each.

Finally, a single-subject treatment design indicates the influence of a specified treatment on the specific patient that was treated at a specific point in time. Generalization of the results to other aphasic patients can only be done logically. For example, the same results may be obtained with other aphasic patients who display the same characteristics— etiology, severity, time postonset—as the patient that was treated. Group treatment results permit generalization to the aphasic population on a statistical basis. If a treated group displays significantly more improvement than an untreated group, then the results can be generalized to that portion of the aphasia population that would have met selection criteria for participation in the study.

Most of us spend more time seeing and treating individual aphasic patients than we spend conducting group treatment studies. Thus, we tend to conduct more single-subject designs. They are appropriate for what we do most often, developing and refining effective treatments. And, they answer our most immediate question—Is my treatment helping Mr. Homer Boomis, the aphasic patient I see at 9:00 A.M. on Monday, Wednesday, and Friday? So, we elaborate here various types of single-subject treatment designs and their practical application in the clinical management of aphasia.

THE DESIGNS

There is, unfortunately, a tendency to think that aphasia treatment is like a globe. You cannot go the wrong way if you travel far

enough. We, like many clinicians, have traveled through treatment with patients farther than we should. We have kept going without getting anywhere. We learned that if what you are doing is not doing any good, doing more of it is probably not an improvement. Our discovery of single-subject treatment design methodology provided direction, kept us from getting lost, and told us whether the trip was worth it. We wish we had found single-subject treatment designs earlier.

Some may pause when we suggest research criteria should guide and order aphasia treatment. We do not, because we have found single-subject designs prevent our treatment from becoming a pastiche. They tell us whether our results are notional or factual. Further, if we find a single-subject design indicates a specific treatment is effective with one patient, we are encouraged to apply the same approach with similar patients—a single case study with replications.

Use of single-subject designs in the daily management of aphasic patients requires knowing about the types and requirements of these designs. Most of what we know and use we have learned from Hersen and Barlow (1976) and McReynolds and Kearns (1983). Three popular designs—the withdrawal or design, the multiple baseline design, and the alternating treatments design—will be elaborated here. In addition, we will discuss two other less frequently used designs—the crossover design and the changing criterion design.

WITHDRAWAL OR ABA DESIGN

The withdrawal design comprises three basic components: one, a pretreatment or baseline period, called the A phase, where a patient's responses to specific stimuli are measured and plotted; two, a treatment period, called the B phase, where the patient is treated and responses are periodically tested and plotted; and three, a withdrawal period, called the A phase, where the treatment is withheld and the patient's ability to retain responses is tested and plotted. The number of measurements in the baseline (A), treatment

(B), and withdrawal (A) periods depends on the consistency of the patient's performance during baseline, whether and how performance changes during treatment, and whether and how rapidly performance deteriorates during withdrawal. Evidence of a treatment effect is indicated by better performance during treatment than in baseline and a drop or leveling off of performance during withdrawal.

An idealized ABA design is shown in Figure 5-2. For purposes of illustration, we display something that seldom happens in clinical practice—a flat baseline, abrupt and marked improvement during treatment, and immediate and continued sag in performance during withdrawal. We also omitted what happens after withdrawal. Each component requires discussion.

First, one attempts to establish a stable or predictable baseline. If pretreatment performance continues to improve, it is difficult to demonstrate intervention with treatment is the cause of continued improvement. Thus, one attempts to establish a flat, deteriorating, or minimally variable baseline. At least three baseline measures are necessary to do this. If performance continues to improve or varies markedly across these three measures, one continues baseline testing until improvement stops or variability is minimal. If neither occurs after about six baseline measures, we select a more difficult behavior to baseline, or we seek the source of the variability—learning as a result of repeated testing, inappropriate stimuli, influences outside the baseline session, inconsistency in our behavior, etc. To demonstrate a credible treatment effect, one must establish a predictable or stable baseline.

Second, after an acceptable baseline has been established, treatment begins. How long treatment continues and how improvement or the lack of it is measured depends on the treatment task. If the desired performance is only slightly more difficult than what the patient can do without treatment, we expect immediate improvement, and treatment sessions are few. Conversely, if the desired performance is markedly different from what the patient can do, more treatment sessions are necessary. Further, the selected criterion performance, for example, 90 percent correct in three consecutive sessions, will influence the length of the treatment period. The patient who attains criterion in the first three treatment sessions is placed in withdrawal. The patient who is climbing steadily toward criterion or hovers around it receives a few more sessions. The patient who does not improve or whose performance is extremely variable across sessions is troublesome. The clinician must determine why the treatment is not boosting performance or seek the source of the variability. Typically, 10 to 15 treatment sessions is the maximum necessary to reach criterion or to decide it is time for a change.

Testing during the treatment phase is done by periodic probes or a criterion run. Probe testing requires inserting or specifying stimuli within the corpus of treatment stimuli. The patient's responses to probe stimuli are

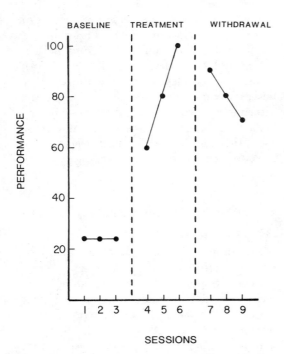

Figure 5-2. Idealized ABA design, showing a flat baseline, improved performance during treatment, and a drop in performance during withdrawal.

calculated, and the result is plotted as the data point for that treatment session. A criterion run is similar to baseline testing. Before or after the treatment session, the patient is tested with a specific set of stimuli and performance is plotted. When testing is done depends on the question to be answered. Testing at the beginning.of a session looks at retention from the previous session. Testing at the end of a session evaluates learning resulting from that session. Regardless of the schedule selected, it should be consistent throughout the treatment phase. Whenever possible, we attempt to make testing unobtrusive. And, we always specify and maintain consistency in who does the testing and under what conditions.

Third, withdrawal, the second A phase, begins after the patient has reached criterion performance or when the clinician decides the treatment has accomplished as much as it can. Approximately three data points are collected during withdrawal. Typically, the patient is tested during withdrawal the same way he or she was tested during baseline. Withdrawal indicates whether the patient retains what was achieved during treatment. Purists insist performance must deteriorate or plateau during withdrawal or one cannot conclude the treatment has helped. This is a reasonable approach if one is testing the efficacy of a medication. Performance is measured during baseline, the medication is administered during the treatment phase, and the patient is taken off the drug during withdrawal. Unless the medication "cured" what the patient suffers, we must see a sag in performance to know that the medication helped during treatment. Treatment of language deficits is not so transparent. Most clinicians want and expect treated behaviors to improve and remain improved even after the treatment ends. A slight sag in performance during withdrawal is acceptable. An abrupt dive to pretreatment baseline performance is unexpected. What happens during withdrawal indicates what one does next.

Fourth, an ABA design may end after withdrawal, more of the same treatment may be administered, or a modified treatment for the same behavior may be elected. If performance during withdrawal continues at treatment levels or does not sag below criterion performance, the clinician may select a more difficult treatment task to push performance further. This requires a new ABA design. If performance improved during treatment but dropped markedly, below criterion, during withdrawal, more of the same treatment is usually selected. This yields an ABAB—baseline, treatment, withdrawal, treatment—design. And, to check retention after the second treatment phase, a second withdrawal is added to yield an ABABA design. If the treatment did not accomplish what was desired, the clinician may change it after withdrawal. Thus, we have an ABACA—baseline, treatment, withdrawal, different or modified treatment, withdrawal—design. Simmon's (1980) use of an A-B-BC-B-BC-A design with a blind patient who suffered aphasia and apraxia of speech illustrates the unlimited creativity possible in single-subject design treatment.

The ABA design, basic or with modifications, is not sterile or stilted or just "research." It is a systematic means for managing aphasic patients. It can tell us what a patient can do, baseline; whether what we do helps, treatment phase; whether what we did is retained by the patient, withdrawal; whether more of the same is needed, second treatment or B phase; whether we should try something else, a different treatment or C phase; or whether we should move on to a more difficult or different task, a new ABA design. It is efficient, all phases are relatively short, and, for chronic patients, it can provide a strong statement about our treatment's efficacy or the lack of it.

Clinical considerations may confound the purity of an ABA design. For example, adding a second B phase to an ABA design creates an interaction between the type of treatment administered and time. Was the second B phase more effective than the first B phase because it increased the amount of treatment administered, or was it more effective because it was offered at a specific point in time; later than the first B phase? More confounding is the ABACA design. This creates a multiple treatment interaction as well as an interaction with time. For example, the C phase cannot be compared with the previous B phase. We do not know whether C treatment was more effective than B treatment because it was a different treatment, or because it was offered at a different point in time, or whether it was just additional treatment. Hersen and Barlow (1976) suggested avoiding an ABCA or ABACA design. We do too if the purpose is research. Nevertheless, we have employed these designs with patients in our clinics. When we do, we remind ourselves of their limitations.

Figure 5-3 shows the results of an ABA design with J. D., a 52-year-old gentleman who had suffered a single, left hemisphere thrombotic infarct. He was seen as an outpatient at 13 months postonset. Overall PICA performance was at the 81st percentile, his WAB Aphasia Quotient was 87, and he was classified as displaying anomic aphasia. J. D. was plagued by word-finding problems, and he was eager to improve these. PICA verbal Subtests showed Subtests I and IX, sentence

formulation and sentence completion, were substantially superior to subtest IV, confrontation naming. So, we developed an ABA design to determine whether his stating the function of the word that eluded him might evoke its name. His ability to name 50 pictures was baselined in three sessions. Performance was scored with the PICA multidimensional scale. Treatment was administered in one-hour sessions three days a week. Each of the pictures was presented in a confrontation naming task, "Tell me the name of this." An error was followed by as many of the following steps as necessary: (1) "Tell me what you do with it, and then tell me the name"; (2) "Finish the sentence, You (clinician provides the function) with a _____"; (3) "I'll say the name and you say it after me, say _____." All 50 pictures were presented again at the end of each treatment session as a criterion run. This consisted of a repeat of baseline, confrontation naming of the 50 stimuli. Criterion performance was set at a mean score of 13 on the PICA scale in three consecutive sessions.

Figure 5-3 indicates a fairly stable baseline, a mean around 10.5 in the three sessions. Performance during treatment shows gradual improvement across sessions and criterion performance after 12 treatment sessions. Withdrawal indicates a slight sag in performance in two of three sessions, but J. D. remained at criterion. Posttreatment Overall PICA performance was at the 87th percentile, and his WAB AQ was 91. J. D. was incorporating the strategy, using function to cue retrieval of names, in his conversation. Thus, we elected to move on to another, similar treatment task, use of the strategy in picture description, rather than enter a second treatment (B) phase. In this chronic aphasic patient, improved naming ability appeared to result from the treatment administered.

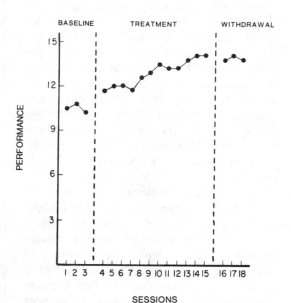

Figure 5-3. Results of a single subject ABA treatment design for improving naming in an aphasic patient.

MULTIPLE BASELINE DESIGN

The multiple baseline design is similar to the ABA or withdrawal design in that it employs an A, baseline, phase and a B, treatment, phase and can employ a second A, withdrawal, phase. But, the multiple baseline design examines performance on a number of target behaviors, whereas the ABA design examines performance on one target behavior. An idealized multiple baseline design is shown in Figure 5-4.

Two or more target behaviors are selected each is baselined. Then, one behavior is treated, and the other or others continue in the baseline condition. All behaviors, treated and untreated, are tested, systematically, and performance is compared. Improvement on the treated behavior and a lack of or less improvement on the untreated behavior or behaviors implies a treatment effect; what is treated improves and what is not treated does not improve. In addition, treatment is systematically introduced for each behavior in the design. If each behavior remains stable during baseline and improves only when it is treated, the multiple baseline design provides evidence that improvement results from treatment.

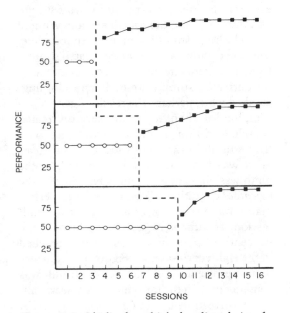

Figure 5-4. Idealized multiple baseline design for three behaviors. Baseline performance is represented by the circles to the left of the dividing line and response to treatment is represented by the squares to the right of the dividing line. Note that performance does not improve on a behavior until it is treated.

For example, four lists of equally difficult printed words may be selected as stimuli. An aphasic patient's ability to read aloud each word in each list is baselined. Then List 1 is treated, and Lists 2 through 4 are not treated. Improvement on List 1 and no improvement on Lists 2 through 4 indicate a treatment effect. Systematically, treatment is introduced on Lists 2 through 4. Again, improvement on each list only after it is treated and no improvement on a list until it is treated implies treatment effects.

Multiple baseline designs provide an advantage over ABA designs if treatment is initiated early after onset of aphasia, because an ABA design will not demonstrate whether improvement results from the treatment administered, spontaneous recovery, or both. A multiple baseline design's ability to compare treated and untreated behaviors frequently permits showing a treatment effect during the period of spontaneous recovery. For example, if three similar behaviors are selected, one is treated, the other two are followed in baseline, and only the treated behavior improves, we have evidence of a treatment effect. If improvement resulted only from spontaneous recovery, we would expect all three behaviors to improve. Warren, Gabriel, Johnston, and Gaddie (1987) have demonstrated the effective use of multiple baseline designs to demonstrate treatment's efficacy with acutely aphasic patients.

A disadvantage in multiple baseline designs is generalization. Treating one behavior may cause other, untreated, behaviors to improve, because the treatment effects are generalizing across stimuli or behaviors. However, this can be reduced by selecting dissimilar targets or some that are significantly more difficult. Nevertheless, we have a clinical conundrum, because we seek generalization. Who has time to treat every word or behavior an aphasic patient needs? But, generalization of improvement to untreated stimuli or behavior dilutes proof of therapeutic effectiveness. Typically, we seek a balance in our selection of targets for multiple baseline designs. The right amount of dissimilarity and difficulty among targets will permit us to detect generalization by an increasing slope in the untreated behaviors' baseline, but this slope is vividly less than the change that results from introducing treatment.

Figure 5-5 shows a multiple baseline design for W. M., a 65-year-old man who was three years postonset from a left hemisphere CVA suffered during carotid artery surgery. He was severely aphasic, 19th percentile overall on the PICA and a WAB AQ of 45. He profiled as Broca's aphasia, but severe auditory comprehension deficits almost dropped him into the upper range of global aphasia. W. M.'s wife reported he "had some speech therapy, but he was too confused to benefit from it." This congenial, retired electrician convinced us he was ready to try again at this late date.

A multiple baseline design was used to see if we could budge his impaired auditory comprehension. Single word comprehension was 32 percent correct. Thirty pictures—10 fruits, 10 animals, and ten items of clothing—comprised the stimuli for a single word comprehension task. Each set was baselined in a matrix of 10 on a "point to the _____"

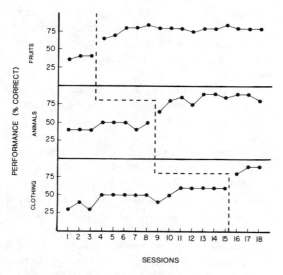

Figure 5-5. Results of a single subject multiple baseline design for improving auditory comprehension in an aphasic patient.

task. Treatment in one-hour sessions, three days a week began with fruits. Animals and clothing remained in untreated baseline conditions. The treatment consisted of four steps on each picture, if necessary: (1) "Point to the _____." (2) if an error was made, the request was repeated. (3) If the error persisted, W. M. was instructed, "Look at each picture. Which one is the _____?" (4) If his response was still incorrect, he was shown the correct picture and asked to point to it. Criterion performance was set at 80 percent correct in three consecutive sessions. When criterion was reached on the first set of stimuli, fruits, we began treating the second set of stimuli, animals. Clothing stimuli were introduced after criterion was reached on animal stimuli. The data points in the treatment phase represent the percent correct responses to step (1) commands, "Point to the _____."

Baseline performance in three sessions was fairly stable; 30 to 40 percent correct, on each set of stimuli. Treatment for fruit stimuli was introduced in the fourth session. Animal and clothing stimuli remained in baseline. Immediate improvement on the treated stimuli, fruit, indicated a treatment effect. Performance on untreated stimuli, animals and clothing, climbed a bit, perhaps the result of generalization, but less than the change seen on treated stimuli. Criterion performance was reached on fruit stimuli in the eighth session, and treatment was initiated on animal stimuli in the ninth session. Clothing stimuli remained in the baseline condition. When criterion performance was attained on animals in the fifteenth session, treatment began on clothing in the sixteenth session, and criterion was reached in the eighteenth session. Figure 5-5 indicates that improvement on each set of stimuli was consequent with the introduction of treatment.

Posttreatment testing with the PICA showed Overall performance at the twenty-ninth percentile, and a WAB AQ of 55. PICA auditory subtests, VI and X, had improved by 20 percentile units, and the WAB Auditory Word Recognition subtest had improved 38 percent. Thus, the auditory comprehension treatment administered appeared to do what it was designed to do. And, the multiple baseline design indicated improvement could be attributed to treatment and not spontaneous recovery occurring at three years postonset.

ALTERNATING TREATMENTS DESIGN

For some aphasic behaviors, we have no effective treatment. For other aphasic behaviors, there may be several effective treatments. For the former, we seek what is not available. For the latter, we seek that which is most effective. The alternating treatments design (Barlow & Hayes, 1979; McReynolds & Kearns, 1983) is a means for determining which of two or more treatments is most effective. For example, an aphasic patient who has difficulty in confrontation naming could be treated with an auditory program—a picture is presented, the clinician says the name, and the patient repeats it; or a reading program—a picture is presented, the printed name is presented, and the patient reads it. These different treatments are presented in different sessions, and performance is measured in or after each session. The results are compared as in the idealized example in Figure 5-6.

As in the ABA and multiple baseline designs, performance is measured pretreatment in a baseline condition. In our example, shown in Figure 5-6, baseline performance is similar for both conditions, auditory and reading. During the alternating treatments phase, treatment 1, auditory, is conducted randomly in sessions 4, 7, 9, 10, and 13. Treatment 2, reading, is conducted in sessions 5, 6, 8, 11, and 12. The idealized results indicate that treatment 1 is clearly more effective than treatment 2. When this was established, an application phase (McReynolds & Kearns, 1983) was conducted to demonstrate continuation of treatment 1 resulted in continued or improved performance.

Alternating treatment designs, based on their appearance in the literature, are less

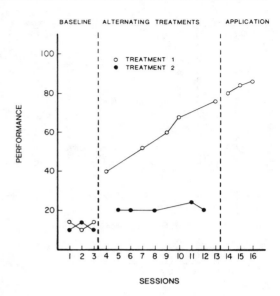

Figure 5-6. Idealized alternating treatments design comparing the effectiveness of two different treatments. Treatment one is clearly superior to treatment two.

popular than ABA and multiple baseline designs. Their value is in allowing the patient to demonstrate by his or her behavior which of the potential treatments available is most effective. Their limitation is that generalization from one treatment to another may make interpreting results difficult. This can be controlled, somewhat, by counterbalancing when different treatments are presented, who presents them, and even the stimuli presented in each treatment. Rubow, Rosenbek, Collins, and Longstreth (1982) reported an alternating treatments design that compared simple imitation treatment with imitation and vibrotactile stimulation treatment for a patient suffering apraxia of speech. Loverso, Prescott, Selinger, Wheeler, and Smith (1985) compared clinician treatment with computer treatment using an alternating treatments design with an aphasic patient.

Figure 5-7 shows the results of an alternating treatments design with D. M., a 37 year old man who suffered a left hemisphere thromboembolic infarct slightly less than one month

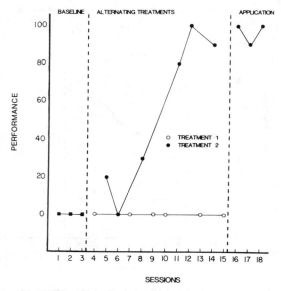

Figure 5-7. Results of a single subject alternating treatments design for obtaining voice in a case of apraxia of phonation. Treatment 2, manual pressure on the larynx, was clearly superior to treatment 1, electrolarynx stimulation.

prior to evaluation. Overall PICA performance was at the thirty-seventh percentile, and his WAB AQ was 16.6. In addition to a severe Broca's aphasia, D. M. displayed severe apraxia of speech and an apraxia of phonation. Otolaryngology reported no involvement of his vocal folds, and this was supported by normal, nonvolitional coughing, throat clearing, and phonation during laughter. The tried and true method for obtaining voice in cases of apraxia of phonation—quick, forceful pressure on the diaphragm during exhalation—achieved nothing but a sore stomach. We demonstrated D. M. could produce an acceptable whispered /ɑ/. Our task was to obtain phonation.

We placed D. M. in an alternating treatments design. Treatment 1 employed an electrolarynx during requests to add voice to his /ɑ/, and treatment 2 consisted of our placing manual pressure in the notch of the thyroid cartilage during his attempts to produce /ɑ/. These treatments used 15 minutes of each of two daily one-hour sessions, one in the

morning and one in the afternoon. The remainder of each session was devoted to treatment for auditory comprehension, reading, and writing deficits.

Three sessions, each composed of 20 attempts to produce /ɑ/, were collected as a baseline. All treatments were administered by the same clinician during the alternating treatments phase. Presentation of treatment 1, electrolarynx, and treatment 2, manual pressure, was counterbalanced across morning and afternoon sessions. Treatment consisted of 50 requests to produce /ɑ/ during the application of the specified treatment. This was followed by 20 attempts to produce /ɑ/ with no intervention, as in baseline. The percentage of correctly phonated productions in the 20 attempts comprised the data point for a given session. Criterion was set at 80 percent correct in three successive sessions for either treatment.

Figure 5-7 shows no phonated productions of /ɑ/ during baseline. Six sessions with treatment 1, electrolarynx stimulation, were effete. Conversely, six sessions with treatment 2, manual pressure, after a shakey start, resulted in rapid acquisition of phonation during /ɑ/. Criterion was reached, and treatment 2 was continued for three sessions in an application phase. Continued performance at or above criterion supported our faith in treatment 2.

Posttreatment testing with the PICA showed D. M.'s Overall performance was at the forty-fifth percentile, and his WAB AQ was 28. Obviously, we had the advantage of a co-clinician, spontaneous recovery, for this patient who was treated at one month postonset. Thus, the gains in PICA and WAB performance must, in part, be shared. The reacquisition of phonation, however, seemed to result from the treatment administered. Of course, one could argue that spontaneous recovery has an affinity for manual pressure and shuns electrolarynx stimulation. But we would not.

CROSSOVER DESIGN

The crossover design (Coltheart, 1983; Howard, 1986; Howard, Patterson, Franklin, Orchard-Lisler, & Morton, 1985; LaPointe,

1984) is similar to a multiple baseline design. Performance on two behaviors or two sets of stimuli is assessed in baseline before treatment. Then, one behavior or one set of stimuli is treated and the other behavior or set of stimuli is not treated and remains in the baseline condition. After a period of treatment for the first behavior or set of stimuli, treatment is stopped, and treatment for the other behavior or set of stimuli is initiated. The first behavior or set of stimuli is now placed in the untreated phase and is assessed periodically, as in baseline, while the second behavior or set of stimuli is treated. Thus, there has been a crossover—what was treated is now untreated, and what was untreated is now treated. Figure 5-8 shows an idealized crossover design.

As shown in Figure 5-8, two behaviors, for example, behavior A, naming pictures, and behavior B, writing the names of pictures, are tested in baseline, sessions 1 through 3. Then, treatment is administered for behavior A, naming pictures, in sessions 4 through 13. Behavior B, writing the names of pictures, continues in baseline and is not treated. Behavior A improves rapidly across sessions, and behavior B shows much less improvement. In session 14, the crossover occurs. Behavior B is now treated in sessions 14 through 23, and behavior A is no longer treated. In the example, behavior B improves during treatment, and behavior A remains unchanged. Thus, there are, essentially, two treatment effects. Both behaviors improve but only when treated.

Howard (1986) pointed out two problems that may occur with crossover designs. First, if only one behavior or set of stimuli improves, it is difficult to conclude there was a treatment effect. It is possible that spontaneous recovery was active during the period of improvement for the one behavior and not active during the period of treatment for the other. Further, the problem could lie in the methodology. For example, the means for measuring improvement were appropriate for one behavior but not for the other, or the behaviors were too dissimilar, or one set of stimuli was easier than the other, etc. Second, if the results indicate improvement in the untreated behavior, claiming a treatment effect is questionable. If both behaviors, treated and untreated, improve, the source of improvement may be spontaneous recovery. Another possibility, of course, is that treatment for one behavior generalizes and results in improvement in the other, untreated behavior. These problems can be avoided by using crossover designs only with chronic aphasic patients who are well beyond the period of spontaneous recovery and by selecting behaviors for treatment that are sufficiently independent to prevent or limit generalization.

Figure 5-9 shows our use of a crossover design with D. L., a 52-year-old man who suffered a left hemisphere thromboembolic infarct four months prior to this treatment. His PICA Overall percentile was 71, and his WAB AQ was 77. He profiled as anomic aphasia, and his word-finding difficulty created constant angst. We attacked this in a crossover design using our modification of a method developed by LaPointe (1984). Forty pictures that D. L. could not name were tested in three baseline

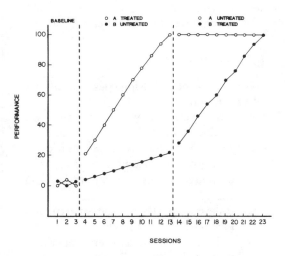

Figure 5-8. Idealized single subject crossover design. Initially, behavior A is treated and behavior B is not treated. In session 14, the crossover occurs; treatment is now administered for behavior B, and behavior A is now untreated. Note that each behavior improves only when it is treated.

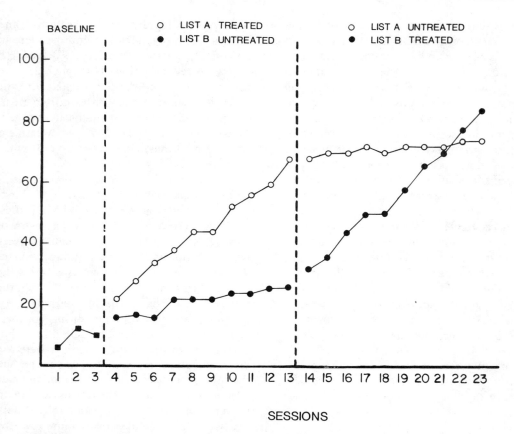

Figure 5-9. Results of a single subject crossover design for improving confrontation naming. List A, treated, improves, and List B, untreated, shows less improvement. After the crossover, List A, untreated, plateaus, and List B, treated, improves.

sessions. Then, the pictures were divided into two equally difficult lists, A and B, of 20 pictures each. List A was treated during sessions 4 through 13, and List B remained in an untreated, baseline condition. In sessions 14 through 23, treatment was given for List B, and List A was placed in an untreated, baseline condition.

The treatment package, adapted from LaPointe (1984), consisted of the following steps:

1. If D. L. named the picture correctly, knowledge of results—"That's right"—was given, and the next picture was presented.
2. If D. L. did not name the picture correctly,

as many of the following cues as necessary were presented:

A. The stimulus was repeated—"Try again. Tell me the name of this."
B. If the error persisted, a semantic cue was given by placing the stimulus in a sentence completion task—"You _____ with a _____."
C. If the error persisted, a phonemic cue was given—"Listen! It starts with a ____."
D. If D. L. continued to err, repetition was used—"I'll say it, and you say it after me. Say _____."

The data point for each treatment session represented the percent of correct responses at step one. Approximately 100 trials were run in each 45 minute treatment session. Baseline testing, confrontation naming, for the untreated list always followed treatment in each session.

As shown in Figure 5-9, D.L. made steady improvement on List A when it was treated. Less improvement occurred on the untreated stimuli, List B. The slight improvement that did occur on the untreated stimuli may indicate expected variability or a generalization of the treatment package. When crossover occurred in sessions 14 through 23, List A now untreated and List B treated, performance on List B began to climb and performance on List A stabilized. D. L.'s tendency to improve on treated stimuli and not on untreated stimuli makes us bold enough to claim a treatment effect. Posttreatment performance on the PICA showed an overall percentile of 89 and a WAB AQ of 86. Anomic aphasia persisted, but its severity was less.

CHANGING CRITERION DESIGN

The changing criterion design (Hartmann & Hall, 1976; McReynolds & Kearns, 1983) is similar to a multiple baseline design or a series of ABA designs. It is particularly appropriate for demonstrating the effectiveness of treatment in shaping a behavior. As shown in Figure 5-10, there are two primary phases; a baseline phase and a treatment phase. In the latter, the criterion for acceptable performance is changed, systematically, across sessions. For example, once a stable or predictable baseline is achieved, treatment is initiated, and a specific criterion performance is set. When the patient achieves that criterion, it is changed, and treatment continues until the new criterion is met. This procedure is continued until the ultimate criterion is met. Thus, each phase in the design provides a baseline for the next phase. If performance changes in the direction desired consequent with the change in the criterion, the treatment is efficacious.

As shown in the idealized changing criterion design in Figure 5-10, baseline

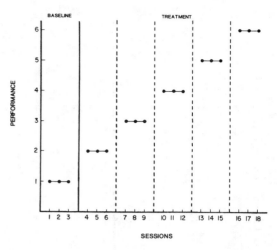

Figure 5-10. Idealized changing criterion design showing a systematic change in criterion performance during treatment.

performance is established for a behavior, for example, mean length of utterance in a picture description task. Then, a treatment package is initiated to shape the behavior, gradually, through five systematic changes in criterion performance. In the example, the initial criterion is a two-word mean length of utterance, and the criterion is changed, systematically, to achieve a six-word mean length of utterance. Rosenbek (1987) reported the successful use of this approach to increase the length of utterance in an aphasic patient.

Another example of the changing criterion design is shown in Figure 5-11. N. B. was a 59-year-old aphasic man who had suffered a single left hemisphere thromboembolic infarct. Six months of treatment and spontaneous recovery had evoked a marked improvement in his communicative ability. At eight months postonset, he performed at the eighty-ninth Overall percentile on the PICA, and his WAB AQ was 91. He profiled as displaying anomic aphasia. N. B.'s oral-expressive language was functional, but occasional word-finding problems resulted in a flurry of verbal intrusions that distracted him and his listeners, called attention to his errors, and eroded the

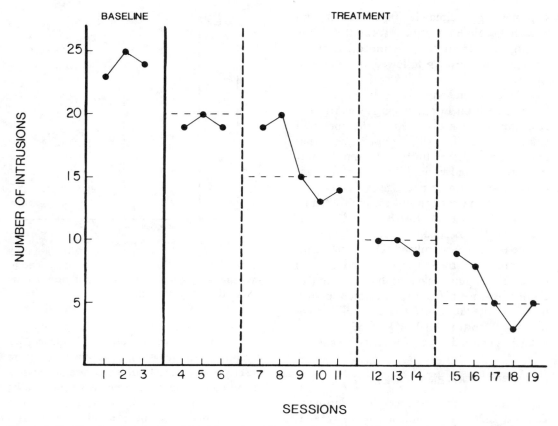

Figure 5-11. Results of a single subject changing criterion design for reducing verbal intrusions in picture description. The number of acceptable intrusions was systematically reduced by five after each preceding criterion had been met in three successive sessions.

performance he was capable of. For example, when he balked in his attempt to retrieve the word "sailboat," the result might be, "There's a boy, I don't know it's a boy, it might be, anyway, he is in a, what do you call it, I know what it is, that's what I keep telling you is the problem, you know what I mean, it's there, but I don't know when it, uh, what was I saying?" Thus, N. B. destroyed what he could do by what he did. And, we decided to see whether we could do something about it.

A changing criterion design was established to reduce the number of N. B.'s verbal intrusions that did not assist in word-finding. Forty pictures showing actions and situations were selected as stimuli. N. B. was asked, "Tell me what is happening in each picture." The

number of intrusions that did not convey the information requested were counted in each of three baseline sessions. He displayed 23 to 25 intrusions on the 40 pictures across the three sessions. In session four, treatment was initiated, and criterion performance was set at no more than 20 intrusions on the set of 40 pictures. Treatment consisted of explaining its purpose and initial criterion, stopping N. B. when an intrusion occurred, and having him use Helm's (1979) pacing board to produce a response without intrusions for the picture that evoked the intrusion. The pacing board appeared to have two influences. First, it slowed, focused, and directed his response. Second, he disliked using it and worked hard not to. Thus, we had his attention, and he was well aware of the desired behavior. The changing criterion was a gradual reduction in the number of intrusions, and three consecutive sessions at the specified criterion were required before the criterion was changed. Each data point in the design represented the number of intrusions on 40 pictures for a given session.

As shown in Figure 5-11, the initial criterion was reached in three sessions. Then, the criterion changed to no more than 15 intrusions on the set of 40 stimuli. Five sessions were required to meet the specified performance at this level. Next, the criterion was changed to no more than 10 intrusions. This was achieved in three sessions. Finally, the criterion was dropped to no more than five intrusions. N. B. achieved it in five sessions. Because he could meet the changing criterion performance by being mute—a fact he pointed out to us, we scored each response with the PICA multidimensional scale to monitor his overall verbal descriptions. PICA scores in baseline ranged from a mean of 9.5 to 11.9, essentially in the "corrected" range on the multidimensional scale. Across the four changes in criterion, mean PICA performance ranged from 11.1 to 13.4, "incomplete delayed" to "complete delayed." Thus, N. B. met each imposed criterion, and he showed a slight improvement in sentence formulation as measured by the PICA scale. Posttreatment performance on the PICA was at the 91st Overall percentile, and his WAB AQ was 92; essentially unchanged from pretreatment performance. Nevertheless, the amount of useless verbiage in his oral-expressive communication was dramatically reduced. He liked saying at least as much by saying less. And, we liked the evidence from the changing criterion design that indicated his intrusive verbalizations were gradually diminished by the treatment administered.

SUMMARY

We have not exhausted the types of single-subject designs available for evaluating treatment's influence on aphasic behavior. More importantly, we have been somewhat superficial in our explanations, applications, and cautions. For those who want more, they will find it in Hersen and Barlow (1976) and McReynolds and Kearns (1983). What we have attempted to demonstrate here is that single-subject treatment designs are good for the patients treated, and they are good for the clinicians who provide the treatment.

Most of us come to aphasia treatment armed with theory and principles. These tell us what we think we are doing. There is nothing more clinically practical than a good theory or a good principle. Both identify the most promising data to collect and how and when to collect them. Both are concerned with explaining, predicting, and changing behavior. Use of single-subject designs provides a means for testing theory and principles, for comparing what we think we are doing with what we are doing.

So, we urge the use of single-subject designs in the treatment of aphasic patients. They provide a balance for how much noticing is necessary—too much and you drive yourself around the bend, but too little and you miss the whole show. Perhaps you need to conduct a few single-subject designs to think them beautiful. But, to those who do, come moments of beauty unseen by the rest of the clinical world—stable baselines, controllable treatment effects. Soon, you become accustomed to these very beautiful sights, and then something comes along that just breaks all of the rules.

DOES TREATMENT WORK?

This chapter has attempted to discuss, not answer, the question of whether treatment works. For, the question cannot be answered unless it is preceded by "For whom." Too few controlled randomized trials have been conducted. Too much variability exists among aphasic patients for the answer to be provided in a single study. Thus, saying treatment works for aphasia is a solecism unless one specifies for whom it works.

Equipped with the evidence discussed in this chapter, the clinician can promise the efficacy of his or her efforts with patients who have suffered a single, left hemisphere throm-boembolic infarct; who are less than six months postonset; and who will receive at least three hours of treatment each week for at least six months. For other patients, the words are as difficult to formulate as the promises they are developed to express. For these patients, however, single-subject designs are available to determine quickly and accurately whether treatment will help. Most of all, we believe that clinical insouciance about the efficacy of our efforts is unacceptable. We do not know what we can accomplish until we do our best to find out. And, it is our privilege to do this thing until it is done.

6

PRINCIPLES IN
CLINICAL APHASIOLOGY

We learned our principles from others—other professionals and the aphasic men and women who have agreed over the years to spend time with us. We have learned the same things over and over from some, and unique things from a few. Like a code for living, the principles governing our daily activities with aphasic people have evolved, sometimes so subtly that they escape our notice until we sit down, as now, and take stock. The three of us do not believe all the same things, but our differences are not great. When we could not agree, we deleted. Not too much ended up in the wastepaper basket. All that did probably would not have helped anyhow.

CLINICAL APHASIOLOGY REQUIRES CLINICAL APHASIOLOGISTS

Part-time clinicians, if they are full-time clinical aphasiologists, can treat aphasic people. But simple caring is not enough. Intellect and a subscription to *Brain and Language* also are not enough. Nor is having earned one's 10 year pin or 10 ASHA-approved CEUs a year. Training in neurolinguistics is not enough nor is knowing how to run a successful private practice from a garage after working all day in the public schools. Aphasic people deserve the care of clinical aphasiologists.

Clinical aphasiologists care about aphasic people; they spend time with them everyday; they read, remember, and integrate what they read; they go to workshops to stay abreast; and they specialize in the understanding, diagnosis, and treatment of aphasia and aphasic people.

APHASIA TREATMENT HAS THREE GOALS

The goals of treatment are (1) to assist people to regain as much communication as their brain damage allows and their needs drive them to, (2) to help them learn how to compensate for residual deficits, and (3) to help them learn to live in harmony with the differences between the way they were and the way they are. The first two goals require skills that are a traditional part of all clinical training, and methods for meeting them are developed in a series of treatment chapters. The third goal requires subtler, less obvious skills, including knowing when education and counseling are necessary and when not to intrude. These skills are harder to acquire and they arrive—when they arrive at all—only after clinicians have accumulated experience with success and failure and after they have abandoned the folly of thinking they they must be all things to all people.

131

THE MOST IMPORTANT GOAL IS USUALLY TO PREPARE PATIENTS FOR A LIFETIME OF APHASIA

Aphasia nearly always continues long after both acute medical care and acute and chronic rehabilitation have ended. Some people have no or little trouble adjusting to their enduring aphasia even if they are never seen for treatment. Others never adjust, despite the clinician's best guidance. Some—probably a majority—adjust and are helped in that adjustment by things their clinicians do. What is it that clinicians do to prepare each patient for a lifetime of aphasia? They can begin by providing a realistic guess about the future, even if that future includes severe, persisting deficit. Most patients are not destroyed by a poor prognosis; they can be irrevocably harmed by unrealistic promises, however. Counseling about the value of life during and after treatment has ended may also help. Equally helpful is for the patient to know that treatment's goal is not normal communication but making the best use of what remains. Clinicians behave differently once they lay down the burden of normal as a goal; patients do too. Perhaps the most helpful thing a clinician can do, however, is keep the patient successful.

It is a harsh paradox that treatment may make a lifetime of aphasia harder to live with than does merely being discharged from the hospital after the acute illness has passed. The clinician, therefore, has to help the patient work to improve deficits without making those deficits seem unbearable. A moment of contemplation reveals the dilemma. Treatment's early portion is often characterized by an emphasis on exploiting what is good and improving what is impaired. Left untreated, people seem to avoid what they cannot do, they do not read, or watch TV, or socialize with friends; and they concentrate on what they can do—walk, bounce the grandkids on one knee, make breakfast. Enter treatment and they are asked to read, or listen, or talk. Only superhuman effort can prevent the connotation of "bad" from coming to cling to activities selected for improvement.

Knowing that superhuman effort is required by one's job makes it easier to get up in the morning and go to work. The result of that effort is usually a patient who looks forward to the sunrise also.

APHASIA TREATMENT SHOULD BE INFLUENCED BY ATTITUDES ABOUT WHAT APHASIA IS

We believe aphasia is a language disorder that, with few spectacular exceptions, crosses all modalities. We believe that both competence and performance are likely to be impaired. We believe that significantly different groups of syndromes of aphasia exist and that the differences have prognostic, counseling, and treatment significance. We believe that aphasia, of whatever type, is accompanied by other sequelae of brain damage such as perseveration and distractability that are influenced by and influence the aphasia. We believe aphasia is a human disorder that alters not only a person's language but also a person's life and relationship to others. We believe aphasia is often modifiable and that an appropriate therapy is one that takes into account all the deficits—linguistic, cognitive, behavioral, social, familial.

We do not believe that everyone else must agree with our view of aphasia or practice the methods consistent with it. Hegemony stultifies. We continue to learn from a variety of clinicians who have primarily linguistic orientations or cybernetic, modality, process, or behavioristic orientations. We do believe, on the other hand, that some view is essential. Atheoretical treatment does harm. Aphasic men and women have been asked to blow out candles and say words backwards. We suspect that such outlandish methods were foisted upon them by clinicians, perhaps even well-intentioned ones, who were more concerned with activities than with treatments and rationales. A theory, or concept, or view of what aphasia is keeps one from doing silly things, but only if the theory, concept, or view is not absurd. So although we would not defend one orientation, we would defend against all weak-minded ones.

ATTITUDES ABOUT APHASIA SHOULD BE INFLUENCED BY WHAT HAPPENS IN TREATMENT

We also believe that methods inconsistent with one's view of aphasia can be admitted into the treatment room. Attitudes, like certain recreational drugs, can sometimes distort one's view. Trying a method that "cannot possibly work," if done carefully, is appropriate and it might even work. If so, conceptual notions about aphasia will have been influenced. Aphasiology's underpinnings need influencing. They do so because too many of them have dropped from researchers' benches and too few from clinicians'. If one merely speculates about aphasia and forces a few aphasic speakers into a variety of experimental paradigms, any concept—and the more creative the better—becomes likely or even possible. Few things mold and temper creativity like spending several consecutive sessions with some aphasic person. Few things have such a felicitous influence on points of view.

APHASIA TREATMENT SHOULD BE INFLUENCED BY AN ATTITUDE ABOUT WHAT AN APHASIC PERSON IS

Aphasic persons do not talk at all or nearly as well as before becoming ill, and all their other communicative acts are impaired in varying degrees as well. In addition, they are likely to be more irritable, scared, depressed, and distractable than before they got sick. Despite these changes, they are often unchanged at the core. If they were loving before, they will be again. If they were irascible, they will remain so. If they were making their ways through life, they will continue to do so. If they were dying, regardless of how subtly, the episode causing the aphasia will not be an antidote. Above all, if they were doing the best they could before, they will set about doing the best they can to adjust to their disability and to the treatments that are likely to accompany it.

All this is not fatalism or resignation. It is applause for the resiliency of aphasic people,

and it is an appeal for aphasiologists to avoid getting in the way of each patient's recovery. It is also the summary of an attitude that profoundly influences what we think aphasiologists should do in addition. Clinicians should reinforce the patients' personal strengths and support their natural processes. They should treat aphasic people and not aphasia. Knowing what to support, what to change, what to accommodate, and what to ignore are marks of clinical maturity.

CLINICAL APHASIOLOGY HAS ITS LIMITS

Aphasiologists must resist trying to be all things to all people. With equal assiduity they must avoid trying to provide services just because no one else on the health care team is providing them. Aphasiologists have been known to give marriage, financial, and sex counseling, psychotherapy, and advice about working, driving, and retiring. The rationale is some form of "Well, someone has to do it, and after all, we are better than anyone else at communicating with aphasic people." Such reasoning is spurious, at least in our view.

More than the illogic, however, it is the potential uselessness and even harm of such an attitude that we fear. Unless aphasiologists are trained as marriage counselors, or psychotherapists, or for any of the other professions, they lack essential skills. Being a good listener is not enough, nor is being able to help the patient understand language. All treatments require, in addition to a knowledge of technique, the ability to separate treatable from untreatable conditions. Bad marriages can sometimes be made worse by a stroke and aphasia, and treatment even by a specialist in marriage counseling may not help. Other times a bad marriage can be more effectively treated after a stroke changes family dynamics than it could have been prior to the stroke. Speech pathologists, even the happily married ones, are unlikely to know how to distinguish between the two. Bad financial planning, poor diet, and alcoholism often resist modification by any professional, but especially by a speech clinician.

Nor is the argument for certain kinds of intervention by the aphasiologist strengthened by evidence that some nonlanguage problems such as alcoholism influence aphasia treatment's techniques, intensity, and outcomes. Asthma and heart disease also influence one another, but the wise cardiologist handles the interaction by referring his asthmatic patients to an allergist. If the cardiologist does not, then wise patients go anyway. Aphasia influences driving, but driving examiners do not practice aphasia treatment. We must be similarly respectful of boundaries and of the limits of our expertise.

The alternatives to attempts to be all things to all aphasic people are hard to tolerate, but tolerate them we must. Referral is one alternative. Trusting in people's ability to survive and to cope and in the powerful salutary effect of natural processes is also crucial. People survive and endure. Time helps. And sometimes what clinicians do creates a problem rather than a solution. If one has had to endure stroke, enduring a bad clinician or one who fails to recognize boundaries is double jeopardy. If associated problems are disrupting treatment, if time and listening do not help, and if referral is impossible, then treatment must be altered to mute the disruptive effects or it must be terminated.

TREATMENT IS NOT LIMITED TO SPEECH-LANGUAGE AND COMMUNICATION

The obverse to the previous principle is the principle that aphasia treatment is more than speech-language or even communication treatment. New clinicians sometimes have difficulty treating severe, ill, very stubborn, demented, or confused patients. This difficulty probably has several sources, one of the most potent, it seems to us, is the common clinical notion that therapy is a set of activities involving clinician and patient and controlled primarily by the clinician. Sometimes of course, it is just that. Usually, however, treatment is much more. It is counseling. It is education of family, friends, peers, and patients. It is standing by and waiting. It is

listening. It is providing a prognosis and helping people accept the implications of the prognosis. It is referral to another more appropriate professional. It is a soupçon of face-to-face treatment at regular but widely spaced intervals to detect change. It is a telphone call from time to time to see how things are progressing, It is periodic follow-up. It is providing a family with a name and number thay can call if they have questions, answers, or fears. It is helping a family order a large print newspaper, computer, or talking book. Thus defined, treatment can more comfortably be provided for a variety of complicated patients for whom formal tests and drill are inappropriate. Thus defined, treatment is easier to stop when it is not helping, and easier to change when it is helping but not enough.

INDIVIDUAL TREATMENT IS APHASIA THERAPY'S CORNERSTONE

We believe that one clinician and one aphasic person are the heart of successful treatment. We also believe in group therapy. Groups can be made up of one or several aphasic people, one or several clinicians, one or several family members, friends, or other professionals. We also believe that groups supplement individual treatments. Groups replace individual treatment only if a patient has never responded or has stopped responding to individual work, but wants to continue treatment. Groups can be used for education, support, carryover, practice, and even new learning. In our view, however, they should not be used to increase a caseload or control one that would otherwise be out of control. Nor should groups be formed out of whomever is around. Organizing groups that work may be one of clinical aphasiology's biggest challenges.

TESTING IS CRUCIAL TO TREATMENT

Finding out what patients can and cannot do are among the first orders of clinical business. Formal tests are best for these tasks. We use them, as was amply shown in Chapter 4. We know, however, that clinicians—as they gain experience—come to rely on the supplemental findings of unstandardized measures, as well. We also use and recommend these, although some of our colleagues (McNeil, 1982) form their eyes into narrow slits when we admit it. We recognize that nonstandardized measures are like bigotry—they can cut us off from certain realities.

We also recognize that they are of limited use in discussions with peers, especially published discussions. For example, if one reports a comprehension score on the Boston Diagnostic Aphasia Examination (BDAE) (Goodglass & Kaplan, 1972), colleagues know how that score was gotten (pretty much) and perhaps even something about how to interpret it. Interpreting a score on a homemade test of comprehension is more difficult, or impossible. Our feeling, however, is that formal tests are an inadequate basis for treatment planning. So, when we talk about our patients, we use formal tests. When we get ready to talk to them we use informal ones. We do not abandon reliability and validity as a result of relying on informal measures, because much of our treatment is conducted within the constraints of single case design research. Clinicians familiar with these restraints recognize that they are as rigorous, and sometimes more rigorous, than those imposed by most tests.

LISTENING IS THE MOST IMPORTANT PART OF TESTING

What a patient has done and endured prior to coming under the speech pathologist's care and what a patient knows and feels about illness and disability may be as important as the test performance. No person arrives at the speech pathologist with a *tabula rasa* for a history. People have had previous strokes, or other debilitating disease. They have had what some might consider a too full (or empty) history of using recreational drugs such as alcohol. Some have never talked as well or as much as their peers. Some have not written a word since signing a marriage certificate, a

social security check, or papers allowing them to enlist in the armed forces. Some have not read, even the newspapers, since quitting school.

Knowing all this simplifies interpreting the test data. Writing errors, for example, are easier to interpret if the clinician knows a patient was an active reader and writer. Speech is easier to evaluate if the clinician can confirm that a patient's speech had previously been normal and plenteous. So we ask them questions about how they used to be and we listen as carefully to the answers as we do to their procedural and narrative discourse and their picture naming.

Listening to patients and families can also result in more appropriate treatment goals and discharge planning. Mildly aphasic persons will tell clinicians about the debilitating parts of their aphasia that might otherwise escape detection during formal tesing. Once these occult parts have been revealed, treatment that might not have been proffered based only on test scores can be structured to change them. In addition, deciding which modalities to treat, what stimuli to select, and what to expect from treatment are all conditioned by what kind of person the aphasic speaker was and is, what kind of family he or she has, what patient and family expect and will tolerate, and how they all get along. Improved reading is not important to a nonreader nor will reading be very useful as a mode for improving something else, such as speaking. Protracted treatment may be rejected by patients who have little use for themselves or others or who want to fish rather than talk. Homework may be harmful to a patient loathed by a spouse. On the other hand, treatment cannot be too long or too intense for those eager to rejoin the talking world.

Just a few more words about talking and human existence. Speech pathologists believe that the first is crucial to the second. Anchorites do not think so, and even a large proportion of people living with other people do not believe nearly so uncritically in the value of taking as do speech pathologists. Some aphasic people, although not hermits before aphasia, do not mind hermitage afterward. Some are willing to rely on what little communication they can accomplish with looks, waves, and head nods, supplemented by their own ambulation. Some want to communicate but not to endure communication therapy. Others want back all that they had and will do anything to get it. Others want the very best a clinician has to offer, regardless of how limnited the gains. These different people all want and need different things from their clinicians. Clinicians who are merely adequate treat all people more or less equally. The superior clinician finds out what each patient wants and needs, balances these against available resources and what testing and experience say will be possible, and then counsels and treats (or does not treat) accordingly.

APHASIA TREATMENT MUST BE STRUCTURED

In our view, treatment is structure. It is not a new activity each day, regardless of how creative. It is not a rush of frenzied or even relaxed activities. It is not limited to communication and understanding. The structure of aphasia treatment is palpable and dynamic. The components of that structure are methods, stimuli, responses, analysis of performance, knowledge of results, repetition, movement, and good humor. Most of these components are treated extensively in subsequent chapters or in subsequent principles. The importance of repetition and of movement will be treated here.

In our view, aphasia therapy, if it is being done with the hope of changing talkers rather than merely keeping them company while they change spontaneously or await discharge, must emphasize the systematic repetition of appropriate activities. There is no right number of repetitions. We do believe, however, that once is not enough. If a single exposure or a few exposures during a day or a week were therapeutic, few patients would visit the clinical aphasiologist, because even severe patients are greeted, queried, entreated, disciplined, and cajoled. Normally they nod, fume, point, and even talk in response. But they do not necessarily get better. Getting

better requires even more. More repetitions. More structure.

The view that aphasia therapy requires repetition is compatible with the view that aphasia therapy should emphasize communication rather than correctness. Repetition refers only to number of trials. It denotes and connotes nothing at all about what is to be practiced nor how accurately something is to be performed. The responses to be produced and the criterion of correctness or adequacy against which they will be judged are determined by the patient's symptoms and needs and the clinician's training and orientation.

Treatment's structure must allow and even foster movement within each session. Most of our treatment time is spent moving aphasic people toward as much independence and functional use of language as they can muster. Hierarchies can create that movement, but only if they are intelligently designed and creatively used. A hierarchy is not good, a priori, even if it features what seem to be graded tasks and begins with activities a particular patient finds easy. Order for the clinician may be chaos for the patient. Steps that the clinician has ordered for sound linguistic, phonetic, and learning reasons may be a gaggle of dissociated activities for an aphasic person. Nonpareil clinicians may profitably remember that all the steps of a hierarchy may not be necessary, some can be skipped or deleted altogether, all patients do not need to remain equally long at all steps, movement along a hierarchy is back and forth and not just forth, and that hierarchies are built to be destroyed.

NO SINGLE SET OF TASKS OR PROCEDURES IS ADEQUATE TREATMENT

Aphasia is not tonsillitis; the acceptable treatments have not been narrowed to a precious few. And although it is not the case that everything goes, it is the case that many things do. Or, many things do potentially, and patients let us know how wisely we have chosen their methods from the list of all possible treatments.

The din created by position papers and

commercial treatment materials and programs can make it hard to hear what one's own patients are saying. In our more brittle moments we long for a time when position papers bolstered by hints of miraculous recovery will be forever banned and treatment materials will be reviewed by peers and by patients prior to their publication. Then we recover our humor and insouciance and turn our attention back to our patients. What happens when we do? Activities that are merely appropriate or logical are replaced by those that work. Treatment becomes a dynamic, eclectic interchange with the patient at the center, and is not allowed to become solely a testing ground for whatever is in vogue.

One of us said "Some treatment tasks (and objectives) must be functional and related to daily living. Some treatment tasks are process directed (designed to improve the process of auditory comprehension, for example) and the stimulus items may not even remotely resemble functional tasks." We are irenic. We seldom choose up sides in the battle over how pragmatic, or how convergent, or how functional treatment should be. Depending on each patient's need and disability, any one of our sessions is a pastiche of specific, limited tasks and more functional activities. A patient in need of more names can profit from specific naming drills as described in Chapter 9 and from activities that allow names (most likely the ones specifically worked on) to spill out into descriptions, conversations, and informal treatment activities. Provincialism has no place in aphasia treatment. If one has an overwhelming need to belong to a school, it should perhaps be a dance school; it should not be a school of therapy.

CONCENTRATE ON ANTECEDENT RATHER THAN CONSEQUENT EVENTS

Good communication is its own reward, therefore, most patients do not rely on our applause or other rewards. They do appreciate that approval and support. They do rely on us for the best materials and methods. This observation, combined with our feeling that good clinicians can—by their stimulus selection,

ordering, and presentation—elicit responses from all but the most severe or sullen patients, causes us to emphasize antecedent over consequent events. Something positive will usually happen every time a good clinician and a good aphasic person sit down together. If patients like what has happened they will willingly do what is necessary to make it happen again. If they do not like what has happened, no reward will make them endure an activity very long.

TREATMENT STIMULI MUST BE ADEQUATE

Despite the obvious importance of adequate stimuli to successful treatment, it is somewhat difficult to decide what adequate stimuli are. Schuell (Schuell et al., 1964) said an adequate stimulus was one that elicited a correct response. She believed that the clinician's duty was to elicit a series of correct responses and that clinicians should restimulate after an error rather than have the patient self-correct. We believe something subtly different, especially about treating chronic speakers or those for whom we predict chronic, severe (but not global) residuals. Such patients can profit from error analysis and correction so long as it occurs in an environment of trust, support, and progress. For us, then, an adequate stimulus is not necessarily one that elicits a correct response. We also believe that a stimulus can be adequate even though it does not elicit any overt response at all as long as it does lead to active—if overt—problem solving. Finally, an adequate stimulus can also be one that elicits only a partially correct or even an incorrect response so long as a series of such responses becomes increasingly more adequate with successive presentations of the stimulus.

Sometimes—sometimes often—patients make errors. An adequate stimulus after the patient has made an error is one that helps self-correction and one that prevents the patient from being diminished by one or several errors, even consecutive ones. An adequate stimulus is also one that grants a speaker all possible independence and makes future independence more likely.

APHASIA TREATMENT EXPLOITS STRENGTHS

An acceptable approach in aphasia therapeutics is to exploit each person's strengths. This means drill or stimulation confined to the most intact modalities and the reinforcement of the best communicative performance. This approach is especially appropriate for acutely aphasic people and for those who have become discouraged. If the strongest performances are of activities not typically used in communication (such as using meaningful gestures), their use and reinforcement in therapy is best preceded and accompanied by counseling. If the patient wants it and the clinician agrees, once strengths have been enhanced, they can be used in combination with weaknesses.

BEWARE DISSOCIATIONS

One of aphasiology's moldiest notions is that a patient's strengths can be paired with weaknesses to improve the weaknesses. The visual is paired with the auditory, writing is paired with speaking, gesturing is paired with speaking, and so on. Sometimes such pairing works, although we suspect the effect is most often like that of a splint. The good supports the bad while the bad is mending naturally. Sometimes pairing fails. One explanation for the failure is dissociation. After brain damage, abilities can be dissociated, which is to say that their relationships are severed. A common example is in that subgroup of Wernicke's aphasic people who can write words but not say them or who can write words while saying the sheerest form of nonsense (Hier & Mohr, 1977). Recognizing dissociations is crucial to long-term treatment, and most dissociations can be revealed—indeed, are often only revealed—by short-term, systematic clinical experimentation.

The clinical necessity is for more than mere recognition and revelation, however. If two modalities are dissociated so that performance in one has no influence on performance in the other, pairing them will not help. Indeed, such pairing may retard treatment regardless of how good one of the dissociated modalities is.

PREPARE FOR RATHER THAN PRAY FOR GENERALIZATION

We hope we are not being sententious in our statement of this principle, but it seems to us that many clinicians feel falsely confident about generalization because at one extreme they see themselves as being good clinicians, or, at the other, they see themselves as nearly powerless to cause generalization. Members of both groups may make clinical mistakes because they assume either that they can do no harm or no good.

Generalization in aphasia has infrequently been studied, but experience confirms that the issues involved in it are not simple. Experience also confirms that generalization must be prepared for with all patients except those benefiting from significant physiological recovery.

Generalization can never be guaranteed, but it is made likely by a series of specific clinical activities. Our list of the most important ones follows: (1) Expose each patient to numerous repetitions of each activity; 10 repetitions are usually too few, and several hundred may be just right. (2) Train a large number of items in a given category; training 100 food items is better than training 10. (3) Teach self-generated cues. (4) Involve the patient and loved ones in treatment planning and (where appropriate) in treatment itself. (5) Extend treatment outside the clinic with specially selected assignments and activities. (6) Provide patients all possible independence by organizing treatment so that patients learn to use their treated responses when they want to rather than when their clinicians want them to. (7) Teach general strategies such as relaxation while simultaneously teaching specific items or skills.

APHASIC PEOPLE NEED TO BECOME THEIR OWN CLINICIANS

We sometimes meet aphasic people who quite innocently expect that treatment will restore them to some approximation of "normal" and that treatment is the clinician's responsibility. In their minds, they bring the problems and clinicians bring the solutions.

A ubiquitous theme in this book is that improvement results from the clinician's insight and support and the patient's total commitment to becoming his or her own best clinician. Aphasic patients find the transition to aphasia clinician easier if they are improving and if they learn self-cueing. Subsequent treatment chapters develop the specifics of how this is to be done.

INVOLVE OTHERS

Aphasia is a family disorder; improvement is a family proposition. So we involve them, if they are willing and available, or we involve friends when families are nonexistent or unavailable. Involvement of significant others begins before, at, or shortly after the first evaluation when we take a history from them, and explain the disorder, the prognosis, and our treatment plan. It continues with their observing treatment, helping us select and modify tasks, and listening to our summaries about progress and changes in the plan. It grows with our enlisting their help in getting each patient to accept certain drills, compensations, and compromises. Sometimes it involves their helping with homework and with monitoring carryover. It ends only when treatment, disposition, and follow-up have been completed.

APHASIOLOGISTS SHOULD RECOGNIZE WHEN IMPROVEMENT MAY NOT BE WORTH THE COST

Clinicians must make hard decisions about the cost of improvement. It is undeniable that "yes" and "no" are responsible for most human actions and reactions. Is it worth the cost and energy of three years of work to get a "yes" and a "no"? Perhaps for some. Probably not for most. This is an extreme example. Clinicians could no doubt recall other less extreme, but very real ones from their own experience. Our point is only that sometimes treatment does not do very much. Treatment that does not do very much, very quickly becomes too expensive and too painful. Medicine can keep terminally ill people alive for long periods. Is it worth it? Many patients and families think not. Surgery

can prolong a tumor patient's life for a few weeks or months. Is it worth it? Many think not. Speech pathology can improve some aphasic people a little. Is it worth it? Many do not think so.

AVOID TREATMENTS THAT MAKE A PATIENT FEEL ABNORMAL

Some of our methods such as gestural reorganization and alternative modes of communication make some patients feel abnormal. Some patients, therefore, reject them. It is as if handicap is more normal than some treatments or treatment tools. Most people remember a neighbor, a friend, or a family member who had a stroke and could not talk or walk very well but who "got along." On the other hand, to talk exclusively with one's hands, or with the help of a communicative board may surprise many potential listeners. That these procedures are therapeutic does not inevitably reduce the stigma. Witness the number of severely aphasic people who continue thumbing through magazines when they can no longer read, or cheerfully nod "yes" or "no" even when they cannot or have not understood. Most of us want to be normal, or at least, to appear to be so. Without adequate explanations and encouragements, therefore, some methods and many materials will be rejected as being more abnormal than the sequelae of brain damage they are purported to change.

TREATMENT'S BEGINNING AND ENDING ARE LAWFUL

Aphasic people are not treated merely because they arrive at the hospitals, are referred, or because a sophisticated advocate prepares the way. Some—probably most—aphasic people in treatment are admitted because clinicians think the treatment will be successful. Other patients are admitted for idiosyncratic reasons such as the clinician's interest or conviction that a particular person deserves contact with a clinical aphasiologist. Such special patients are informed about these special reasons and their consent is secured before treatment begins.

Treatment stops, unless the patient decides to leave prematurely, for equally sound reasons. As one of us said, "Treatment has an end. When it occurs should be considered before treatment begins." We use a number of criteria for ending treatment. If learning never begins or ceases despite the clinician's best efforts, treatment (under ordinary conditions) should stop. In addition, if treatment effects do not generalize, if gains are not maintained, at least a little, and if the cost of teaching every response becomes too great, treatments should stop. Treatment stops also when patients have had enough regardless of how well they may be doing.

We know that treatment decisions are sometimes personal. Depending on a clinic or a clinician's mission, patients with little hope of improvement may be entered and continued in treatment. We see some people for years if they continue to teach us or our students, and if they agree. Our apparent obduracy about criteria for beginning and ending treatment is only to reinforce our message that speech pathologists must assiduously avoid the image which in surgery is called "being a hack." We can work away at selected aphasias and aphasic people; we should not hack away at all.

COMMON SENSE AND GUILT SHOULD INFLUENCE CLINICAL EXPERIMENTATION

Clinical practice and clinical experimentation can often occur simultaneously. When they can, they should, because aphasiology has much to learn about its methodology. However, each patient's treatment need not conform to the strict requirements of a single case design nor should such a structure be forced on each treatment. Some patients, because of their severity, psyches, or for other reasons, may simply be impossible to treat with more than the general structure that prevents sessions, regardless of how resistant the patient or the disorder, from being merely harmless social occasions or capricious flurries of activity. At other times, clinicians may have too little energy or spirit to do the work necessary to meet rigid experimental requirements.

Looming over all, however, are two realities. The first is the reality that all aphasic people can teach us things as we treat them. To the degree that our treatments of them are structured, their teaching of us will be too. The second reality is that clinical aphasiologists are weary of responding to cynicism about treatment's efficacy and appropriateness, especially during the period of physiologic recovery and with severe patients. A decade of data collection within the restraints of single case design will produce sufficient data to silence the questioners if journal editors will treat such designs with the same respect traditionally reserved for studies with one or more subjects in each group. Clinicians and editors both are obliged to do their parts.

EVEN SUCCESSFUL TREATMENT CANNOT IGNORE MODERN DEVELOPMENTS

What works today will be replaced by tomorrow's better treatments. Computers, for example, will help change the face of aphasia treatment. In the hands of competent clinicians, computers will improve clinical precision, save time, reduce the burden of providing as many systematic repetitions as aphasic people need, and simplify data collection and analysis. Positron emission tomography, magnetic resonance imaging, and other developments will expand and modify what we know about brain function and the correlation of lesion, behavior, and recovery. Eventually, surgery and medication may prevent stroke or reduce its effects, and aphasic people may pass from an endangered species list to extinction. Until that time, clinicians need to profit from what is new and work as successfully as dentists to abolish their own jobs.

GAIETY HAS ITS OWN PLACE

Clinicians and aphasic people deserve to laugh. Laughter breaks the tension, makes errors easier to accept, and rewards a job well done. It may even be good treatment. Treatment can too easily become ponderous, dull, and deathly serious. The requirement for repetition, the frustration of failed communication, the easy fatiguability that accompanies brain damage, the daily routine and sometimes slow progress, and most of all, the realization that very little will be the way it was before are all potentially deadly forces. Laughter will not change them—or perhaps not change them much. It may make these forces easier to bear and serve as proof that they are being borne with peace. We have the impression that many patients take their moods from clinicians. Clinicians consumed by the enormity of their therapeutic responsibility will seldom be greeted by a smile from across the table.

CLINICIANS NEED TO BE PROTEAN

Clinicians plan their clinical activities and one of the things they plan to do is change. Long- and short-term goals and a treatment plan are essential because they force clinicians to think about test results, patient needs, and what both mean for specific treatment sessions. They give structure to treatment's overall course as well as to the initial moments of individual sessions. But lesson plans exist primarily so that clinicians will recognize when to abandon them. Hierarchies and stimulus lists are the same. They exist primarily to be changed. Patients improve, they fatigue, they get depressed, they get news of an impending weekend pass. Clinicians respond to the accompanying changes. If they do not, treatment becomes confinement.

FINALLY

These are the principles that guide our daily clinical activities. They are not unique, exhaustive, or even very durable. They were written as an exposé of the attitudes that led us to write what we have in the rest of this book.

7

TREATING AUDITORY
COMPREHENSION DEFICIT

uditory comprehension deficit is the veiled disorder of aphasia. The most dramatic and obvious signs of aphasia are oral: convoluted syntax, quirky word selection, and telegraphic speech, among other oral manifestations. But the link between perception and production has been carefully documented in human communication and degradation of auditory processing and comprehension has been recognized by several careful observers not only as a primary deficit, but perhaps also as the occult, indirect cause of output deficit.

Therefore, treatment of the person with aphasia must rely heavily on a proper appreciation of the quality and severity of comprehension impairment. In fact, certain approaches to treatment are steeped in auditory stimulation. Schuell and colleagues (1964), for example, believed the auditory mode to be crucial, and stated, "Probably because of the great dependence of language on the auditory system, there is almost always demonstrable impairment of auditory processes in aphasia" (p. 115).

Although a precise definition of auditory comprehension deficit is not universally accepted and a good deal of controversy exists regarding the necessary components, levels, and stages of comprehension, most clinical aphasiologists would agree that aphasic auditory comprehension deficit is a deficiency

in the ability to process or understand spoken language that cannot be accounted for by peripheral sensory deficit, generalized cognitive deficit, or primary disturbances in attention or arousal.

Although much contemporary research attention is directed at a better understanding of aphasic auditory impairment, for many years the output of aphasic individuals was much more frequently studied. Perhaps, as Boller, Kim, and Mack (1977) suggested, the study of comprehension has lagged because comprehension can never be observed directly, but must always involve a level of inference. Whereas spontaneous production of language can be observed directly for paraphasia, agrammatism, or neologistic jargon, the act of comprehension must rely on some mode of output response and therefore, runs the risk of being confounded with output deficits. This chapter deals with treating aphasic deficits in auditory processing and comprehension. In order to develop or reinforce an appreciation of the complexities of treating this modality, it will be necessary to discuss the nature of the impairment, methods of assessment, and a sampling of classic and contemporary research.

The year 1874 proved to be a turning point in the study of aphasia. In that year, Carl Wernicke, a 26-year-old German neurologist, reported his discovery of a second speech area;

Auditory Comp. deficit = a deficiency in the ability to process or understand spoken language that can't be accounted for by peripheral sensory deficit, generalized cognitive deficit or primary disturb. in attention or arousal.

a center responsible for sensory aspects of speech. Thirteen years earlier, in 1861, Paul Broca fueled brain-behavior debate among European scholars by providing evidence on the localization of cerebral speech function, but the picture of aphasia was incomplete. As Eggert (1977) has pointed out in a monograph that traced Wernicke's life and contributions and translated his major research, Wernicke's 1874 report *Der Aphasische Symptomen-komplex* (The Aphasia Symptom-Complex) supplied a missing ingredient for a cohesive theory of aphasia. In this study, in addition to the major impact of focusing attention on the problem of language comprehension impairment and its localization in the left temporal lobe, Wernicke synthesized the diverse and seemingly contradictory features of aphasia and organized them into a coherent framework. He also explored the symptom-triad of what he called sensory aphasia that included auditory comprehension deficit, paraphasia, and word-finding difficulty (Eggert, 1977).

Wernicke discussed in detail the effects of destruction of the area of the temporal lobe he labeled A_1 (which subsequently would be relabeled after him), and stated that the "sound images of the names of possible objects will be lost" (Boller et al., 1977, p. 9). Wernicke also noted the indirect effects of damage to the "sensory speech area" by observing that patients have aphasic manifestations in speaking because of the "absence of the corrective function exercised unconsciously by the sound images" (Boller et al., 1977, p. 9).

Wernicke was not the first to report auditory comprehension deficits in aphasia. As early as 1770, Gesner described a patient who complained of difficulty understanding other people's language (Boller et al., 1977), but Wernicke triggered a roman candle of clinico-pathological studies in aphasia, many of which paid careful attention to observation and testing of comprehension status. For example, one of Wernicke's assistants, Heilbronner, stressed the necessity of testing the hearing of aphasic patients so that losses of acuity could be differentiated from higher levels of auditory comprehension impairment (Eggert, 1977).

Wernicke's contributions are firmly entrenched in the field of aphasia and no discussion of auditory comprehension impairment is complete without acknowledgment of his landmark research that began at age 26. Unfortunately, his brilliant life as a scholar was to be prematurely terminated on June 15, 1905. A cycling excursion with a colleague along a narrow forest road ended in tragedy when he fell under a timber cart, and the rear wheel crushed his chest (Eggert, 1977).

NATURE OF AUDITORY COMPREHENSION

MODELS, LEVELS, AND PATTERNS

In a very general sense, auditory comprehension refers to the piecing together of meaning from sounds. Clark and Clark (1977) stated that it "denotes the mental processes by which listeners take in the sounds uttered by a speaker and use them to construct an interpretation of what they think the speaker intended to convey" (p. 43). But, as McNeil and Kimelman (1986) pointed out in their essay on the information processing structure of auditory comprehension and processing in aphasia, no single formalized model or theory of auditory comprehension exists that considers each and every level from initial vibration of the tympanic membrane by sound waves, to electrochemical transfer in the cochlea and brainstem, through the complicated association and abstraction processes that result in interpretation of a speaker's intent. Nevertheless, the clinician who works with adults with aphasia must develop an appreciation for the overall hierarchical arrangement of behaviors and processes involved in language comprehension.

PERIPHERAL AUDITORY FUNCTION

As indicated earlier, Heilbronner stressed the need for evaluating auditory function of people with aphasia many years ago. Audiological assessment continues to be recognized as an important aspect of evaluation. Wilson,

Fowler, and Shanks (1981) presented a useful overview of audiological assessment in aphasia, including modifications in routine procedures necessitated by aphasia. The application of site-of-lesion and evoked response measurement is stressed as well.

The causes and age distribution of hearing dysfunction in aphasia were reported by Boehme (1984). In a population of 1,138 aphasic patients with cerebrovascular disease, 100 subjects were randomly selected and 41 (41 percent) showed sensorineural hearing impairment on tonal audiograms.

COMPONENTS, STAGES

Florid argument has been known to erupt during discussions of what stages or components are necessary for successful auditory comprehension of language. Yet, despite disagreements, consensus is beginning to emerge on general components of the process. Aten (1972), among others, has indicated the following stages as essential:

1. *Stimulus detection*—Includes awareness of the stimuli, not only in terms of auditory acuity but also in terms of "set to attend" and attention over time (auditory vigilance).

2. *Discrimination of stimuli*—Involves the act of recognizing minimal differences among auditory stimuli, as in phonemic discrimination.

3. *Retention*—Includes the act of storage and retrieval of auditory material on both a short- and long-term basis.

4. *Categorization*—Includes the complex process of retaining then comparing or associating new stimuli in stored material.

5. *Sequential retention*—The process of organizing successive auditory stimuli over time.

PATTERNS OF IMPAIRMENT

The observation that several stages or components of auditory function have been recognized has led researchers to speculate on the possibility of identifying distinctive patterns of impairment in aphasia. This is an attractive speculation as it implies that differential intervention strategies may be more efficacious as well as more economical than traditional approaches to treatment. The suggestion that it is an oversimplification to view "auditory reception" as a unitary disorder was advanced by Goodglass, Gleason, and Hyde (1970), who explored some factors contributing to auditory comprehension in aphasic individuals, and these researchers concluded that standard diagnostic groups may have different types of comprehension difficulty. Green and Boller (1974) also studied features of auditory comprehension in severely impaired aphasic subjects and they implied that the cortical mechanisms underlying comprehension do not simply work as a single component, but have various functions that clinical testing may identify.

In the 1970s Brookshire (1972, 1978b) discussed varieties and attached labels to several patterns of impairment. LaPointe, Horner, Lieberman, and Riski (1974) found this speculation so attractive that they set about trying to sort out patterns of impairment by observing performance on an array of auditory measures. The following patterns of impairment were postulated:

1. *Slow Rise Time*—Represented by the aphasic individual who misses the first few units of information then performs efficiently. The patient "tunes in" slowly when asked to respond to auditory commands and responds correctly only to the final portions of a message. Short commands may be missed entirely.

2. *Noise Build Up*—More accurate performance on the first part of a message with increasing difficulty in series of words or commands.

3. *Information Processing Lag*—Alternately accurate and inaccurate performance within a message. Better performance on first and last portions apparently caused by inability to receive and process at the same time.

4. *Intermittent Auditory Imperception*—Fading in and out in apparently random fashion.

5. *Capacity Deficit*—Limited number of units that can be processed. Performance seems to drop off at about the same point in longer messages.

6. *Retention Deficit*—Difficulty in holding material over time. Best tested by presenting material, imposing a delay and then requiring a response.

LaPointe and colleagues (1974) collected data with a variety of auditory tasks on 12 aphasic subjects, four nonaphasic right hemisphere damaged subjects, and six subjects who were free of neurological pathology.

Analysis of patterns of impairment for the aphasic subjects revealed a mixture of pattern components. Some patients presented a predominant pattern and secondary patterns in lesser degrees. Capacity Deficit and Noise Build Up emerged as the most frequent predominant patterns, though all six categories occurred at least as secondary patterns. The stability and validity of these patterns has not been confirmed by subsequent research. However, other researchers soon picked up the trail and began generating and testing other hypotheses regarding inter- and intrasubject variability on auditory tasks.

In order to gain insight into subject variability and perhaps the very nature of aphasia, McNeil and his associates undertook a careful study of performance fluctuations on measures of auditory comprehension. Using the Revised Token Test (McNeil & Prescott, 1978), four patterns of auditory performance were studied (McNeil & Hageman, 1979) including flat, tuning-in, tuning-out, and intermittent. McNeil (1982) speculated that the internal state's responsibility for the intermittent pattern of response might be reduced and/or inefficient allocation of effort or attention. He refined his view of this aspect of variability in aphasia even further and postulated a revision in the nature of linguistic deficit in aphasia in a recent work (McNeil & Kimelman, 1986).

A bit of water has been dashed on the early fire that surrounded the search for distinctive patterns of auditory impairment, however. In a study of reliability of patterns of auditory processing deficits, Hageman, McNeil, Rucci-Zimmer, and Cariski (1982) reported that little reliability of subtest patterns of the Revised Token Test were found across individuals. They caution against treatment strategies that attempt to make use of these patterns.

The existence of reliably measurable patterns of auditory impairment related to type of aphasia and/or location, extent, and type of lesion remains an attractive speculation, if somewhat dimmed. At this point, research has been unable to demonstrate unequivocal patterns of dysfunction that lend themselves to type-specific treatment, but perhaps further sophistication of our measurement techniques will re-open the issue, and with it rekindle the promise of economical and efficient clinical intervention that will allow focus on less global impairment of comprehension.

ANATOMY OF AUDITORY COMPREHENSION

In his landmark discovery in 1874, Wernicke not only described the role of auditory comprehension loss in certain types of aphasia, but also was the first to try to delimit the anatomic correlates of auditory comprehension. He implicated lesions involving the posterior superior aspect of the left temporal lobe and its posterior extension. Advances in brain imaging techniques, such as those outlined in Chapter 2, are contributing much more. Selnes, Niccum, and Rubens (1982) reported CT scan correlates of recovery in auditory comprehension in a series of 31 patients. These patients were tested at approximately 30 days postonset and retested at monthly intervals for five months. Auditory comprehension performance from months one and six were compared. A summary of their findings included the following:

1. Degree of auditory comprehension impairment at one month postonset is not predictive of lesion location (i.e., lesions outside the posterior superior temporal lobe [PST] may cause impairments as severe as those directly affecting PST).

PST = posterior superior aspect of the left Temporal Lobe

2. Presence of a PST lesion is associated with poor prognosis for auditory comprehension; conversely, absence of a PST lesion is associated with good prognosis—even in cases with severe initial comprehension deficits.

3. Aphasic subjects without PST lesions show very rapid improvement such that most of their recovery occurs before three months postonset. Subjects with PST involvement show a much more gradual recovery rate.

Six of the seven most severely impaired subjects in this study had lesions in the PST that extended into the infrasylvian portion of the supramarginal gyrus as well. Studies such as this one by Selnes and colleagues (1982) appears to contribute solely to our understanding of the brain and how it relates to language loss. The careful clinician, however, notices that the prognostic and recovery implications can have very real translation to clinical management. The problems we encounter in answering the questions of family members about recovery of selected functions will be lessened considerably by advances in our understanding of the relationships between recovery and site/extent of the lesion.

PHONEME IMPERCEPTION— REAUDITORIZATION

Few clinicians who have experience with a large number of aphasic individuals report difficulty with phoneme discrimination to be a fundamental problem in aphasia. Schuell included a section on phoneme discrimination in her test battery (the "peas-bees" subtest) but few aphasia batteries since the development of the MMTDA have considered it necessary.

Some researchers remain convinced, however, that difficulties in auditory comprehension can be traced to the phoneme level. Varney (1984), for example, isolated 14 aphasic subjects with impaired phoneme discrimination from a larger population of 100 patients with left hemisphere lesions. All patients with impaired phoneme discrimination were significantly impaired in aural comprehension, but many demonstrated intact sound recognition and some showed normal reading comprehension. Defects in phoneme discrimination typically were seen in the acute stages of aphasia resulting from stroke; in most cases, no longer than four months postonset. All patients who recovered normal phoneme discrimination also made significant improvement in aural comprehension. These findings by Varney (1984) support the concept that some auditory comprehension defects result from a specific disturbance in phoneme discrimination, though, if his sample is representative, we can expect only 14 percent phoneme discrimination problems and those 14 percent to resolve early (within four months).

Reauditorization is another problem. Schuell emphasized lingering problems in an aphasic person's ability to reauditorize. The concept is a bit ambiguous, but appears to be related to poor performance on auditory tests other than single word recognition. In fact, Schuell and colleagues (1964) reported that of the 107 patients who recovered speech, 103 revealed impairment on tests of understanding spoken language, even though they had no difficulty in recognizing single words. Perhaps further research on Schuell's idea would clarify both the nature and extent of so-called reauditorization deficit.

MODALITY-STIMULUS INFLUENCES

A variety of modality variables and stimulus forms were used in a study of comprehension in severe aphasia by Lambrecht and Marshall (1983). In addition to examining auditory and auditory visual presentation modes, these researchers presented commands, yes/no questions, and informational questions to eight severely impaired aphasic adults. Subjects performed significantly better when stimuli were presented in an auditory-visual condition than in an auditory condition. No differences were found among the three stimulus forms; however, in analyzing trends, the authors suggested that commands appeared to be the easiest stimulus form for the severely aphasic subjects. The authors suggested further that the various yes/no questions within aphasia test batteries are not of equal difficulty.

LEXICAL-SYNTACTIC ASPECTS

Lexical versus syntactical errors in both reading and listening comprehension were studied in 10 Broca's aphasic subjects by Gallaher and Canter (1982). They found that subject-object reversal errors occurred significantly more frequently than lexical errors. What is unclear is whether this pattern of error is unique to Broca's aphasic subjects or characteristic of any group of aphasic subjects with mild to moderate comprehension impairment.

COMPREHENSION IN CONTEXT

Comprehension involves more than just deciphering material from a message. Several research studies have shown that semantic knowledge or a more general knowledge of the world is sufficiently preserved in at least some aphasic individuals to allow them to use this information to decode messages. Deloche and Seron (1981), for example, found that some aphasic patients can use knowledge of the world to improve their comprehension.

Manipulation and utilization of context also has been studied in order to explore effects on comprehension. Redundancy appears to help comprehension. The inclusion of a semantically supportive word improved comprehension of target words in a sentence in a study by Gardner, Albert, and Weintraub (1975), and this form of redundancy can be applied by clinicians during treatment. Waller and Darley (1978, 1979) studied contextual influences as well. In one study (Waller & Darley, 1978) comprehension of relatively noncohesive paragraphs was improved by preceding the paragraph with a verbal context. Cohesive paragraphs produced no such improvement. Conversely, Waller and Darley (1979) reported in a subsequent study that comprehension of a variety of syntactic structures was not improved by contextual sentences. Context may not have been facilitating in this study as the subjects were functioning at a reasonably high level, and the contextual sentences used to facilitate understanding may have been too general.

Perhaps it is the aphasic person with lower comprehension skills who benefits most from contextual prompting or cues. Pierce and Beekman (1985) studied 20 aphasic subjects and compared their ability to comprehend target sentences presented in isolation with sentences that were preceded by either a single sentence or a picture that predicted target information. The results revealed that subjects who performed at lower levels on standard tests of auditory comprehension performed better when target information was preceded by contextual information than when it was presented in isolation.

Much is yet to be learned about contextual facilitation of comprehension. But, this study and several others suggest that because language is typically processed in context, the ability of aphasic persons to comprehend brief messages, as assessed by most tests, may not reflect how accurately they can comprehend in more natural communicative environments (Pierce & Beekman, 1985).

Not all aphasic subjects benefit from contextual cueing, however. Nicholas and Brookshire (1983) found that nonfluent aphasic adults benefited from both simplification of complex sentences and from hearing such sentences in context. Clear benefit from simplification and context cues were not as apparent with fluent aphasic subjects.

ESOTERIC TYPES OF AUDITORY IMPAIRMENT

The terminological web in aphasia in general assures extension into the auditory realm. Many labels are unclearly defined or used interchangeably. "Cortical deafness" and "pure word deafness" are good examples. Although some writers are careful to distinguish both the salient characteristics and associated sites of lesion, others are less clear. Rubens (1979) described pure word deafness as the inability to comprehend and discriminate spoken language although the ability to read, write, and speak is relatively intact. As Rubens indicated, the dividing line between cortical deafness and mixed verbal- and nonverbal-sound auditory agnosia is poorly defined.

The very low incidence of pure word deafness is attributable to the fact that it takes an unusually placed, very circumscribed lesion of the superior temporal gyrus to involve Heschl's gyrus (the primary cortical auditory location) or its connections and still selectively spare Wernicke's area (Rubens, 1979).

Reports from patients with pure word deafness reveal that they feel that speech sounds muffled or like a foreign language. Various patient descriptions collected by Rubens (1979) include the comments that "voices come but no words"; "[speech is] an undifferentiated continuous humming noise without any rhythm"; and "words come too quickly [and] sound like a foreign language."

These conditions occur much more rarely than the traditional type of auditory disorders associated with aphasia, but seem to crop up in the literature with inordinate frequency because of their novelty and because they sometimes have explanatory utility.

A case of cortical deafness was described and has been connected to the work of Kneebone and Burns (1981), in which the disorder was associated with mild aphasia due to bilateral temporo-parietal infarction in a 70-year-old man. These authors reported partial return of hearing acuity after one year with continued difficulty in speech discrimination and continued inability to recognize music. Cortical auditory evoked responses were initially absent despite intact brainstem auditory evoked responses. Cortical evoked responses returned after one year.

Another esoteric type of auditory disorder was described by Michel and Andreewohy (1983), who proposed "deep dysphasia" as an analog to deep dyslexia in the auditory modality. They report on a patient with two left hemisphere lesions, a small one in the prefrontal lobe and a larger one in the temporal lobe. The unusual syndrome they reported is a massive deficit for comprehension and expression of oral language contrasting with fairly good preservation of written language. A remarkable feature of this syndrome was the unusual frequency of semantic paraphasia during attempts at repetition.

Occasionally, the ingenuity of clinicians is sorely tested by the demands of such patients. We are asked to design a plan of treatment for those difficult problems, and we find that we have difficulty even conducting an appropriate assesment. As Burger and colleagues (1983) have stated, "Cortical deafness has been observed more than it has been managed. And when it has been managed, treatment did not focus on improving auditory comprehension" (p. 127).

Two treatment studies that focused on teaching sign language as an alternative means of communication were reported by Kirshner and Webb (1981), and Doyle and Holland (1982).

Burger and colleagues (1983) treated a 66-year-old man with bilateral CVA's resulting in mild to moderate aphasia and severe cortical deafness. He failed to respond to any auditory stimuli without visual cues. A multiple baseline ABA design was instituted to evaluate treatment effect. Treatment consisted of systematically manipulating and repeating elements from Level IV of the Revised Token Test. Treatment was highly structured and redundant. The patient showed significantly improved performance on the treatment task and no improvement on other measures of aphasia such as the Western Aphasia Battery (WAB) and the Porch Index of Communicative Ability (PICA).

ASSESSMENT OF AUDITORY COMPREHENSION

EARLY TESTS

As far as is known, one of the earliest special tests for the assessment of auditory comprehension was the Proust-Lichtheim Test, which was reported in 1872 (Boller et al., 1977). With this test, the person suspected of auditory comprehension impairment was asked to raise his or her fingers, to squeeze the examiner's hand, or to blink or breathe out as many times as there were syllables in the name of objects presented. An excellent chronicle of early contributions to the testing of comprehension is provided by Benton (1973).

One early effort to test comprehension was proposed, perhaps unexpectedly, by Liepmann, a name more frequently associated with apraxia. Liepmann presented a test consisting of a series of comments both meaningful and absurd, with the patient nodding agreement or disagreement (Boller et al., 1977).

The most famous early comprehension test is that designed by Pierre Marie in the early 1900s. Marie developed a series of commands designed to assess comprehension, but his Three Papers Test is the one that is most quoted. Comprehension was evaluated by observing the response to the following command: "Here on this table are three pieces of paper of different sizes; give the largest one to me, crumple the middle-sized one and throw it on the floor; and as for the smallest one, put it in your pocket" (Boller et al., 1977, p. 12). Obviously, such factors as memory load, production deficits, and educational level served to confound the results of these early tests, just as they must be a concern today.

Henry Head (1926) described a series of comprehension assessment tasks in his two-volume work *Aphasia and Kindred Disorders of Speech*, including several that sound as though they were part of a carnival act (i.e., the Coin and the Bowl Test; the Hand, Eye, and Ear Test; and the Man, Cat, and Dog Test).

Apparently, Goldstein, in 1948, was one of the first to stress the importance of noting the context in which difficulties occurred (Boller et al., 1977). Perhaps Goldstein's was a pioneering gesture to assess some of the pragmatic aspects of auditory comprehension in the natural communicative environment. He suggested examiners attempt to judge if a patient understood everyday questions better if they related to the patient's own personality or interests. This may be a shadow of the pragmatic emphasis that was to permeate language analysis in the 1970s.

CONTEMPORARY MEASURES

Just about every comprehensive aphasia battery published since the 1950s has a section designed to evaluate auditory impairment. The Minnesota Test for the Differential Diagnosis of Aphasia (MTDDA) contains tasks for evaluating auditory disturbances that are typical of standardized batteries. These include Recognizing Common Words, Discriminating between Paired Words, Recognizing Letters, Identifying Items Serially Named, Understanding Sentences, Following Directions, and Understanding a Paragraph. Some standardized aphasia batteries are not nearly as comprehensive.

TOKEN TEST

DeRenzi and Vignolo introduced the Token Test in 1962 and since that landmark publication in the journal *Brain*, the test not only has spawned extensive research in a dozen countries, but also has produced many offspring and mutations.

Generally, studies have found that the Token Test has been an accurate and sensitive indicator of the presence of aphasia. In fact, the designers of the test intended for the measure to be relatively uncontaminated by situational, intellectual, or redundant linguistic factors. In the Token Test, 20 tokens that vary in size, shape, and color are placed before the person to be tested in a standardized array. The examiner then presents a series of spoken commands that require the person to point to or manipulate the tokens. Scores of theoretical, clinical, and linguistic studies have been reported using data gathered with the Token Test and several chapters (Boller et al., 1977; Riedel, 1981) and even a book (Boller & Dennis, 1979) have focused on the responses of aphasic subjects to the test.

Although the test has engaged researchers worldwide, it is not without its detractors, and an important concern is whether or not the measure can be considered a valid or relatively pure measure of verbal comprehension. The influence of nonlanguage factors such as memory load, color discrimination, and visual-spatial skills may influence Token Test performance. The precise extent of that influence continues to be studied.

A frequently used offspring of the test is the shortened version reported by DeRenzi and Faglioni (1978). Thirty-six commands are presented in six sections corresponding to increasing levels of difficulty.

REVISED TOKEN TEST

The Revised Token Test (RTT) was developed by McNeil and Prescott (1978) and was introduced as a standardized, commercially available measure that used a multi dimensional scoring system. The RTT presents more control over the manipulation of syntactic variables, and performance can be plotted graphically to reveal variance in performance patterns across subtests. Performance norms are provided and reported administration time ranges from 15 to 75 minutes.

Attempts to shorten the test and economize continue. Even revised tests are further revised. For example, the 1985 Clinical Aphasiology Conference witnessed a report on two shortened versions of the (RTT) (Arvedson, McNeil, & West, 1985). In this study, 20 adult aphasic subjects were tested on three consecutive days with (1) a standard version of the RTT, (2) a five-item version (the first five items of all 10 subtests), and (3) subtest six alone. Results revealed the five-item version predicted the mean overall RTT score accurately.

AUDITORY COMPREHENSION TEST FOR SENTENCES

The Auditory Comprehension Test for Sentences (ACTS) (Shewen, 1979) was developed to evaluate comprehension in more detail at the sentence level. The sentences in the ACTS gradually increase in length, lexical difficulty, and syntactic complexity. The examiner reads the sentences aloud and the person being tested responds by pointing to the correct picture from a field of four. Performance norms are provided and responses can be qualitatively analyzed by observing error type. The ACTS can be a valuable aid to treatment planning in that syntactic deficit areas can be isolated and treatment tasks constructed to remediate specific problems.

Attempts to understand the nuances of sentence comprehension in aphasia have taken several approaches. One is the sentence verification procedure. With this method, spoken sentences are presented with pictures that either do or do not represent the pictorial meaning. Subjects are then requested to respond "yes" if sentence and picture match or "no" if no match is apparent. Brookshire and Nicholas have used this strategy with some frequency, and a study of sentence verification of verbs (Brookshire & Nicholas, 1982) is representative of their programmatic probing of this issue. Generally, these researchers have found that verbs take longer to comprehend than subjects or direct objects, and that some verbs take longer to comprehend than other verbs. Further research may provide explanations as to when and why some verbs appear to be easier than others for the aphasic listener. Verbs are pivotal to understanding and answers to these questions of differences in difficulty will aid our selection of treatment materials.

FUNCTIONAL AUDITORY COMPREHENSION TASK

The protocol and test format of the Functional Auditory Comprehension Task (FACT) was described by LaPointe and Horner (1978). The various versions of the Token Test have been criticized for their abstract and acontextual nature and a frequent complaint of clinicians is that performance on the Token Test underestimates the aphasic person's functional comprehension of language in context. The FACT was designed to incorporate some features of performance that might be more related to the demands of daily living auditory comprehension, while retaining some control over the stimulus variables. A carefully controlled hierarchy of length difficulty was maintained and the test is composed of one-part commands (20 items), two-part commands (15 items), and three-part commands (20 items). Stimulus items also reflected a balance of action and object categories in that equal distribution of verb and noun form classes was maintained. The test requires 12 readily available objects, six of which are movable and comprise a "closed set" (coin, key, pencil, paper, cup, spoon) and six of which comprise an "open set" (ceiling, floor, table [or desk], door, chair, pajamas [shirt or blouse]).

The 10 actions selected were judged to be familiar and used relatively frequently in functional communication (point to, tap, shake, pick up, give me, turn over, lift, move, hand me, touch). Responses can be analyzed relative to the precise level of breakdown (one-part, two-part, three-part commands) as well as to relative impairment of action-object manipulation at varying levels of difficulty. Supplemental analysis can be conducted to determine if three-part commands are differentially impaired at the beginning, middle, or end of commands.

In a study that attempted to clarify the relationship among two measures of auditory comprehension (Token Test, Functional Auditory Comprehension Task) and a measure designed to sample communication under more naturalistic circumstances (Communicative Abilities of Daily Living), LaPointe and colleagues (1985) found moderate significant correlations ($R = .64$) between the FACT and the Token Test, a strong correlation between scores on the FACT and CADL ($R = .82$), and no significant correlation between performance on the CADL and Token Test.

DISCOURSE *or Connected Speech*

Extension of evaluation of auditory comprehension skills to types of communication more representative of the interchanges we conduct during daily living situations has been scanty. The evaluation of discourse or connected speech skills has assumed greater importance in recent years, and Bond and Ulatowska (1985) described a methodology for assessing auditory comprehension of discourse with aphasic persons. The strategy of these researchers was to attempt to separate discourse problems related to inability to process aspects of reference from other problems. Much remains to be refined on the application of discourse analysis to assessment in aphasia, but the area promises to disclose subtle or residual communication problems that other analyses miss.

Although there appears to be a consensus among clinicians that careful assessment of spoken language comprehension is necessary in aphasia, there appears to be a growing concern about what to make of it. Investigations of short-term memory, emotional factors, nonverbal disorders, and the confounding of production impairment increasingly support the notion that disorders of speech comprehension are associated with factors that transcend spoken language (McNeil & Kimelman, 1986; Riedel, 1981). Yet, the assertion that a fundamental core, or at least a primary component, of the difficulty in aphasia is a failure at some stage of auditory processing remains an attractive idea to many who toil daily with aphasic individuals and observe their auditory comprehension performance on a variety of tasks.

While ongoing effort attempts to clarify the precise role of comprehension disorders, clinicians will continue meticulous appraisal of apparent breakdown in auditory function, interpret the significance of these disorders and relate them to the overall picture of aphasia, and intervene vigorously in an effort to reduce comprehension barriers that stand in the way of a return to an acceptable quality of communicative life.

Stop   Go to 163

TREATMENT OF AUDITORY COMPREHENSION DEFICIT

PRINCIPLES

We are guided, in our clinical management of aphasia, by a set of principles that have been overtly stated in Chapter 6. Like dolphins shadowing a shrimp boat, these principles have surfaced and resurfaced throughout this book. An important principle that has a good deal of relevance to this chapter is that we believe aphasia is primarily a linguistic-symbolic disorder that crosses and interacts among the modalities of production and reception, and affects all of the linguistic processes including the lexical-semantic, morpho-syntactic, and phonological spheres. But we recognize equally strongly that cognitive, processing, and cybernetic factors manifest themselves in such activities as association, categorization, recognition and recall, memory, vigilance, and arousal-attention and also are vital to adequate linguistic function. To separate these factors from linguistic processes is as fruitful as trying to separate two sides of a coin. Therefore our treatment, particularly of auditory comprehension deficit, considers and addresses both linguistic and cognitive-processing factors.

We also feel that aphasia is not solely a performance deficit but, particularly in global aphasia, may degrade language competence as well. Maybe someday more sophisticated measurement will allow us to unveil previously cloaked language competence, but with today's techniques, for some severely impaired patients, we are unable to discern a glimmer of behavior that suggests competence for selected language behaviors is retained. This affects our treatment. It affects task selection, clinical objectives, and procedure. Other principles relate more specifically to auditory function.

SCHUELLIAN PRINCIPLES

Hildred Schuell was enthralled with the auditory system. She conceived of the language system as dependent upon auditory control not only for processing information directly, but for mediating and regulating language through feedback loops.

Schuell and her colleagues stated, "We think that in aphasia one of three conditions may be observed, reflecting damage to some part of the interacting auditory and language systems" (Schuell et al., 1964, p. 126). Schuell postulated reductions in auditory discrimination, auditory memory span, and sometimes in learned auditory patterns. She also recognized a more severe involvement of the auditory mechanism in aphasia in which she described patients who behaved as though they did not hear, although no impairment on pure-tone audiometric testing could be demonstrated. She indicated this condition had been labeled "word deafness" but stated, "we have no quarrel with the label 'partial auditory imperception' to describe this condition" (Schuell et al., 1964, p. 127).

Her belief in the eminence of the auditory system in language and her clinical observation

that there "is almost always demonstrable impairment of auditory processes in aphasia" (Schuell et al., 1964, p. 115), led her to generate principles of treatment that are quite consistently, steeped in auditory emphasis. For example, effective therapeutic techniques, she said, must be based on two principles:

First, the patient must hear language, and secondly, he must grasp what he hears. To insure the latter he must always be asked to respond in some way. If hearing speech alone were enough, as it may be in some cases, spontaneous recovery would soon occur, for people hear language all day long. But what most aphasic patients learn from the barrage of stimuli is not to listen. (Sies, 1974, p. 202)

Darley has been a staunch advocate of many Schuellian principles, and in a review on maximizing input and output in aphasia (Darley, 1982) he quoted and elaborated upon one of Schuell's principal therapeutic beliefs, that of so-called auditory bombardment: "The first principle of treatment for aphasia should be use of intensive auditory stimulation, although not necessarily stimulation through auditory channels alone" (p. 187).

Others espoused the primacy of auditory stimulation as well. Eisenson (1984) suggested that most aphasic patients recover considerable auditory comprehension in the early stages of their aphasic involvement, but stated, "The first principle of training for a patient with auditory disturbances . . . : *patients must learn to listen if they are to learn to understand what they hear*" (p. 213).

Davis (1983) emphasized that for most cases exercising auditory comprehension assumes primary emphasis during early treatment and stated, "At any linguistic level, the patient should demonstrate comprehension before he or she exercises verbal expression at that level" (p. 265).

Others (Duffy, 1981; Marshall, 1981) have reviewed principles underlying controlled, repetitive auditory stimulation and its role in facilitating language and heightening auditory comprehension.

Although we feel that auditory comprehension training retains an important role in treatment, we are not as willing to accept it as prescription, uncritically and without caveat, or without a careful assessment of each aphasic individual's specific problems and response to treatment.

A CAVEAT

Rosenbek (1979) has suggested that our strong reliance on auditory comprehension training may have generated unmet expectations and that the assumptions underlying "auditory bombardment" are in need of testing and perhaps revision. Others (Gardner & Winner, 1978; Prins et al., 1978) have suggested that in certain forms of aphasia, comprehension and production may become dissociated. This observation would raise serious questions about the economy or effectiveness of expecting auditory comprehension training to exert an indirect beneficial effect on other language modalities.

Marshall and Neuburger (1984) reported on four aphasic subjects who were given "extended comprehension training." All of their subjects improved in comprehension performance, and two of the four demonstrated a correlate change in production of the same items. Although their sample is hardly large enough to engender flights of generality to the aphasic population as a whole, Marshall and Neuburger concluded that the notion of auditory bombardment and particularly its effect on production tasks is in need of reconsideration.

We are not ready to abandon emphasis on auditory comprehension and processing in aphasia treatment, but we are not as willing to approach it with the less critical eye of our early years.

INFLUENCES ON TREATMENT DECISIONS

Just as with other processes, a host of factors influences treatment decisions. Aphasia type, relative severity of impairment across the modalities, psycholinguistic interactions, communicative need, occupational-educational differences, and amount of nonlanguage involvement are all important. Deciding on targets or therapeutic objectives and the subsequent preparation of tasks or activities deemed to be appropriate to those objectives is one of the most crucial jobs of the clinician. These decisions are fused to and molded by the unique characteristics of each human who comes through the clinic door. Tasks must be designed, refined, and custom tailored to suit the idiosyncratic pattern of deficit and communicative need that has been revealed by careful appraisal. Treatment planning and task construction is hard to teach and born of experience, and few resources are available to the beginner as topographic maps to guide the hike. But the clinician must be aware of the myriad of variables that can influence auditory performance in order to select and order stimuli during treatment.

Darley's (1982) chapter on maximizing input and output is a comprehensive collection of factors extracted from clinical research in aphasia that can aid the clinician in controlling variables that can facilitate language performance. The elements that comprise the antecedent event in the treatment process, and that can be most readily manipulated to affect language performance, are discussed as well by LaPointe (1985). The most potent aspect of control over the antecedent event in treatment is in stimulus manipulation. As clinicians we can control what we stimulate a patient with and how we present it. Thousands of variables exist along those two dimensions; and manipulation of each can make tasks easier or more difficult. The introduction, pattern and duration of presentation, hierarchical arrangement of stimulus sets, and our techniques of shaping, correcting, and stabilizing patient responses is the stuff of therapy. Knowing the influences that work to vary the capacity of stimuli to arouse, evoke associations, and elicit responses is crucial to good intervention. Table 7-1 lists some of the principal aspects of auditory input that can differentially affect language performance.

TABLE 7-1.
Auditory Input Features That Facilitate or Degrade Comprehension.

Feature	Explanation	Effect
Repetition, Redundancy (Gardner et al., 1975 LaPointe et al., 1978)	Restimulation	Improvement
Saliency (Goodglass, 1973	Prominence, significance, affective value	Varies, depending on saliency value
Loudness (McNeil, 1977)	Intensifies input	No improvement
Selective Binaural Stimulation (LaPointe et al., 1978 McNeil, 1977)	Selects, channels intensity input	No improvement
Masking Noise (Wertz & Porch, 1970)	Covers or distracts	Poorer performance or marked variability
Background Noise (Skelly, 1975)	Covers primary signal	Poorer
Directness of Wording (Green & Boller, 1974)	Length, nonsubstantive wording variations	Some improvement
Speaker Position (Albert & Bear, 1976)	Face visible	Improvement
Emotional Content (Boller et al., 1977)	Emotional content vs. neutral content	Improvement
Modality Combination (Lambrecht & Marshall, 1983)	Live, audio, videotape	No differences
Telephone Presentation (Raymer & LaPointe, 1983)	Live auditory, live auditory and visual, telephone	Degradation in some
Alerting Signals (Loverso & Prescott, 1981)	Warnings, tones	Some improvement
Syntactic Complexity (Shewan & Canter, 1971)	Grammatical manipulations	Greater complexity degrades
Rate Reduction, Pause (Lasky et al., 1976; (Salvatore, 1974)	Slower rate, more pauses	Improvement for some subjects

RATE MANIPULATION, PAUSE INSERTION

Our patients tell us we speak too fast for good comprehension. They tell us, "Slow down!" "Where's the fire?" "That goes in, and before I figure it out, it's gone." One of our patients made the classic remark, "You speak in books, and I can only understand in pages." Skelly (1975) and others who have catalogued suggestions to others by people with aphasia have shown that speech rate is near the top of the list in practical suggestions for improving communication. At least a dozen studies of the facilitating effects of speech rate have been completed with aphasic subjects, and most demonstrated positive effects of either rate reduction or appropriate pause placement. Many of these studies were reviewed or summarized by Darley (1982), Marshall (1981), or LaPointe (1985).

The relative speech rate of health care professionals when conversing with nonaphasic and aphasic hospital patients has also been studied (Gravel & LaPointe, 1982, 1983, 1984). Generally, health care professionals do not spontaneously slow their speech rate in discourse with aphasic individuals with known auditory comprehension impairment. In fact, some professionals talk faster to people with aphasia, although other linguistic facilitating effects may be used such as length reduction and increased redundancy.

Some writers have questioned the consistency of rate manipulation effects, however. In a report by Nicholas and Brookshire (1985) aphasic, right-hemisphere-damaged, and non-brain-damaged subjects listened to 10 stories. This study used half fast rate manipulation, in that half the stories were presented at a slow speech rate and half at a fast speech rate. Comprehension and retention of stated and implied main ideas and story details were tested after each story. For both stated and implied main ideas, only aphasic subjects with low comprehension showed a significant decline in performance for the fast rate. All subject groups performed worse on story details at the fast rate. Despite the caution by Nicholas and Brookshire that consistent facilitory effects are not always seen, the consensus of a considerable amount of clinical research and the voluminous pleas of our patients suggest that judicious and appropriate rate reduction and pause insertion is worth incorporating.

"GET READY, GET SET, GO": ALERTING SIGNALS

An attractive parameter of stimulus manipulation has been the span of time before a verbal message is presented. Because so many theories of aphasia recognize the contribution of attention-arousal problems to impairment of comprehension, an intuitive intervention strategy seems to be to alert the receiver prior to message delivery. "Get ready, Mr. Babcock! Here it comes. . ." is a clinical trick that, on the surface at least, appears to have some validity as a facilitator of auditory comprehension. After all, nonaphasic subjects benefit from a warning signal, and reaction time measurements have demonstrated that an alerting signal causes faster reaction time. Allowing a person to get ready for a signal enhances detection of that signal. These and other aspects of the manipulation of alerting signals were reviewed by Loverso and Prescott (!981), who also studied the use of alerting signals on the ability of aphasic subjects to make "same-different" judgments. Loverso and Prescott reported that both nonaphasic and aphasic subjects' accuracy and reaction times were facilitated by the use of a 750 Hz tone presented bilaterally. An important point seemed to be the closeness in time of the alerting signal to the visual stimuli presented. Aphasic subjects were slower than nonaphasic subjects and did not benefit from the full effect of the forewarning until it was spaced one to three seconds before stimulus onset. The aphasic subjects, then, seemed to require more warning time for optimal facilitation to take place, and Loverso and Prescott (1981) concluded that this appears to support Wepman's "shutter principle." The speculation that aphasic subjects may not be able to move the processing system to an active state as quickly as nonaphasic subjects is the basis for the so-called shutter-principle.

Although Loverso and Prescott's report offered some evidence in a comforting direction, much remains to be studied on the facilitating effect of alerting signals. Clinical usefulness of such strategies must be explored carefully with individual clients with aphasia. Clinically, the alerting signals can take many forms. They can include saying the person's name, a touch on the hand or arm, saying "ready," "listen," or "here it comes," or, as in an example provided by one of our friends and a master clinician, the raising of the hand to signal a change in topic (P. Holtzapple, personal communication, 1985).

OBJECT-PICTURE STIMULUS VARIABLES

Interpretation of auditory comprehension can sometimes hinge on the stimulus items used for assessment or on factors unrelated to auditory function alone. For example, pointing to objects in the room may place more demand on visual search, and a variety of selectional, attentional, and memory skills than pointing to objects in an array of items. Helm-Estabrooks (1981) noticed a difference in auditory comprehension scores of the same severely impaired aphasic patients when asked to point to environmental objects as opposed to pictured objects. She studied 21 subjects and found that, as a group, subjects scored significantly more accurately when pointing to pictured objects than when pointing to the same real objects located in their natural setting. This might seem a surprising result to those of us who expect the more natural, commonly dealt with context to be optimally facilitating.

Helm-Estabrooks (1981) reported that a few individual subjects performed unlike the rest of the group. She suggested that some patients might have difficulty *finding* objects rather than merely recognizing them, and that therapy might be directed more economically toward improving visual search skills.

Darley's (1982) summary of the effects of auditory input manipulation on facilitation of language is a guide not only to task preparation and treatment planning but also to conversational interaction with aphasic persons. We should try to make auditory stimuli as salient, prominent, unambiguous, and clear as possible. Increasing our loudness, as we tend to do to non-native speakers of our language, probably will not help, but freedom from background noise and distractions will. Direct rather than indirect wording and uncomplicated syntactic complexity helps, as does repetition, manipulation of timing variables, live presentation, and emotionally arousing content (Darley, 1982).

THE TREATMENT SEQUENCE

Our treatment takes many forms, depending upon the needs of the patient and the moment. Sometimes it is casual and conversational and serves as an opportunity to check connected speech and discourse skills. Most of the time, however, it is more structured than unstructured. We like to have a firm grasp of our goals and in reports and treatment plans will write down both short-term and long-range objectives in fairly operationally defined terms. The overriding objective of just about every session is to attempt to facilitate maximal return of volitional control of communication by the aphasic person. This goal crosses modalities, linguistic processes, and levels of severity. In treating auditory comprehension, as in treating speaking skills, we like to keep track of responses and graph progress by some sort of session by session recordkeeping system that preserves samples of patient performance but can be carried out online and relatively unobtrusively. The BASE-10 Response Form (LaPointe, 1977a) is one way to do this and helps us organize and present our stimuli, keep track of progress, and answer clinical questions that relate to generalizations of nontrained items.

No unalterable format of a typical structured treatment session exists, but once we have decided on our clinical targets (e.g., the ability to follow short commands), selected and ordered stimuli, decided on how to score and preserve patient responses, and measured base rates of performance, we are ready to attempt to modify, shape, or facilitate inadequate responses. The sequence presented in Table 7-2 is typical of a clinical interaction or treatment sequence for many, but not all, tasks. Not all steps are utilized with each patient and flexibility must be preserved to work with each individual at the level appropriate at the time. This sequence of therapeutic interaction occurs frequently enough for both input and output tasks to suggest that it can be used as a broadly conceived model for many therapeutic activities.

This treatment sequence has been adapted from the work of many clinicians and researchers, principally Vignolo (1964) and Basso (1978) and has been presented previously by LaPointe (1982).

It takes much longer to write or read this sequence than to actually practice it. The clinician-patient interaction should be dynamic and paced to the level of the patient, and frequently resembles a rapid interchange liberally sprinkled with modeling, shaping, prompting, cueing, and large doses of appropriate, genuine, positive reinforcement.

TABLE 7-2.
The Treatment Sequence.

Step	Activity	Example
1.	*Isolate the error*	Picture cards scored as incorrect separated (Polaroid photographs of family members).
2.	*Indicate, explain nature of error* (semantic, syntactic, phonologic, other)	"You pointed to Gene, your son, on this one. I asked you to point to Jane."
3.	*Model corrected version* A. Produce correctly B. Contrast correct-incorrect	 "Watch me. Here's Jane. This one is Jane." "Gene is over here. That's not what I asked. Here's Jane. This one is Jane."
4.	*Patient produces corrected response* (reinforce) A. With clinician B. Alone (cues, prompts to facilitate response)	 "Point with me. Show me Jane. Where's Jane?" (Fade clinician's gesture) "Point to Jane. Where's Jane?" "Good. That's right, you've got it."
5.	*Repetition-stabilization* (reinforce) A. Immediate B. With delay	 "Point to Jane. Show me Jane. Good. Three times now. Show me Jane. Show me Jane. Show me Jane. Good." "Point to Jane. Wait. Not yet..." (3 to 5 second delay). "Watch my signal. Now. Good."
6.	*Transition to volitional control* (laddering: increase length, complexity, naturalness)	"Show me your daughter. Good. Which one of these pictures is your first-born? Good. Show me Jane and show me your wife. Great! Way to go!"
7.	Restimulate in original form (optional)	"Point to Jane. Show me Jane."

From LaPointe (1982).

SPECIFIC TREATMENT TECHNIQUES

Relatively few books in aphasia have been written from the perspective of the clinician charged with management of the aphasic person. Many more pages have been devoted to discussions of the symptomatology and localization of auditory comprehension impairment than to how to improve it. The clinician interested in specific treatment techniques can find them in a few sources, however. Darley (1982), Marshall (1981), and LaPointe (1985) have presented specific examples of intervention strategies. Davis (1983) presented some exercises for auditory problems and gave advice on task construction and intervention strategies for specific problems as did Shewan and Bandur (1986). From our clinical experience and from a variety of other sources we have gleaned the following suggestions that relate to specific disorders.

ATTENTION

Inattention is common in fluent aphasia resulting from posterior lesions. Distractibility and short attention span are characteristic of poor "therapeutic set." Patients tend to talk when listening is appropriate, fade away from instructions, and not accept readily the demands of a task. Treatment suggestions include:

1. Listen to auditory stimuli and make differential response between two choices.

2. Discriminate among nonverbal, environmental sounds.

3. Imitate modeled pointing responses to pictures representing environmental sounds.

4. Listen for and discriminate among target words.

5. Listen for numerals and signal target in numeric sequence.

6. Alter number and order of response arrays with single target.

7. Auditory vigilance drills—words and numbers are taped randomly and target is signaled. Attempt to increase spans of vigilance with low error rates.

SEVERE COMPREHENSION DEFICIT

The programs for global aphasia described in other chapters are applicable to severe comprehension deficit, such as Helm-Estabrooks and colleagues' Visual Action Therapy (VAT) (1982). Marshall's Auditory Comprehension Training (ACT) (1981), has levels appropriate to the severely involved patient.

1. *Picture-object pointing:* Instructions are uncomplicated or able to be gestured. Stimuli are frequent, concrete, functional, and repeated.

2. *Picture-object pointing:* Manipulate parameters of rate, familiarity, emotionality, form class (noun, verb, etc.), number in response array, imposed delay.

3. *Yes/No questions:* Body parts and necessary functional environmental objects can be used to stabilize yes/no responses. We have used a two-color light box to aid consistency of head nodding/shaking as well. Stable and reliable yes/no response is sometimes crucial to communication in patients with severe verbal impairment.

4. *Whole-body commands:* Axial or midline body movements and whole-body commands are easier for some patients. Short, concrete commands using these movements can be incorporated into drills with some individuals. As with all suggested activities,

expansion and gradual movement toward more complex, functional language use should be incorporated.

PHONEMIC DISCRIMINATION

Few aphasic patients seem to present or remain at a level of impaired phonemic discrimination. Eisenson (1984), in suggestions to improve discriminative hearing, stated, "The patient must direct attention to the overall meaning of an utterance, to visual components of articulation, to inflection, stress, and intonation [in order] to compensate for impaired phonemic discrimination" (p. 214). If recovery or compensation do not take care of the problems, the clinician can try:

1. *Minimal pair distinction:* Live voice or tape-recorded stimuli can be presented and the patient responds by pointing to appropriate pictures ("peas-bees," "nail-mail," "Aunty Rose-panty hose").

2. *Phonetic fusion:* With some agraphic or alexic patients with peculiar dissociation syndromes, spelling a word aloud may help them recognize it. Though we have not observed the analog of this condition in the auditory mode, occasionally patients benefit from breaking down and reconstructing the phonetic elements of a difficult word.

FLUENT APHASIA, WERNICKE'S APHASIA

The combination of reduced comprehension and inattention due to press of speech can create a real challenge for the clinician faced with task construction for fluent aphasia. For Wernicke's aphasia and other types of disruption, a number of clinicians have attempted to train comprehension skills by using Token Test–like training procedures. West (1973) treated mild to moderately involved patients and found they improved on her treatment task, but did not display significant change on portions of the Minnesota Test for Differential Diagnosis of Aphasia (MTDDA).

Holland and Sonderman's (1974) mild to moderate patients made gains on their Token Test treatment task, but moderate to severe patients made no gains. Neither group showed improved posttreatment on selected MTDDA subtests.

Burger and Wertz (1984) described a token treatment paradigm with a 73-year-old man with Wernicke's aphasia, who underwent twice a week, 60 minute sessions for 34 sessions. They reported erratic, variable performance across treatment and generalization phases. The patient's family reported that he "participates more in conversations and understands them better following the Token Test treatment" (p. 179), but Burger and Wertz expressed disappointment with the lack of change in treatment phase data points.

No disappointment, however, can be expressed over careful attempts to measure performance change using cautious single-subject treatment designs. Burger and Wertz demonstrated a sound design that can be replicated with other subjects to try to add more to what we understand about specific treatment packages. Other techniques with fluent aphasia include:

1. *Stop strategies:* Signals to stop talking (especially gestures) and structured and allocated response times help some fluent aphasic patients relearn the pragmatics of turn-taking in discourse.

2. *Re-statement or paraphrasing:* Tasks that paraphrase or restate can be directed at reduced self-monitoring abilities, if a series of original utterances are tape-recorded, played back, and paraphrased. Error or off the topic awareness may be improved in patients who demonstrate reduced recognition of their difficulty.

SHORT-TERM MEMORY—INFORMATION PROCESSING DEFICIT

Davis (1983) suggested ways to differentially exercise short-term memory and comprehension processes. We are not so sure of our attempts to dissociate these processes, but clinical experience has suggested that tasks can be constructed along the following lines:

1. *Capacity:* Digit or unit span can be measured (number of units that can be

immediately recalled or indicated in some fashion) and tasks constructed that attempt to gradually stretch capacity.

2. *Retention:* Impaired delay tasks with gradual increase in delay times can be used to attempt to decrease decay.

3. *Rehearsal:* There is some evidence to suggest that aphasic patients with verbal formulation problems cannot or will not rehearse; and we know from the literature on normal verbal learning that rehearsal is necessary for storage and retrieval of material. Nevertheless, tasks can be constructed to prompt rehearsal of incoming stimuli (e.g., phone number, grocery list drills).

4. *Memory tricks:* Mnemonics, pegging, linking, chunking, and clustering are all strategies from the literature on training normal recall and retention. Few of these strategies have been attempted in aphasia and those few that have been tried have met with limited success. They deserve to be tried, though, and formulated into testable hypotheses about the recall and retention of people with aphasia.

SENTENCE, DISCOURSE COMPREHENSION

As Davis pointed out (1983), tasks for exercising sentence comprehension are very similar to those used for evaluating this function. Syntactic and semantic manipulations with a control on length can be accomplished by selection of stimuli similar to those in the Auditory Comprehension Test for Sentences (ACTS) developed by Shewan (1979). Other tasks include:

1. *Pointing to pictures:* Pictures can be collected, assembled, or purchased that vary semantic, syntactic, spatial, or transformational information.

2. *Following instructions:* The token tasks described for fluent aphasia can be used for following instructions. Flowers and Danforth (1979) described such programs as did the previously cited researchers.

3. *Sentence verification:* Verification of correct sentences where a picture is used with

two verbally presented sentences (e.g., a picture of a baseball player being hit by a pitch is presented. The patient indicates which sentence applies: "The baseball player is hitting the ball," or "The ball is hitting the baseball player").

4. *Answering questions:* Questions must be designed to fit the verbal capabilities of the patient. They can be yes/no, short answer, or more elaborate. These can be easily customized or tailored to the individual (e.g., "Do you have a golden retriever?" "Do you drive a beat-up 1964 Buick Skylark with one fender missing?" "Were you born in Sagola, Michigan?"). Memory demands can be manipulated by a format that uses a statement followed by a question (Davis, 1983) (e.g., "The ore train leaves Iron River at 3:00 and arrives at Channing at 5:45. What time does the train leave Iron River?").

LISTENING SKILLS FOR MILD COMPREHENSION IMPAIRMENT

The mild aphasic patient has been generally neglected in aphasia research. Raymer and LaPointe (1986) presented a viewpoint on the importance of intervention in mild aphasia, and discussed the nature and assessment of the so-called mildly impaired patient. Very little has been written about the improvement or enhancement of listening skills in aphasia, mild or otherwise. Considerable information is available on the development of general listening skills in nonaphasic people. Wolvin and Coakley (1985) discussed factors influencing the listening process, methods of improving the generation of feedback, skills involved in listening and auditory discrimination, types of listening (critical, appreciative, therapeutic, comprehensive), and strategies for improving listening skills. Application of these concepts to aphasia are untested but worthy of consideration if we are to discover techniques that are appropriate to improving auditory comprehension in aphasia.

APPLIED PRAGMATICS

Conversational structure is incorporated into the treatment program developed by Davis

and Wilcox (1985). Promoting Aphasics' Communicative Effectiveness (PACE) was introduced by these clinical researchers in 1978 and the development of the system was traced in their 1985 publication. The program will be elaborated upon in subsequent chapters, particularly those that deal with treating verbal impairment (Chapter 10). Several pragmatic components are built into PACE therapy, including expression of a wide range of speech acts, turn-taking between participants, hint-and-guess sequences when communication breakdown occurs, opportunities to express and comprehend given and new information, and opportunities to use paralinguistic and extralinguistic contexts.

One of the four fundamental principles of PACE therapy is that the clinician and the client participate equally as sender and receiver of messages. PACE treatment allows the client to serve as a respondent, and this role emphasizes a very different set of communicative behaviors. Davis and Wilcox (1985) suggested that these skills are based largely upon receptive processes, in that the client is required to decode relevant contextual information and apply given and new conventions to the message that is received. Several examples of treatment that concentrate on receptive skills are provided and one strategy that is emphasized is that of attempting to increase client use of contingent queries. Contingent queries are simply requests for clarification or additional information. Contingent queries might take the form of:

1. *Nonvocal contingent query:* Any nonverbal indication that further information is desired (e.g., raised eyebrows, an inquiring look).

2. *Vocal contingent query:* Vocal indication that further information is desired (e.g., "huh?" or "humm?").

3. *Verbal contingent query:* Production of appropriate linguistic response (e.g., "Say what?" "What's that?" "What do you mean?").

Contingent queries have been studied with aphasic subjects by Apel, Newhoff, and Browning-Hall (1982) and by Prinz (1980). In addition to specific prompting, the clinician can serve as a model for increasing an aphasic

TABLE 7-3.
Tasks for Auditory Comprehension.

Tasks—Activities
Understanding words–body parts
Understanding words–objects
Understanding words–pictures of objects
Understanding words–food items
Understanding words–room objects
Understanding words–action pictures
Understanding words–pages of advertisements, products
Understanding descriptions–body parts
Understanding descriptions–objects
Understanding descriptions–pictures of objects
Understanding descriptions–pages of advertisements, products
Understanding descriptions–photographs from magazines
Understanding shorter questions–yes/no questions (factual)
Understanding shorter questions–yes/no (absurdities)
Understanding shorter questions–yes/no (general facts)
Understanding sentences–yes/no (true-false)
Understanding sentences–yes/no (definitions)
Understanding questions–yes/no (family photographs)
Understanding questions–point to (family photographs)
Understanding shorter directions–("blink eyes," etc.)
Understanding shorter directions–objects
Understanding shorter directions–pencil and paper directions
Understanding sentences–read sentences and questions
Response switching
Listening to taped newscasts
Sentence verification tasks
Responding to questions
Structured token tasks
Attention-alerting tasks
Capacity increasing drills
Retention drills
Imposed delays
Syntactic manipulation with length control
Syntactic manipulation with lexical control
Alerting signal tasks
Associational pausing
Discriminative listening (main idea)
Discrminative listening (story details)
One, two, three stage commands
Sequential assembly

person's ability to disambiguate messages by making a special point of producing contingent queries during message reception. PACE format provides a good means of developing this communicative strategy. "Tell me that again," "Slow down, please," "I didn't get all of that," "Run that by me again," are all very appropriate attempts by the aphasic listener to gain more control of a communicative situation and can be used profitably during PACE interaction.

MANUALS AND PROGRAMS

An increasing number of manuals and programs are becoming available for use with auditory comprehension disorders, including the use of microcomputer assisted instruction. The disadvantage of most workbooks or manuals is that they neglect the idiosyncrasies of the individual patient, they do not ensure entry at the appropriate severity level, and many are quite expensive. The major advantage is that they provide a spectrum of stimulus materials in the format of pictures, questions, and commands in degrees of difficulty. The astute clinician can pick and choose those items that are appropriate to each patient. Programs and workbooks we have used with varying degrees of success include *Clinician Controlled Auditory Stimulation for Aphasic Adults* (Marshall, 1978), *Language Rehabilitation: Auditory Comprehension for Patients with Aphasia* (Martinoff, Martinoff, & Stokke, 1980), *Graduated Language Training for Patients with Aphasia* (Keith, 1980), *The Aphasic Patient: A Program for Auditory Comprehension and Language Training* (Baer, 1976), and *Sourcebook for Aphasia* (Brubaker, 1982).

THE INEVITABILITY OF THE COMPUTER

Treatment of auditory comprehension impairment by using the microcomputer may prove to be a means of extending the number of individuals that can be seen for treatment, or of providing greater amounts of therapy for selected appropriate problems. A microcomputer program that uses a digitized speech production peripheral attachment was reported by Mills (1982). He used this equipment to study the effectiveness of an auditory comprehension training program with an aphasic subject who was 16 months postonset. Mills reported improvement on all three difficulty levels of a word recognition task as well as correlate improvement on Token Test and PICA auditory subtest scores. The conclusions of this study on the effectiveness of the training on changes in comprehension must be tempered by limitations of the study design, as no withdrawal or multiple baseline single-subject research strategies were used, but, at the very least, this study points the way to future use of the computer for treatment. The reading and writing modalities appear to be more adaptable to computer use at this stage of technological development, as will be demonstrated in subsequent chapters.

We finish this chapter on treating auditory comprehension by presenting a summary table of tasks that have been mentioned, studied, or used in aphasia treatment (Table 7-3). Most of the work on relative effectiveness of different treatment strategies is yet to be done, so we present these without endorsement or evaluation but rather in the spirit of shared clinical suggestions that sorely need testing. We leave it to the judiciousness and clinical sense of the reader to pick and choose those which may be useful and discard those which prove to be unworkable.

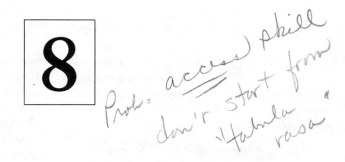

Prob: access skill
don't start from
"tabula rasa"

8

ACQUIRED DYSLEXIA:
TREATING READING PROBLEMS
ASSOCIATED WITH APHASIA

J udging from the lack of literature and the relatively meager research effort afforded to the subject, at the prom of aphasia, reading impairment has achieved the popularity of a bird in the punch bowl. Certainly in relation to its younger cousin, developmental dyslexia, the adult, acquired version of reading impairment has been sorely neglected. At least this apathy has resulted in fewer misconceptions than the popular myths that dog childhood dyslexia. As Vellutino (1979) suggested "[A] number of prominent people, such as Albert Einstein, Nelson Rockefeller, and Lee Harvey Oswald, suffered from dyslexia in early childhood. Disorders that affect the famous and infamous are somehow accorded a degree of status and notoriety that inevitably breeds folklore and misconception" (p. xi).

Perhaps one of the few misconceptions about acquired dyslexia is that it is a trivial residual of aphasia and should be mopped up last, if at all. In our view, that attitude is counterproductive. Certainly, not every person values the gift of reading equally, but to neglect its assessment and intervention equally across those who suffer aphasia is to lose the opportunity to restore what some would consider to be a primary ingredient in what constitutes the good life.

CONTRASTS BETWEEN ACQUIRED AND DEVELOPMENTAL DYSLEXIA

Fundamental differences exist between the child and the adult. Differences are apparent in reading disability, too. Although a vast literature exists, much of it equivocal on nature and remediation, the principles and approaches used in dealing with developmental dyslexia may or may not be appropriate to the adult. Some of these differences are important to consider, including:

Adults, unless illiterate, were once able to read, and had an intact as opposed to a developing language system.

This means that we are not beginning with a blank slate or a partially filled slate, and that we are more likely dealing with an access problem instead of a learning problem. Treatment approaches may focus to a large extent on facilitation strategies instead of the gradual accumulation of new skills and bits of information. If an aphasic patient is illiterate, reading disability probably should not be a part of the clinician's intervention plan, as other communicative deficits will be crying for attention and will no doubt be more amenable to change.

Reading impairment that accompanies adult aphasia is rarely the only difficulty.

One could argue that this is true in children as well, but the dramatic convolutions and distortions of syntax and semantics that cross many language modalities in aphasia confound reading problems enormously in adults. This means that morphosyntactic problems, paraphasias, reduced auditory comprehension, motor speech impairment, and other components or concomitants of aphasia may get in the way of a direct attack on reading and careful priorities of attention and strategies of circumvention must be formulated.

Most reading materials useful with children are not directly suitable or appropriate to adult interests.

Most adults have outgrown their unbridled curiosity about Little Sally's Surprise and the adventures of Spot and Puff. This is not to suggest that adults do not find delight in occasionally picking up the threads of childhood, but to confront an educated, mature, aphasic adult with reading materials that are filled with Bozos, balloons, and space monsters is to risk serious insult to that person's sensibilities. Enough harmful residual

stereotypes about the nature of aphasia exist (Plumridge, LaPointe, & Lombardino, 1985) without reinforcing the myth that aphasia is a regression to previous developmental stages of language use. Aphasic adults must not be infantilized, and attention to the materials we select for evaluation and treatment is a good place to start.

MODELS OF READING: PHONICS OR LOOK-SEE?

In the thrilling days of yesteryear, when most people in the authors' generation were learning to read the boringly repetitive antics of Dick, Jane, Sally, Spot, and Puff, an issue began to emerge among educators as to whether or not "phonics" or "look-see" methods were necessary for reading skill acquisition. The controversy surrounding that issue has remained alive and vigorous for several decades. In fact, analysis of the reading impairment of acquired dyslexia has both fueled the controversy and shed new light.

The primary argument revolved around whether the acquisition or disruption of reading involves phonological recoding, recognition and appreciation of the visual forms of printed material, or both. Figure 8-1 (adapted from Coltheart, 1980, p. 202) is a schematic representation of processes that have been postulated to be involved in the comprehension and/or pronunciation of printed letter strings. In this model, comprehension is assumed as soon as a printed letter string (if

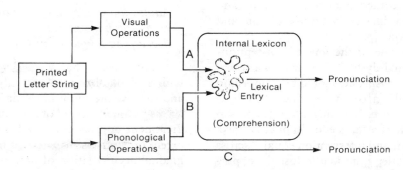

Figure 8-1. Schematic representation of processes thought to be involved in comprehension and/or pronunciation of printed letter strings. Adapted from Coltheart (1980, p. 202).

it is a known word) reaches the operation of lexical entry.

Some theories of reading processes propose that access to a specific lexical entry within the internal lexicon *requires* a phonological recoding process (letters are converted to sounds by grapheme-phoneme conversion rules). Others have disavowed the need for phonological processes and claim that reading only requires visual processes. "Dual-access" theories propose that both pathways exist and can be called upon for different purposes.

The symptom patterns of Japanese dyslexic patients have provided some evidence on the issue of reading processes and pathways. The Japanese orthography symbol systems, *kana* (phonetically based syllable symbols) and *kanji* (nonphonetic, logographic symbola for lexical morphemes), are used in combination. Because of this dual nature of Japanese writing, various types of dissociation have been reported in brain damaged subjects. A series of careful studies of the relative impairment-intactness of *kana* versus *kanji* processing was summarized and reported by Sasanuma (1980), and she concluded, "The findings obtained in the present study would seem to be in accord with a tentative conclusion that the dual access model of reading provides a useful, as well as valid framework" (p. 86).

UNDERLYING MECHANISMS

Other possible mechanisms that result in acquired dyslexia are not precisely understood at this time and no doubt vary across individuals with changes in etiology, site and extent of lesion, and a host of subject variables. Both single factor and multifactor theories have been proposed and these have been reviewed by Vellutino (1979). Single factor explanations postulate a rather vague general deficiency in "visual-spatial organization" whereas multifactor theories implicate deficits in linguistic processing that involve both auditory and visual systems. Four fundamental deficiencies postulated to be central to the disorder include the areas of: (1) visual

perception or visual memory, (2) crossmodal association or intersensory integration, (3) serial order recall or attentional factors, and (4) lexical-semantic or morphosyntactic processing. Time and continuing research effort may reveal the validity of these postulates or reveal others equally important.

Certainly, reading is a more complex process than the rather simplistic models would lead us to believe, but they allow us at least to gain a rudimentary appreciation of the fundamental processes involved. Ultimately, understanding of the reading process may point to treatment or strategies of compensation.

TERMINOLOGY AND TYPES

A rich variety of labels and classification schemes have been used to describe reading problems. Benson (1979a) and LaPointe and Kraemer (1983) have catalogued a few of these attempts. Such terms as *pure word blindness*, *strephosymbolia*, *occipital alexia*, and *tertiary alexia*, *agnostic alexia*, and *motor alexia* are but a few. Dejerine's pioneering efforts in his carefully crafted reports of the early 1890s laid the groundwork for the eventual acceptance of two primary types of acquired reading deficit: *alexia with agraphia*, associated with a dominant parietal lobe lesion, and *alexia without agraphia*, associated with damage to the dominant occipital lobe and a specific portion of the corpus callosum. Benson (1977) contended that a third clinically distinct variety of alexia is related to damage to the frontal language areas and is associated with Broca's aphasia. Finally, the entity of *deep dyslexia* has attracted a good deal of attention, particularly from neurolinguists, and will be considered here in appropriate depth.

ALEXIA WITH AGRAPHIA disturbance of reading + writing

Alexia with agraphia is the clinical variety of reading loss that is most frequently noted in the evaluation of aphasia.

The primary features are disturbances of both reading and writing. Cerebral pathology is most evident in the dominant posterior language areas of the cortex, and for that reason, Benson and others have referred to it as *parietal-temporal alexia*. Site and extent of the lesion determine the exact nature of the impairment as well as the course of recovery. Generally, individuals will be able to produce letters and letter combinations that resemble words, and the comprehension deficit sometimes appears to be at such a basic symbolic level that even numbers or musical notation cannot be deciphered. Of course, gradients of the disorder exist and depending on neuropathogenic factors, a wide variety of severity levels can be seen across patients.

ALEXIA WITHOUT AGRAPHIA

As in all types of neurogenic reading disturbance, a variety of neuropathologies such as tumor, vascular disruption, head trauma, disease, and toxic processes can create a language problem, and it takes a very specific and clearly defined interhemispheric disconnection to create alexia without agraphia. As reviewed in some detail elsewhere (LaPointe & Kramer, 1983), this syndrome has been associated repeatedly in the literature with cerebral infarction in the distribution of the dominant *posterior* cerebral artery. Most commonly, the disconnection necessary to create the syndrome occurs from damage to the left medial occipital lobe of the cortex and in the splenium or posterior section of the corpus callosum, that rich bundle of fibers that allows information to be transferred from the left to the right hemisphere. Benson (1979a) called the syndrome *occipital alexia*, and, in essence, the primary underlying reason for reading impairment is disconnection of the visual-verbal pathways (occipital association cortex from the dominant angular gyrus). The damaged dominant (usually left) occipital visual association area prevents appreciation of written or printed material and the coexisting lesion in the splenium of the corpus callosum prevents transfer of information and blocks participation by intact visual association areas of the nondominant hemisphere.

No identifiable cluster of reading errors has been associated with alexia without agraphia. The singular feature that makes the syndrome unique is the remarkably preserved ability to write in the context of impaired reading. One of the most frequent clinical observations is that the afflicted individual will produce a string of legible written words and then be unable to read what was just written.

ASSOCIATED DEFICITS. Several associated neurologic and behaviorial deficits have been reported to be associated with alexia without agraphia. Because the etiology that creates the syndrome is usually vascular, other areas within the distribution boundaries of the posterior cerebral artery can be and frequently are affected. Neighborhood deficits are well documented. Many patients also show right visual field deficit. Paralysis and hemisensory loss is usually absent, but often color agnosia is present. This manifests itself in an inability to name colors presented visually, although no problem is experienced with color names in conversation or by auditory comprehension (e.g., "What color is a dog's tongue?").

Other accompaniments to the syndrome include verbal memory impairment, mild anomia or word retrieval difficulty in speech, abnormal written calculation, difficulty in number naming and sometimes impaired musical notation reading (in those who could read music, of course).

FRONTAL ALEXIA

Frontal alexia, which Benson called the third alexia, is reported to be associated with Broca's aphasia. According to some reseachers, the frontal reading disturbance differs from the other types in that the individual comprehends lexical-semantic words better than "relational" or syntactic structures. Four factors have been cited to explain frontal alexia, including: (1) an optic factor relating to paresis of gaze, (2) the inability to maintain appropriate sequence of verbal material, (3) the inability to comprehend syntactic structure (the well-recognized agrammatic disruption associated with anterior lesions [e.g., Zurif, Caramazza, & Myerson, 1972]), and (4) literal alexia, or a selective problem in recognizing or naming individual letters of the alphabet.

As Benson (1977) suggested, although it

is possible to consider the process of reading as a holistic, universal function (and recent evidence from cerebral regional blood flow studies lend support to this notion), clinical evaluations demonstrate definable variations in reading breakdown apparently dependent on location of underlying neuropathology in the central nervous system. This notion is another reason why careful and comprehensive evaluation is being seen increasingly as vital to understanding neurogenic reading impairment.

DEEP DYSLEXIA

Not infrequently, advances in our understanding of aphasia have been made after the impetus provided by careful description of a single case. The area of reading disorders seems to have benefited from the misfortune of the subject G. R., described first by Marshall and Newcombe in 1966. The most striking aspect of G. R.'s behavior after sustaining left hemisphere injury was the large number of semantic errors during attempts to read aloud. Analysis of G. R., along with a subsequent flood of inquiry with similar objectives, not only provided a description of specific types of reading error, which are useful to effective clinical focus, but also "insinuated" the existence of a specific symptom-complex labeled *deep dyslexia*.

Semantic error was the primary feature of this disorder. For example, when G. R. read aloud, the following errors occurred:

act	"play"
close	"shut"
dinner	"food"
afternoon	"tonight"
uncle	"cousin"
tall	"long"

Follow-up study of G. R. (Marshall & Newcombe, 1973), as well as retrospective inspection of the reading errors described in six earlier studies in the literature, resulted in a refined description of the components of deep dyslexia (Marshall & Newcombe, 1980). Four additional components seemed to be part of the disorder. They included derivational errors, visual errors, inordinate function word impairment, and inability to read aloud pronounceable nonwords.

Derivational errors are misreadings of adjectives or verbs for the related nominal (or vice versa). For example,

wise	wisdom
strange	stranger
entertain	entertainment
calculation	calculator
employ	employers
truth	true
birth	born

Patterson (1980) studied derivational errors further and discovered that most derivational paralexias occurred on words with suffixes; that suffix deletion (i.e., hardest → hard), was the most frequent error, followed by suffix substitution (i.e., projection → projector); and some suffixes were more susceptible to error than others (i.e., -*ing* and -*er*).

Patterson raised the point that the existence of a separate category of derivational errors has been guaranteed by some, as these errors are so visually similar to the target. She stated however, "To the extent that root and bound morphemes can be shown to receive separable processing, there is some independent justification for maintaining the derivational classification of paralexias" (1980, p. 304).

In deep dyslexia subjects, errors in which there is a clear visual or shape similarity between the target or stimulus word and the oral response also are common. For example,

stock	shock
saucer	sausage
crowd	crown
crocus	crocodile

Syntax and form class also appear to be important variables in that concrete nouns are missed least frequently; adjectives, verbs, and abstract nouns were of intermediate difficulty; and function words were missed nearly every time they occurred. Even though errors on function words are common in aphasia, they are so frequent in deep dyslexia as to deserve a vital role in the symptom complex. For example,

for ————→ and
the ————→ yes
in ————→ those

The final category of error initially proposed by Marshall and Newcombe (1980) was that of inability to read pronounceable nonwords. As they put it, "Finally, we note that G. R. can never read aloud a non-word—an orthographically legal character string which happens not to have found a semantic niche in the English language" (p. 2). Examples of this disability include:

dup ————→ damp
zul ————→ zulu
wux ————→ "don't know"
jun ————→ jump

Evidence is accumulating that deep dyslexia may very well exist as a separate syndrome caused by some yet undiscovered single underlying mechanism. Coltheart (1980) and Saffran, Bogyo, Schwartz, and Marin (1980) have proposed involvement of the right hemisphere in the creation of the observed symptom complex in deep dyslexia. However, as Marshall and Newcombe (1980) cautioned, "But we must not ignore the possibility that we are studying an accident of anatomy and sampling, whose consequences have misled us by their tantalizing appearance of order" (p. 20).

Perhaps we will learn that the proposed cluster of symptoms of deep dyslexia is merely a reflection of the broader linguistic impairment that affects the other modalities as well; or that it may exist in relative isolation from other aphasia or modality effects.

The clinician's responsibility will remain, however, whether or not the syndrome is validated. That responsibility involves careful specification of intact and impaired skills, along the conditions across which these skills vary. The existence of a syndrome may lead to explanation and better understanding of the deficit or offer a shorthand approach for economical communication about deficit clusters, but careful individual evaluation and delineation of areas of difficulty still will be needed for adequate treatment planning and intervention.

READING AND THE ANGULAR GYRUS

In most models of reading and related cognitive function the posterior and lower area of the dominant parietal lobe (angular gyrus and immediate neighborhood) is suggested to be of critical importance. As mentioned by Hynd and Cohen (1983), some authors deny the uniqueness of this area in humans, but a strong case is made for its importance by a host of researchers who have constructed and refined conceptual models of reading (Geschwind, 1974; Pirozzolo, 1979). Geshwind (1974) argued that the cortical area around the angular gyrus is uniquely suited to the reading process because it lies between the association cortexes responsible for vision, audition, and somesthesis. Therefore, it is strategically placed to act as a processing center for associations that come from modalities vital to reading. Geschwind went so far as to call the angular gyrus the "association cortex of association cortexes" (p. 99).

Simplistic, schematic line drawings and diagrams of the brain and neural processes are doomed to inadequacy and have led more than one clinical researcher down the primrose path of the self-deluded belief that the arrows and boxes and "centers" truly represent how the complex nervous system operates. Recent advances in regional cerebral blood flow studies and other ingenious methods of brain imagery have underscored the complexity and synergy involved in even relatively simple higher cortical processes. This is not to negate the concept of relative localization of function, but only to underscore that the most frequent mistake of the box-drawers is to forget to remind us often enough that although simple models may help explanation, schematics are inherently simplifications, and that the multilevel complexity of the central nervous system sometimes does not lend itself well to hardwired, Radio Shack representations of complex cross-modal functions. As long as the student of higher cortical function is reminded of this caveat and accepts it, diagrams and schematics can and should be used efficiently as explanatory shortcuts of tentative hypotheses and theories. With these cautions in mind, the role of the angular gyrus in reading and the proposed pathways and sequences of transmission of the visual signal can be more accurately integrated into a system that no doubt includes a good deal of cortical and subcortical function.

A simple illustration of the implication of the angular gyrus in reading may be appreciated from the following example adapted from Hynd and Cohen (1983). Suppose an adult reads the sentence, "As soon as his fingers traced the silken skin of the contours of her face, the blinded Mr. Rochester realized that his beloved Jane had returned." In order to appreciate this bit of Brontë high drama, the visual impressions created by the print must be passed along the peripheral optic tract and pathways to the medial aspects of the occipital lobes (both left and right). Short association fibers transmit the perception to the association areas immediately adjacent to the primary visual zones, and the words take on some rudimentary meaning. A rich network of connecting fibers running to the area of the angular gyrus make associations available for cross reference and integration with impressions from other modalities. Thus, "silken skin," for example, may take on meaning as associations are formed by fibers connected to the sensory cortex. Similar associations may be made with the words "contours" or "face" by connections with other parietal cortex areas. Comprehension of these written images probably occurs by transmission to the cortical region incorporating Wernicke's area as well as the angular gyrus. If the passage were to be read aloud, Broca's area would become involved via the connecting fibers of the arcuate fasciculus. This example demonstrates the involvement of the angular gyrus and a single explanation of possible modes, or at least primary routes, during reading.

Figure 8-2 illustrates these possible cortical routes and it can be seen why such a variety of intramodal, crossmodal, or perceptual deficit types could result from lesions at various sites or levels.

EVALUATION

Assessing the reading of a person with aphasia is not easy. Just as problems exist in the general area of test construction in

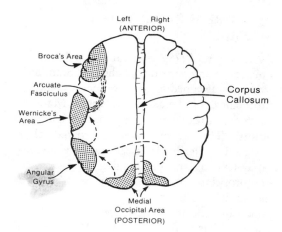

Figure 8-2. Cortical routes and areas thought to be involved in reading. Adapted from Hynd & Cohen (1983, p. 59). Reprinted with permission from The Psychological Corporation, Orlando, FL.

aphasia, there are compelling reasons for encountering difficulty in constructing tests of reading for people with aphasia. Failure on a reading task may not be due solely to the impairment of the fundamental process of reading. A variety of conditions can mimic or secondarily cause alexia. First, what appears to be a reading comprehension problem may reflect instead speech production difficulty, and an aphasic person may not be able to explain a passage because of motor speech or morphosyntactic output problems. Benson (1979a) has called this inability to read aloud or to verbally explain a passage "pseudo-alexia." Second, lengthy passages may reflect fatigue, impaired attention-arousal, or reduced attention span. Third, a variety of associated factors such as visual neglect or visual field defect may interfere.

Although these factors contribute problems, thorough evaluation is essential. Porrazzo (1975) suggested several reasons for testing: (1) to obtain baseline data so that change can be documented, (2) to assist the clinician in selecting appropriate treatment, and (3) to determine whether or not the patient's reading level is functional.

Other reasons exist as well, not the least of which is to determine the distribution of error type, and to attempt to determine pattern of impairment.

ADULT READING EVALUATION MEASURES

Prior to 1979, clinicians had a limited number of assessment tool choices. Standardized tests designed for developmental reading problems could be used or adapted. Many of these measures are inappropriate for use with adults. The array of standardized tests designed primarily for discerning developmental dyslexia or emerging reading skills are often inappropriate to adult interests. Standardized measures that have been used with aphasic adults include the Gates-MacGinitie (1965), and the Nelson Reading Test (1962). Not all tests and materials designed for developmental dyslexia are filled with puppies and piggies, but confronting an adult aphasic person with such content can undermine the best of intentions. Occasionally, some of the principles designed for developmental dyslexia are suitable for use with aphasic adults. Brown (1982), for example, outlined strategies of "diagnostic reading assessment" that are adaptable.

Both Brookshire (1978a) and Schuell and colleagues (1964) have commented on principles important to the evaluation of reading in aphasia, as well as caution in the use of standardized tests not specifically designed for use in aphasia.

Brookshire (1978a) suggested critical evaluation of available standardized tests is crucial, if they are to be used with adults, and he presented guidelines for evaluation.

First, tests should allow evaluation of both reading vocabulary and reading comprehension at both the sentence and paragraph level. They should allow evaluation of both the speed (how much material can be processed in a given time) and power (the complexity level at which comprehension breaks down with no time constraints). Also, tests should include a wide range of reading levels, as we can expect to find reading levels that represent the range of overall language severity in the distribution of aphasia.

Additionally, Brookshire (1978a) suggested modifications of standardized tests for use with aphasic individuals. Changes in the test task are usually appropriate, and in some

cases, vital. Instructions can be simplified in order to minimize the demands on memory, cognitive abilities, and manual dexterity. To this point, perhaps "machine scored" answer sheets should be avoided, as the task requires reading the stimulus item, choosing the correct answer, noting the number or letter of the correct choice, finding the corresponding number on the answer sheet, remembering the correct item, and then filling in the correct choice. A pointing response, which the examiner records, has less potential artifact.

The concept of individualized diagnosis for the purpose of fitting remediation to the patient's pattern of strengths and weaknesses has great face validity and clinical appeal. Hildred Schuell and colleagues (1964), in their clinical wisdom, put it another way when they discussed the goals of reading evaluation. They suggested we attempt to discover not only the general level of reading comprehension, but also why reading breaks down when it does.

Schuell and colleagues posed several questions which should be considered during the course of a careful reading evaluation. Not only will answers to these questions aid us in fulfilling the objectives of evaluation, but they can point to remediation as well. Answers to these questions will foster our grasp of the problem and what to do about it, and they can be grouped into three main categories. First, questions about *peripheral-perceptual factors:*

1. Does visual acuity account for the difficulties?
2. Does a field defect interfere? Does the patient compensate for it?
3. Can the patient match forms, letters, pictures, and words?
4. Is there difficulty following a line?
5. Is there any evidence of visual neglect?

Second, questions about *reading vocabulary:*

1. Can the patient match printed words to pictures?
2. Can he or she match printed to spoken words?
3. Does confusion exist on words with the same visual configuration?

4. Is vocabulary commensurate with education and vocation?

Third, questions related to *retention span deficit*:

1. Does there seem to be an attention or vigilance problem?

2. Do errors increase in proportion to length?

3. Is word recognition slow?

4. Is re-reading evident because of poor retention?

SUBTESTS OF APHASIA BATTERIES

Those sections of traditional aphasia batteries that focus on reading skills generally have limited breadth and do not allow an adequate view of type or degree of reading impairment. With one or two exceptions, these batteries devote only cursory attention to reading skills and are useful more for screening purposes than for revealing a complete picture of impairment. Table 8-1 summarizes the nature and extent of reading subsections of several aphasia batteries.

READING COMPREHENSION BATTERY FOR APHASIA (RCBA)

In 1979, LaPointe and Horner published the Reading Comprehension Battery for Aphasia (RCBA). The test was designed to provide systematic evaluation of the nature and degree of reading impairment in aphasic adults. Clinical experience with children's reading tests and with aphasia batteries were deemed less than adequate, and the RCBA was designed with both the peculiarities and regularities of aphasia in mind. The measure was developed primarily to serve as a springboard from which appropriate treatment could be planned and implemented. It was hoped as well that the test would have potential for furthering understanding of the acquired reading disruption seen in aphasia.

TEST CONSTRUCTION

Guidance for the construction of the RCBA was provided by a body of literature on aphasia and on the reading process and also by the limited number of studies on characteristics of reading by aphasic adults. Material

TABLE 8-1.

Reading Subsections of Aphasia Batteries.

Test	Number of Reading Subtests	Number of Items	Nature of Subtests
Examining for Aphasia (Eisenson, 1954)	6	40	Letter recognition through paragraph comprehension
Minnesota Test for the Differential Diagnosis of Aphasia (Schuell et al., 1964)	9	160	Form matching through oral reading
Boston Diagnostic Aphasia Exam (Goodglass & Kaplan, 1972)	4	46	Symbol-word discrimination through paragraph comprehension
Aphasia Language Performance Scales (Keenan & Brassell, 1975)	1	10 parts	Single word through multisentence comprehension
Western Aphasia Battery (Kertesz, 1982)	2	14	Sentence completion through reading commands
Communicative Abilities in Daily Living (Holland, 1980a)	Integrated	17	Functional tasks
Porch Index of Communicative Ability (Porch, 1981)	2	20	Reading commands

was selected to be suitable to adult interests, so that the test would not insult the adult reader. Items were selected to represent a variety of vocabulary and reading levels. A variety of other factors that could influence reading performance were identified as well, and attempts were made to control them in item and subtest selection. Table 8-2 lists some of the factors identified and controlled in the RCBA.

The RCBA contains 10 subtests that range from matching printed words and pictures to paragraph comprehension. One hundred items provide for a quantitative analysis of performance on the primary dimensions of accuracy and speed. Scores across subtests can be plotted on an RCBA Profile sheet to answer questions on performance configuration or relative impairment across subtests. Table 8-3 lists the RCBA subtests with features of each.

RELIABILITY AND VALIDITY

Two studies related to the psychometric factors of reliability and validity of the RCBA have been accomplished. Pasternak and LaPointe (1982) reported on test-retest reliability over a seven day interval and reported a test-retest correlation coefficient of $r = .99$. Intertester reliability was determined by comparing the scores of four judges to those of the original examiner. Scoring agreement was reported on 90 percent (180 of 200) opportunities for agreement. Pasternak and LaPointe (1982) also reported the mean performance of two groups of normal readers on the RCBA. Sixth grade students ($N = 20$) reading at grade level had a mean score of 92.8 on the text (range = 84 to 97), whereas non-brain-damaged adults aged 47 to 71 years ($N = 20$) ranged in scores from 96 to 100 with a mean of 96.6.

VanDemark, Lemmer, and Drake (1982)

also reported reliability as well as validity data on the performance of 26 aphasic subjects on the RCBA. They, too, found comforting levels of psychometric soundness on the measure. Their findings are summarized as follows:

The data gathered in the present study demonstrate that the RCBA has high levels of test stability, internal consistency and concurrent validity. As an instrument for measuring reading comprehension in aphasia, the RCBA appears on the basis of our data to be psychometrically sound. It measures a wide range and variety of reading skills with subtests which can be arranged in a gradual, orderly progression of difficulty. Such data is an effective adjunct to treatment planning. (VanDemark et al., 1982, p. 291)

A comparison of performance on the RCBA with a modified cloze procedure task was reported by Bogdanoff and Katz (1983). They found that subject performance on the two measures was predictable. Although the authors suggested further investigations to determine the reliability and validity of the modified cloze procedure, they provided a potentially useful conversion table for converting RCBA scores to approximate reading grade levels. The conversion scores they reported were:

RCBA Overall Score	Approximate Grade Level
100-91	8th & above
90-88	7th
87-85	6th
84-82	5th
81-79	4th
78-75	3rd
74-73	2nd
72-70	1st

TABLE 8-2.
Factors Controlled in the RCBA.

auditory	picturability	word length
visual	frequency of occurrence	phrase length
semantic	imageability	test length
form class	concreteness	morphosyntactic context
familiarity	functionality	readability index

TABLE 8-3.
RCBA Subtests.

I. Single Word Comprehension (Visual)	Visual similarity of foils
II. Single Word Comprehension (Auditory)	Foils rhyme
III. Single Word Comprehension (Semantic)	Foils from same semantic field
IV. Functional Reading	Daily living reading stimuli
V. Synonyms	Varied form class, length, concreteness
VI. Sentence Comprehension (Picture)	Varied frequency, imageability
VII. Short Paragraph Comprehension	Varied reading levels, same length
VIII & IX. Paragraphs: Factual, Inferential	Varied levels, cognitive demand.
X. Morphosyntactic	Lexical control, varied syntactic complexity

TREATMENT OF ACQUIRED DYSLEXIA

TREATMENT PLANNING

Treatment planning is a crossroads in clinical decision making, but very few clinically-derived empirically tested suggestions exist to guide us. Because our judgments of whether or not to treat, where to begin, and what targets to select must not be capricious, we value careful appraisal and evaluation in our clinics. As detailed in earlier sections, we need to know what is impaired, what is not, and the types and proportions of errors that are scattered across the behavior of our patients. Differences across the major types of acquired dyslexia will dictate certain constraints, or perhaps suggest avenues of treatment. For example, in alexia without agraphia, intact writing can be exploited by designing tasks and presenting stimulus items that exploit intact modalities. Careful analysis of the profile that emerges from assessment with a standardized measure, such as the Reading Comprehension Battery for Aphasia (LaPointe & Horner, 1979), will allow us to pose a series of questions that will provide a framework for the development of treatment subgoals and subsequently construct specific treatment tasks. Because most of our treatment takes the form of language drill, consisting of error identification, error awareness, and response modification and stabilization, task construction can be guided by answers to questions such as:

1. Does a deficit exist in silent reading comprehension?

2. What is overall performance level?

3. How does performance vary across tasks and subtests?

4. Does simple word comprehension vary relative to visual, auditory, or semantic foils?

5. Is word comprehension better or worse than sentence comprehension?

6. Is functional reading better than nonfunctional reading?

7. Is factual comprehension better than inferential comprehension?

8. Is reading across material with varying levels of imageability differentially affected?

9. Is early versus late acquisition material differentially affected?

10. Does word length affect performance?

11. Can reading grade level be determined to aid in selection of practice material?

12. Does performance vary across morphosyntactic character of sentences?

Generating answers to these and other questions about performance among and within subtests can aid greatly in creating meaningful treatment subgoals, carefully tailored to each person's specific needs.

PRINCIPLES OF TREATMENT

Good language treatment must be driven by a group of principles or a theory on the nature of the breakdown. We find that our general principles for treating reading are remarkably similar to those for other language skills in aphasia. These principles were presented by LaPointe (1977b) and are outlined here.

1. *Find the ability level or level of breakdown; explore the communicative needs of each person.* Aphasia therapy is labor intensive, and we prefer not to waste our time or the time of our clients by attending to tasks that do not need fixing or are trivial. Communicative needs of each individual must be considered with great caution. A patient of one of the authors made it painfully evident after several sessions of different drills on reading tasks, when he remarked, "I never did like reading much. Sometimes I look at the funnies in the paper, but I never have read a book and I'm just going back to live with my brother in that trailer by Jacksonville, and don't expect I'll start reading much. Why do we have to work on this junk?" In this anecdote can be found a prime example of unintentional clinical error caused by not exploring communicative need adequately and by not putting the patient's piece into the treatment equation. Once discovered, the patient's desire was respected.

2. *Build a sight vocabulary if needed.* Particularly for reading survival skills and the ability to deal with daily living reading needs, a sight vocabulary is frequently necessary. This means that a core vocabulary must be selected and drilled upon, particularly with severely involved individuals. It is appropriate as well as a treatment goal with those, for example, who have inordinate difficulty with function words, as in deep dyslexia.

3. *Avoid the phonic approach if confounded by significant dysarthria, paraphasia, or auditory problems.* Motor speech impairment and distorted speech production can impede the use of the phonic approach, which calls for an attempt to "sound-out" or translate graphemes into their phonetic code. The production distortions can create confusion that only amplifies the reading problem. Likewise, the production of nonintended words (paraphasia), or depressed ability to comprehend can add barriers to reading attempts that rely on phonic strategies.

4. *Emphasize comprehension, not oral reading.* Very few adults are called upon to read aloud, so reading treatment should focus on skills of comprehension. Further, oral reading frequently is degraded by concomitant impairment of verbal production skills in the brain damaged population and conclusions about comprehension can be influenced negatively.

5. *Use materials compatible with adult interests.* This principle is so important it becomes a theme, and is repeated in our work because it is vital. Most remedial reading material is designed for elementary school aged children. A grave clinical error can be perpetrated by not expending the effort necessary to gather material suitable to adults, but at the appropriate reading level. Articles, books, and other self-reports in recovery from aphasia are replete with instances of the intelligence and self-image of an adult in treatment being assaulted with material about Cinderella or other topics associated with developmental reading material. The results of such clinical insensitivity can be disastrous, especially superimposed upon an already fragile self-identity that holds regression as a plausible explanation for impaired performance.

6. *Construct a reading task continuum; upgrade level of materials with progress; plot performance change.* The components of this principle are appropriate to most clinical rehabilitative efforts. Ambiguity may still exist about the precise nature of the model from which we work in aphasiology. Some hold fast to the educational framework of skill acquisition and relearning, whereas others embrace the medical model of appraisal, diagnosis, and intervention. Both, or rather, some amalgamation of appropriate pieces of both, probably are relevant to our work. At any rate, rehabilitative progress can be gradual and the duration of our intervention is generally longer than the course of a 10 day prescription of antibiotics. Therefore, we must pay careful attention to matching task and material with changes in reading level. The organization of our reading tasks in a hierarchy of complexity or difficulty allows adaptation to the changing needs of those we treat.

Likewise, task definition and a clinical record of session by session change can be monitored by performance charting and plotting systems such as that afforded by the

BASE-10 approach (LaPointe, 1977a). The use of microcomputers for clinical data management and prediction of eventual performance levels is particularly relevant to reading tasks.

7. *Focus on functionality.* In aphasia, the influence of Holland (1980a) and a host of others who have emphasized the vital role of pragmatics in the study of language has strongly colored the nature of remediation.

In the past, a large portion of our therapeutic effort seems to have been driven by the belief that if some "process" is worked upon, the result will translate to a wide variety of associated tasks. Today, clinicians recognize that, although we retain the goal of attempting to modify performance on language "processes," we cannot ignore the inextricable association of process with the context of language use. This realization guides not only the selection of treatment stimuli but the environment of treatment also.

After a good deal of clinical wheel spinning with a patient who wanted very badly to regain his reading ability, it occurred to one of us in midsession to request two bits of information from the patient regarding reading objectives. He was asked to prepare, with the aid of a family member, two lists to be brought to the clinic on his next visit. One list was to be composed of daily reading items that he would most desire to be able to read; the other was to be composed of functional items he would like to be able to read but could get along without. Table 8-4 presents the lists from this person.

TABLE 8-4.
Patient-generated Functional Reading Lists.

Would Most Like to Be Able to Read	Would Like to Read But Could Do Without
Mail	Messages
Checkbook	Signs
Medicine Labels	Newspapers
Maps	Magazines
Phone Book	TV Guide
Elevator	Menus
Calendar	Bible
Product Labels	Playing Cards

Several items and/or tasks were suggested by these lists that had not appeared in our reading treatment sessions of the past. This client presented a compelling argument for wanting to be able to sort through and read his own mail. This task had been integrated into his daily routine for years, and in his mind, ability to do it would signal a significant return to a degree of familiarity and normalcy in his daily routine. Other tasks might be equally as important to other patients. Exploration of individual functionality is worth the effort.

TARGETS OF REMEDIATION

Keeping in mind that specific targets of remediation will vary across subtypes of acquired dyslexia and across individuals, a number of fundamental reading skills must be acquired if functional literacy is a goal. Some of these skills are frequent targets of remediation in developmental dyslexia as well as in the dyslexia associated with aphasia. These targets include perceptual deficits, sight vocabulary, word analysis skills, contextual cues, fluency, rate modification, and pragmatic skills.

PERCEPTUAL DEFICITS

Perceptual deficits in acquired dyslexia are not well explored. An impressive literature exists on parietal lobe dysfunction and on a host of visuo-perceptive impairments that accompany aphasia, but little research has been accomplished on specific effects of these deficits on reading. This is a fruitful area for clinical research.

Many of the perceptually based deficits seem to involve the processes of scanning, tracking, and appreciation of material in the entire visual field. Hence, the remediation strategies are compensatory. LaPointe and Culton (1969), for example, described a series of compensatory activities with a patient who suffered reading disability and perceptual problems.

Another intriguing compensatory strategy was applied by Carmon, Gordon, Bental, and Harness (1977). They described an adult patient with impaired sequential skills but intact pattern recognition. Therapy concentrated on forming an association of the complete word visual pattern with the retained auditory pattern. With this strategy, the patient learned to read several hundred words and short phrases, although little generalization across untrained words was noted.

Some perceptually oriented specific techniques exist in the developmental dyslexia literature and deserve to be tried or tested with adults, particularly those with global aphasia. One example is described as the object-imaging-projection (OIP) method for teaching disabled readers to associate the sound of a grapheme with a grapheme's appearance. In one report (Isgur, 1975), 10 subjects with disabled reading were studied, one a 29 year old with developmental dyslexia. At the beginning of the study, seven subjects knew no letter-sound associations. Instead of pictures, common household objects were used, one for each initial sound. Each object had the general shape of the letter (i.e., key for "k," pan for "p").

The method included the following steps:

1. Object named and initial sound produced by clinician.
2. Similarities in shape between the object and letter pointed out (Identification).
3. Object traced (Object).
4. Object traced again in space (Imaging).
5. Printed letter traced (Projection).

Five to 10 minutes per letter were required for subjects to learn each. The OIP method was suggested for use with brain damaged persons, but no data were presented on the effectiveness of the strategy with this population. This is the type of technique that may be useful with literal alexia or individuals with a memory or perceptually based impairment. It deserves to be tested.

Another specific technique that appears to be applicable to reading impairment that reflects scanning or tracking difficulty was presented by Gheorghita (1981). In this rather unorthodox approach, words, syllables, and sentences were presented in a vertical rather than a horizontal format to 60 aphasic subjects. Thus, subjects were asked to read:

Words	Syllables	Sentences
T	DI	HOW
A	PLO	IS
B	MA	THE
L	TIC	WEATHER?
E		

Significantly more word errors were recorded with the horizontal mode than the vertical mode.

This deserves further study, particularly to determine whether or not the improvement is merely the result of a novelty effect. The strategy certainly has limited generality to presented material in English, but perhaps the enhanced ability that the vertical mode affords would be a significant compensatory strategy for selected severely impaired readers.

Further recent work on neglect and perceptually based impairment can be gathered from the literature on right hemisphere involvement. Myers (1984) described intervention strategies for perceptually based deficits that include attention to disorders that are caused by neglect of half of the visual fields, visuospatial deficits, and other "lower-order" perceptual impairments.

Stanton, Yorkston, Talley-Kenyon, and Beukelman (1981) also presented a verbal cueing strategy that may have some utility with aphasic readers, particularly if perceptual problems are present. Tasks such as matching sight with left handed columns of stimuli (digits, letters, two-letter combinations, five and six letter words); reading sentences and paragraphs; and a systematic hierarchy of clinician generated cues were used with two individuals who presented visual-spatial-perceptual problems but were able to become functional, independent readers.

A disorder resulting from visual-spatial neglect and perceptual impairment was treated by LaPointe and Culton (1969) using a variety of practical strategies. Drills that focused on drawing from copy and drawing from memory were used, as were step by step strategies of tactile retracing and compensatory rechecking of work previously read or produced graphically. After several months of treatment, the disorder was still quite evident, but the compensatory strategies that were learned enabled the individual to minimize reading errors so he could perform a portion of his job responsibilities more adequately.

SYNTACTIC DEFICITS

We have no data-based studies on the prevalence of syntactically based reading deficit, however, the literature is sprinkled with reports that implicate impaired syntactic facility. In a study on decoding syntax by aphasic readers, Pierce (1983b) suggested that comprehension improves when additional surface structure markers are available. Treatment approaches that focus on syntactic deficit have been developed by Helm (1981) and by Pierce (1983a). Practice material in workbook form is available as well in material prepared by Martinoff, Martinoff, and Stokke (1983).

RATE MANIPULATION

Reading rate as well as accuracy can be diminished. Sometimes rate is only slightly impaired, whereas at other times, reading is laborious and painfully slow. In the so-called mildly impaired aphasic person, reading rate may be one of the final residual deficits. Normal reading rate ranges from 50 to 500 words per minute in moderately educated adults. Professional newscasters, for example, read at a rate of 220 to 344 words per minute (Moyer, 1979).

Techniques for increasing reading rate are largely based on the concept of repeated practice and drill against the backdrop of prompting, or on the use of pacing devices. Pacing drills of recognition of words on flash cards are easy to construct, as are devices that simply uncover a portion of the material by clinician-controlled rates. More sophisticated pacing devices can be arranged with filmstrips or carousel slide projectors that have timed exposure rates. The Reading Accelerator® is listed in catalogs of educational materials and characterized as a pacing device specifically designed to increase reading rates. Desired reading speed can be set and the objective is to read ahead of a shutter as it passes down a page. This serves to push the reader to read faster without backtracking. Reading speed is adjustable from 16 to 3,000 words per minute.

Manipulation of reading rate in aphasia has been demonstrated in at least one experimental study. Moyer (1979) used a treatment strategy she called Multiple Oral Rereading (MOR). In this study, progress on an aphasic subject's ability to read a 600 word passage was charted and timed. Thirty-minute sessions were held daily during which a passage was re-read aloud. A new passage was selected each week and at the end of a three month course, Moyer reported a 42 percent rate increase. Studies such as this deserve to be replicated and extended using today's more sophisticated single-subject research designs. The clinician must be aware of the constant interaction of speech and accuracy on reading tasks. Prompts to increase speed nearly always result in degraded accuracy or comprehension.

As Brown (1982) pointed out, the by-product of fluent reading is added comprehension. Fluent oral (as opposed to silent) reading usually is not one of our primary therapeutic goals, although reading aloud can be a useful means to monitor fluency change and uncover word attack skills or specific error types. Brown's advice on reading rate is that good readers usually read faster than poor readers, but sometimes they are flexible and read more slowly. The following table, adapted from Brown (1982), illustrates not only normal rates for a variety of reading purposes, but also the interaction of rate and comprehension. The trade-off between speed and comprehension is illustrated in Woody Allen's familiar observation on his newly acquired speedreading ability: "I read the entire novel *War and Peace* last night in one and a half hours," he said. "It's about Russia."

TREATMENT TO IMPROVE COMPREHENSION

Most of the techniques to improve reading comprehension have been taken directly or adapted from materials used in

TABLE 8-5.
Normal Reading Rates and Comprehension Levels.

Reading Approach or Purpose	Rate	Comprehension
Intensive, reflective	Rate unimportant, may be 50–150 wpm	Near 100%
Study	125–300 wpm	Above 90% necessary to satisfy reader's purpose
Casual enjoyment	Rate unimportant, may be 125–300 wpm	Comprehension of limited importance; only important to serve enjoyment needs
Rapid	250–600 wpm	60–80%
Rapid survey	400–4,500 wpm	35–45% overall comprehension (90–100% main idea; 75–90% supporting ideas; 30–40% specific details)

Adapted from Brown, D. (1982). *Reading diagnosis and remediation*, p. 35. Reprinted with permission from Prentice Hall, Inc., Englewood Cliffs, NJ.

developmental remedial reading programs. Those used with adolescents are sometimes appropriate, but most of the time material must be selected or adapted to the aphasic adult with careful attention to the specific predominance or pattern of errors presented by each individual. Graded programmed materials such as the Readers' Digest remedial reading series or the Sullivan series of graded workbooks are rich sources of reading passages for treatment. Recent emphasis on functional literacy drills and "survival reading" also provides a lode of material that aphasic adults find interesting and useful. Huizinga's book on American signs (1982) contains photographs of signs taken in a variety of settings such as restaurants, airports, freeways, and movie theaters. Survival reading handbooks, frequently noted in educational materials catalogs, include suggestions and drills on how to find specific information and extract meaning from newspapers, the telephone directory, timetables, television programming guides, motel and campground guides, maps, advertising, menus, package labels, recipes, and meters or gauges.

When reading is severely impaired, an early objective might be to focus on the development of a core or essential vocabulary. During this stage, tasks that serve to increase word-picture association, phrase picture association, or the store of words in sight vocabulary will be practiced.

Of course, there is an interrelationship between basic sight vocabulary, word attack or analysis skills, and reading fluency. Without a basic sight vocabulary, most readers would have difficulty developing word attack skills and comprehension would suffer from deficiencies in both areas.

WORD ATTACK OR ANALYSIS SKILLS

In aphasia, these skills are occasionally important, but not always. Aspects of word attack or word analysis arc phonic analysis, structural analysis, syllabication, and blending. These skills are more appropriate to the moderately involved aphasic adult. The memorization of phonic or syllabication principles or rules may be of limited value, particularly because so many notable exceptions occur in English, but rich sources of advice for developing word attack skills are available (Brown, 1982; Rubeck, 1977).

CONTEXT CLUES

Comprehension is directly related to the ability to utilize context clues. Linguists may refer to the use of context as the use of syntax and structure to facilitate comprehension. As Brown (1982) indicated, context clues become increasingly important as readers become more capable, even to the point that context could overrule analysis or sight vocabulary.

In a paper on the visual characteristics of words, Dunn-Rankin (1977) provided an interesting example. When asked to read the following sentence which has been printed backwards,

.rat eht saw tac ehT

most people read from right to left and decode either "The cat saw the rat" or "The cat was the rat." Based on context, their expectation rejects the correct reading, "The cat was the tar."

Although context and structural analysis skills are important, reading comprehension has been divided into four categories of sub-skills: understanding vocabulary, understanding details, understanding the main idea, and the ability to infer or imply. Each of these sub-skills can be attacked directly during treatment if they are determined to play a significant role.

In aphasia, Waller and Darley (1978) studied the effects of context on reading comprehension. They concluded that simultaneous presentation of picture and verbal introduction significantly helped patient comprehension.

In an experimental analysis of a treatment program for alexia without agraphia, Simmons (1984) used a multiple baseline design across behaviors to investigate two questions:

1. Will training through intact graphic and auditory-verbal modalities result in an increase in reading of trained words in an alexic patient?

2. Will such training result in an increase in reading performance on untrained items?

Results suggested that the treatment yielded improvement in reading trained words. The aphasic subject quickly met 80 percent criterion on each training set during treatment phases, and improvement resulted from training, as untreated sets remained relatively stable until training was initiated.

SPECIFIC TASKS AND TECHNIQUES

The creative clinician, for the most part, will have to custom design tasks for reading treatment. However, a wide variety of commercially available materials can save time, if modified appropriately. Graded reading materials with questions to determine comprehension that are readily adaptable to the aphasia clinic include a number of items from Educational Insights (150 W. Carol Street, Compton, CA 90220). Included in this series are the following materials:

1. Understanding Sentences (#7110)
2. Reading Phrases (#7108)
3. Making Inferences (#7127)
4. Getting the Main Idea (#7105)
5. Noting Details (#7106)
6. You'd Better Believe It (100 individualized reading exercises) (#9131)
7. World of the Future (#9106)
8. The World of Entertainment (#2536)
9. The World of Sports (#2535)
10. Milestones in Life Sciences (#3462)

THE UBIQUITOUS COMPUTER

The computer is present at grocery checkout lanes, on our automobile dashboard, in our bedrooms, and in our clinics. With suitable expressions of caution, it has become increasingly used with aphasic persons, and the treatment of reading lends itself to the advantages of the computer much more readily than other modalities of language. We can expect to be flooded with software that purports application to the language problems of aphasia, and careful critique and analysis of software appropriateness will become increasingly important.

Rushakoff (1984) traced the application of microcomputers to problems of evaluation and treatment. He expressed optimism, "The potential for clinician-independent therapy and for home therapy is enormous and dazzling to imagine" (p. 168), and appropriate caution, "If [the computer] is told in the program to divide the wrong numbers, it will do so over and over again with pitiless glee" (p. 167), and presents synopses of several software packages designed for use with aphasic persons.

One of the most active researchers in the study of computer applications to clinical problems in aphasia has been Richard C. Katz. The work of Katz and his colleagues can be traced by following reports at the Clinical Aphasiology Conference over the past several years. In 1982, Katz and Tong Nagy reported on a program designed to test and treat reading ability in aphasia. They named their program the Computerized Aphasia Treatment System (CATS), and it was composed of a diagnostic reading test, five reading treatment tasks, and one mathematics task. Katz and Tong Nagy reported on the results of 8 to 12 weeks of treatment (2 to 4 sessions per week) on five aphasic subjects. They reported little change in pre- and posttreatment reading tests, but observed improved accuracy, decrease in response latency, and an increased number of attempted items with some subjects.

The following year, Katz and Tong Nagy (1983) reported on a computerized approach for improving word recognition in chronic aphasic patients. This program is designed to accomplish a task difficult to undertake by a clinician and utilizes the advantages of the microcomputer. The program drills 65 words that are presented at varying and controlled exposure rates. This is the type of program that can greatly aid the expansion and stability of an aphasic reader's sight vocabulary.

In a 1985 study, Katz and Tong Nagy reported on a self modifying computerized reading program for severely-impaired aphasic adults. The objective of this study was to improve functional reading, and a program was developed to teach three subjects to read single words without intensive clinician involvement. The program also generates homework activities that are correlated with performance during treatment. Four of the five subjects demonstrated pre- to posttreatment change that ranged from 16 to 54 in percentage of correct responses.

Available software programs designed for reading impairment in aphasia include:

Aphasia I: Noun Association (Weiner, 1983a). Twenty lessons designed so it can be used without the clinician present. Stores and prints session data.

Aphasia II: Opposites and Similarities (Weiner, 1983b). Stores data from up to 28 trials and can report performance in bar graphs.

Understanding Questions (Katz, 1983a).

Understanding Sentences: Absurdities (Katz & LaPointe, 1983).

Understanding Stories (Katz, 1983b). Reading drills for mildly to moderately impaired aphasic adults.

Micro-Lads (Wilson & Fox, 1983). Uses graphics, text, speech output to teach fundamental rules of grammar, syntax.

Computerized Reading for Aphasics (Major & Wilson, 1985). Self-pacing drills in reading comprehension and recognition (nouns, categories, modifiers, synonyms, antonyms, nonassociated nouns, closure, yes-no questions, definitions).

As most experienced consumers of computer software have found, the buyer must beware. Faulty and inadequate software can thwart carefully conceived treatment objectives. Communication with other users plus the careful reading of software reviews can prevent wastes of time and money.

The computer will play an increasingly important role in the treatment of both reading and writing disorders in aphasia, but the clinician need not fear being replaced. In many adults, sudden and prolonged disturbance of reading can be a devastating part of aphasia. A source of enlightenment and enjoyment that flowered during the first grade of school can be severed and denied. The German neurologist Kussmaul wrote about his revered teacher Lordat, who was stricken with aphasia and could no longer read. Kassmaul lamented the fact that the treasures of writing were closed to his teacher as with seven seals. Continued efforts to understand and treat acquired dyslexia will assure removal of those seals and restore the pleasure of reading the printed word.

9

TREATING NAMING

Every aphasic person has difficulty recalling names, but we agree with Benson (1977b) that the problem is not a single or unitary one. We do not agree, however, with those who say that naming disorders cannot be or should not be treated. In our view, the varieties of naming disorder can be identified and the symptoms modified by treatment.

Admittedly, naming programs for aphasic people must be more than "Point to the _____" and "What's this? It's a _____." Many of them are. All have the potential to be more, because models, concepts, and data about both aphasic and normal naming performance abound. Clinicians charged with helping aphasic people with naming deficits do not necessarily need to know about these models, concepts, or data, because deceptively simple programs to improve naming are ubiquitous in the literature. Just as it is possible to pluck sound from a cello without knowing anything about music or stringed instruments, it is possible as well to evoke names from aphasic people without knowing concepts or data. Just as the ignorant plucking of a cello is not pizzicato, however, neither is the ignorant application of a canned program treatment. Treatment requires knowledge of the conceptual underpinnings of specific deficits and the procedures that are suggested to remediate them. Therefore, the first part of this chapter reviews selected concepts and data that support the

specific naming programs that are reviewed in the chapter's final section.

WHY APHASIC PEOPLE CANNOT NAME

A major clinical issue about aphasic naming—perhaps the major clinical issue—is whether aphasic people have a disturbance in the way their words are organized and stored or whether they have problems with accessing otherwise intact information. A mountain of data on aphasic naming disturbances has accumulated, much of it prompted by a desire to discover whether aphasic errors reflect impaired storage or impaired access. How a clinician decides this issue for each patient influences the patient's treatment. Therefore, a review of the experimental data from groups of patients need not deflect us from our clinical orientation.

ERRORS APHASIC PEOPLE MAKE

Buckingham (1979) categorized what he called the "manifestations of blocked access to the lexicon" (p. 273) made by aphasic people with posterior lesions. He discussed (1) definitions, (2) pauses, (3) field errors, (4) unrelated lexical errors, (5) indefinite anaphora, and (6) neologisms and confabulations. His discussion deserved to be read in the original, thus, we will confine ourselves primarily to summarizing some clinical hypotheses. As Buckingham stated, these six error types suggest "lexical retrieval deficits" with at least partial "lexico-semantic structure" (p. 273) intactness. He based his argument in part on a clinically useful differentiation of semantic field and lexical set. The semantic field "subsumes hierarchical (superordinate) paradigmatic relations" (p. 275) such as the relationship of animal to dog to retriever. The lexical set, on the other hand, includes close relationships such as synonyms, antonyms, and like objects. He posited that aphasia is a disturbance of sets rather than fields. Hierarchical relationships are preserved but close relationships are disturbed. As a result, providing the anomic person with numerous members of lexical sets—antonym, synonym, related word—is not good treatment. He seems to be right. Data (Podraza & Darley, 1977) even suggest that such stimuli can cause performance to degenerate, a finding to be recalled when designing or reviewing naming programs.

The variety of aphasic errors, as described by Buckingham, provides other clues to aphasic performance and potential treatments. Some aphasic people define or gesture the words they cannot retrieve. Buckingham said that definitions often contain the superordinate (when trying to provide the word "Jerusalem artichoke," the patient might say, "It's a native American vegetable.") This performance suggests that "the definitional structures can be separated from the labels" (p. 274) and this dissociation may be a reasonable explanation for the frequent failure of definitions as treatment cues. Similarly, the presence of adequate gestures in the absence of specific names may suggest considerable lexical knowledge while simultaneously confirming a dissociation of knowledge about shape, size, and function and the label. Gestures, like definitions, may be poor cues for some patients, and confirming evidence is accumulating (Thompson & Kearns, 1981).

Buckingham called pauses evidence of a profound inability to retrieve. We agree with Buckingham, and instead of teaching our patients to pause, we try to teach them what to do during the pause. Otherwise, it is our experience that simple pausing is likely to produce nothing more than silence and to be accompanied by nothing more than frustration. Finally, Buckingham pointed out that some unrelated substitutions may be symptomatic of nonaphasic deficits such as perseveration. Errors resulting from perseveration and from aphasia co-occur, but individual errors can often be classified as one or the other. The proportion of each in a patient's speech has therapeutic uses. If the patient's major deficit is perseveration, the clinician may want to use a wide variety of unrelated stimuli and present them only once or twice rather than several times consecutively. If the problem is aphasia, the clinician may want to repeat the same stimuli several times in a row.

APHASIC ERRORS COMPARED TO NORMAL WORD ASSOCIATIONS

Rinnert and Whitaker (1973) compared aphasic word finding errors to normal word association responses. They gathered the data "to infer—rather than merely attempt to verify or question—semantic processing and structure: including the specifics of lexical categories, the nature of hierarchical organization of the lexicon, and details regarding semantic distinctive features and how they relate to one another" (p. 59) in aphasic lexicons. Their analysis of word substitution data from several sources led them to conclude that "word association experiments on normal subjects and semantic confusions by aphasic patients follow analogous semantic organizational patterns of the lexicon" (p. 80).

They developed a series of interesting and clinically useful hypotheses about aphasic substitutions: (1) features that differentiate the target word and the substituted word are missing or unavailable, (2) the substituted word is "hierarchically more 'important' " (p. 60), and (3) naming requires some kind of "multiple search routine" (p. 60) with checks against short-term memory, and errors result because of impaired short-term memory. Other hypotheses are that the substituted word is easier to produce for motor, frequency, or hierarchical reasons; the target word is gone;

or access to the target but not to the substitution is impaired. They said that the processes (or explanations) may differ for different patients.

The treatment implications of one of their hypotheses about naming is especially intriguing. They stated it may be that naming by normal speakers means evoking several features and that context inhibits the wrong features. In aphasia, the inhibition fails to operate adequately and words representing the features rather than the target word appear. In treatment, clinicians often attempt to stimulate a name by providing synonyms, antonyms, and so on. It may be that for some aphasic people, such stimuli should not be provided and the patient's production of them during attempts to retrieve should be inhibited rather than encouraged. This is not tantamount to saying that association cues have no place in naming treatment. It is to say that some superficially respectable cues may actually be disruptive.

Caramazza and Berndt (1978) discussed the word associations of aphasic speakers. They observed that aphasic errors often are within category but that specific functional details are confused. They said the similarity of aphasic errors and normal word associations suggest a disturbed lexicon in aphasia. If they are right, their data can be added to data already reviewed to fuel the argument that aphasia is not merely impaired access to intact forms.

APHASIC WORD ASSOCIATIONS

Howes and Geschwind (1969) took a different approach to understanding aphasic naming by studying the specific word associations of anterior and posterior aphasic patients. Among their clinically relevant findings are (1) anterior and posterior patients produce different associations, and (2) posterior patients have a more severe, and perhaps a different, problem with the lexicon than do anterior patients.

Wyke (1962) also reported on the word associations of four aphasic and three nonaphasic adults. This study is an excellent one for clinicians because the author used a variety of tests resembling therapeutic activities. For example, subjects were asked to supply synonyms, antonyms, rhymes, opposite analogies (brother is a boy/sister is a _____), usage associations (Mom and _____), and sentence completion. All patients also completed a traditional word association task and tests of object and picture naming.

The aphasic people did worse than the nonaphasic people on all tests and significantly so on word association, usage association, object naming, and picture naming. Wyke said, "The verbal reactions displayed are those which usually lie at the periphery of the semantic system" (p. 685). One interpretation of these data is that the aphasic people's deficits are not merely those of accessing otherwise normal information. On the other hand, aphasic performance was influenced by certain stimulus conditions because the aphasic people performed more poorly but similarly to the nonaphasic people on some tasks. Variability across tasks is more comfortably explained by the notion of impaired access than it is by any other notion. Wyke, however, was content to describe the variability as lawful and to observe that correct responses were most likely to be forthcoming if the response choices were narrowed. All such narrowing is not equally effective, however. The aphasic people performed well on opposite analogies but poorly on the usage associations, for example. She also noted that aphasic people can be helped if the clinician has them assume a "set" and provides them with syntax. The clinical dividends of her study are that her experimental tasks can become diagnostic tasks and her conclusions can be used to help select treatment material and to help explain the reasons for certain patterns of aphasic errors.

ASSOCIATIONS IN THE SEMANTIC FIELD

Goodglass and Baker (1976) investigated the integrity of semantic fields in 16 non-disabled adults, 14 brain damaged adults without aphasia, and 32 aphasic adults divided into low and high comprehension groups. Their method employed 16 picturable nouns, 8 high frequency and 8 low frequency. All subjects had to name the targets prior to the semantic field testing. For semantic field testing, each of the nouns was placed in turn before the subject, who then heard a pre-recorded list of 14 words, six related systematically to the target, seven unrelated to the target, and the target itself (called identity). The related words were (1) superordinate, or the class or category to which the target belonged; (2) attribute, an adjective describing the target; (3) contrast coordinate, another member of the same category; (4) function associate, verb specifying the action of the target; (5) function context, environment in which the target occurs; and (6) clang, a "sound-alike" word. Latencies and number of errors were recorded.

The results were extensive, but of interest to the eager reader. Of greatest importance to our clinical discussion is the finding that the low comprehension aphasic persons (based on performance on four auditory comprehension subtests of the Boston Diagnostic Aphasia Examination [Goodglass & Kaplan, 1972]) showed disturbed semantic fields despite being able to identify the target itself when named. Goodglass and Baker concluded that low comprehension aphasic people "know what an object is, but not about it. There appears to be a constriction of the semantic field around a concept and it is not a random constriction" (p. 367). They also discovered a relationship between ability to name and semantic field integrity, most obvious for the low comprehension aphasic subjects, but also apparent in the response latency data even for the high comprehension subjects. According to Goodglass and Baker, the associations within an aphasic person's semantic field, as determined by their experimental procedures, seem to be organized in a nonrandom way. The field's inner circle contain the label, the superordinate, the most common attribute (adjective), and "terms related by situational contiguity" (p. 371). Verbs and other members of the same superordinate are toward the outer ring. Examples of the data supporting these notions include the greater than normal difficulty severe aphasic

patients had with verbs denoting the action. In addition, even nondisabled speakers and the high comprehension aphasic speakers were somewhat less responsive to verbs.

The study was described in detail because it raises interesting clinical issues. Because verbs and functional context are at the fringes of the field for severe patients, how useful are they as cues? The answer may be "not very," especially if the clinician's aim is merely to facilitate correct responses. On the other hand, if the clinician's goal is to re-establish field integrity, verb and functional context may be attributes in need of specific treatment. An even more crucial issue, albeit one that goes well beyond this one study, concerns the relationship of naming and semantic fields, especially in treatment. It may be that naming can occur in the presence of disturbed fields, that naming can be treated with little regard for field integrity, and that field integrity does not guarantee adequate naming. Such issues continue to be studied, and clinicans may be able to provide helpful data from their treatment of aphasic people.

BOUNDARIES OF THE SEMANTIC FIELD

Whitehouse, Caramazza, and Zurif (1978) took an equally creative approach to studying the semantic field integrity of five Broca's aphasic and five anomic aphasic people. They used drawings of a glass and a cup that were systematically different in height and width. Faced with each drawing, the aphasic people were to report whether each was a glass, bowl, or cup. The choices of the Broca's aphasic people were reasonably normal. The anomic aphasic people made distinctly abnormal choices. The Broca's aphasic patients were helped by environmental cues, such as when a cup was pictured with coffee. The anomic aphasic speakers were not helped by environmental cues or associations. The authors concluded that the anomic people but not the Broca's aphasic people had a number of problems, including being "insensitive to category boundaries" (p. 71). The authors also posited "It seems that the Broca's internal lexicon is more richly elaborated and better structured in terms of practical or functional information than is the internal lexicon of the patient suffering posterior damage" (p. 72). Broca's and anomic aphasic people may require different treatments, an inescapable conclusion of most of the literature.

CENTRALITY AND THE SEMANTIC FIELD

Grossman (1981) has also contributed to our understanding of semantic field integrity in aphasia and therefore, to treatment of aphasia. He used nine nonfluent, seven fluent, eight right hemisphere damaged nonaphasic, and five nondisabled control subjects. He wanted "to determine the names of things to which a patient thought a word could refer" (p. 316). Subjects were given 60 seconds to respond with examples of each of 10 superordinate terms. He scored the number of responses, their "centrality," and the frequency of occurrence of words supplied.

All aphasic people produced significantly fewer words than the other two groups. The fluent aphasic people produced a high proportion of "out-of-set" responses, or responses whose relationship to the target was hard to fathom. On the other hand, the nonfluent aphasic people stayed close to the center of each superordinate's field.

Of special treatment significance are his conclusions about the semantic fields of fluent and nonfluent aphasic people. The fluent speakers seemed unsure "about the borders around a superordinate's referential field, [but] they apparently do possess at least a rough idea about the nature of a superordinate's referents" (p. 323). The nonfluents, on the other hand, show "dependence on highly representative instances of a superordinate" (p. 321). Again, the difference between fluent and nonfluent aphasic people is suggested, and the thoughtful clinician cannot help but wonder how these differences might influence methods, stimuli, and prognosis.

SEMANTIC FEATURES AND THE SEMANTIC FIELD

Zurif, Caramazza, Myerson, and Galvin (1974), working from a semantic feature view

of the lexicon, compared the way anterior and posterior aphasic patients grouped words such as "trout," "turtle," "woman," "cook," and "mother." The anterior aphasic patients were similar but not identical to the nonaphasic subjects in their groupings of words. Because of the way these anterior patients grouped the animal names, the authors concluded that their "lexical structure . . . is more restricted in its range of conceptual integration" (p. 179). They made the interesting observation, perhaps useful clinically, that "verbal concepts in anterior aphasia appear to be more tightly tied to affective and situational data" (p. 179). For example, the anterior aphasic people grouped the dog with human terms more than did the nonaphasic control subjects. The posterior aphasic patients, perhaps predictably, failed to sort like either the nonaphasic or anterior subjects. Their groupings were more random. This finding the authors took to indicate a "disruption of the underlying lexical organization" (p. 181). They added that a portion—but not all—of their results could reflect a general deficit in problem solving.

Like other studies already reviewed, this one understandably fails to outline a specific clinical approach. It does, however, hint at testable clinical hypotheses. It may be that affective and situational cues will help some aphasic people name. With others, such cues may be feckless or even harmful. For example, some aphasic people (likely to be severely impaired Wernicke's in our experience) may be led even farther away from their target by such cues. It can also be hypothesized that simple facilitation will more likely succeed with nonfluent Broca's type people than with fluent, Wernicke's type people.

PARALLEL DEFICITS IN PRODUCTION AND COMPREHENSION

Another way to think about the semantic field is to see it as a "lexical-semantic component of the language system" (Berndt, Caramazza, & Zurif, 1983, p. 10). The assumption of such a view is that a lexical-semantic disorder would be present in both comprehension and production. Gainotti (1976) studied the single-word expressive and receptive abilities of 113 aphasic patients classified by severity. The data seem "to prove that the signs of semantic impairment observed in verbal production and in language comprehension are strongly reciprocally related" (p. 59), independent of severity. Gainotti admitted that this relationship "does not necessarily mean that the semantic competence of these patients is impaired" (p. 60). "What our results doubtless demonstrate is that not all the aspects of the aphasic disturbance can be considered as due to the impairment of one or more components of the system of performance capabilities" (p. 60). He and his colleagues (Gainotti, Caltagirone, & Ibba, 1975; Gainotti, Caltagirone, & Miceli, 1979) have made similar observations in other studies. These data add to those demonstrating a competence rather than a performance deficit in at least some aphasic people's attempts at naming.

TIP-OF-THE-TONGUE PHENOMENA IN APHASIA

Some aphasic people seem to have words they cannot say on the tips of their tongues, an impression that researchers have used to bolster their feelings that the aphasic problem is merely one of retrieval. Goodglass, Kaplan, Weintraub, and Ackerman (1976) tested 42 aphasic speakers (13 Broca's, 8 Wernicke's, 12 conduction, and 9 anomic) to see what they had on their tongue tips. The authors determined each of these patients' ability to predict the first letter and number of syllables of words that were in error on a confrontation naming task. They then asked the patients to produce any associated word that they thought was related to the target and to select the target from a group of three. Once they got each word correct they were again asked for an association. Forty-eight words, 12 each of one, two, three, and four or five syllables, were used as the test stimuli.

All the aphasic groups except those with anomic aphasia found that longer words were the hardest to name, despite being higher frequency than the shorter ones. The conduction aphasic people were better than all other

groups at predicting first sound and number of syllables. Broca's aphasic people were second. The anomic and Wernicke's aphasic people were worst and not significantly different from each other. Wernicke's aphasic people were least able to predict correctly whether or not they had knowledge of the word. All groups were about equally good at identifying the word when given a choice.

The study has considerable clinical relevance. The authors stated "that word finding is usually an 'all or none' process for Wernicke and anomic patients, in the sense that they either recover a name well enough to produce it or they can give little evidence of partial knowledge" (p. 152). These patients then may be slower to respond to cueing hierarchies than Broca's and other aphasic people, may need different hierarchies, may need more extensive, intensive treatment, and may profit very little from having their behaviors while trying to name identified as strategies (Marshall, 1975) and subsequently reinforced.

SEMANTIC PRIMING AND THE SEMANTIC FIELD

All researchers do not agree about the semantic field deficit in aphasia, however. Blumstein, Milberg, and Shrier (1982) were not so convinced of the presence of a disturbed lexicon even in severe aphasia, for example. Both their method and their reluctance to mount the disturbed lexicon bandwagon make their study interesting. Their experimental method is one of auditory priming of the semantic field. Patients were required to indicate by depressing a switch whether the second of two words presented one-half second apart was a real word or a nonword. They used five experimental conditions. In the first three, the second item in the pair was a real word. In the other two, the second item was a nonword (e.g., "ank"). The real words were either preceded by a related word, an unrelated word, or a nonword. The nonwords were preceded either by a real word or by a nonword.

Subjects were seven people with Wernicke's, three with Broca's, four with transcortical motor, five with conduction, and four with global aphasia, representing a wide range of severities. Because some of the patients were severe, considerable time and effort was spent in teaching the task, and criteria were established for repeating some of the test stimuli if a subject seemed to lose the task's requirements. Accuracy and latency were both measured.

This study produced considerable data. The finding of greatest significance to the question of semantic field integrity is that the aphasic patients, regardless of severity of comprehension deficit or diagnostic group, showed evidence of a priming effect. This means that they made fewer errors and were more responsive when real words were preceded by semantically related words. The subjects were also required to make decisions about the semantic relatedness of selected word pairs. Blumstein and colleagues' hypothesis was that aphasic speakers might have difficulty with conscious decisions in essentially metalinguistic tasks such as determining the relatedness of two words but would have less difficulty with "automatic activation of semantic features" as is sampled with the "priming" experiment.

They developed the notion that word processing involves "automatic activation of semantic information in memory" (p. 314). They stated further, "The distinction lies between the relatively less constrained process of automatic or unconscious activation in which the semantic features of a lexical entry are 'activated' versus the constrained process of conscious or voluntary access to a word in which these semantic dimensions must be appropriately categorized" (p. 314). Predictably, they concluded that it is the conscious access rather than the automatic which is impaired. To the argument about semantic field integrity in aphasia, they added this, "Semantic organization, at least at the level of semantic relatedness, seems to be relatively spared in aphasia" (p. 314). An earlier study (Milberg & Blumstein, 1981) led to the same conclusion, based on aphasic performance in visual priming in which patients made decisions about written words.

SOME OF THE THINGS ALL THIS MAY MEAN

Four findings seem to emerge from the data thus far reviewed. First, anterior, usually Broca's, and posterior, usually Wernicke's and anomic aphasic, people have different naming deficits. Second, these differences may have something to do with the integrity of semantic fields, with the fields being more or differently involved in the posterior patients. Third, a lexico-semantic deficit is more likely in more severe patients. Fourth, ability to recognize a name may be independent of semantic field integrity.

These data are important clinically. They highlight the complexity of naming and warn the clinician about the hazards of its management. Anomia is not like a broken arm. Deficits differ in type and no single approach will be universally acceptable. The data make legitimate the construction of individual naming programs and the rejection of generic programs. They provide any number of clinical hypotheses about which patients are likely to benefit from facilitation and which from didactic programs. They urge clinicians to make the clinic a laboratory. Although the critical experiment for differentiating impaired access from impaired semantic field has not and perhaps cannot be created, structured treatments will make speech pathologists and other scientists smarter about aphasic naming disorders. Simultaneously, treatment will become progressively better.

CLASSIFICATION OF NAMING DEFICITS

Benson (1979b) has provided us with an attractive clinical classification of naming deficits. Like Geschwind (1967), he differentiated aphasic anomia from the naming deficits associated with generalized cortical dysfunction and severe mental illness. Unlike Geschwind, however, who distinguished only two types of aphasic anomia, Benson divided aphasic misnaming into six types. Because he has tested patients extensively, he has been quick to admit that his groupings may be arbitrary, that they overlap, and that many aphasic speakers present with a mix. Clinicians should remember Benson knows this. It will keep them from expecting too much of the system.

WORD PRODUCTION ANOMIA

Benson's first type is word production anomia. As the name suggests, this deficit may result from motor speech deficits. The patient knows the word, recognizes it, and represents it in all modalities, but cannot say it or can say it only with difficulty and after delay and struggle. Benson has suggested that another cause of such an anomia may be difficulty in initiating a response. Finally, he has identified a subtype of word production deficit in a subgroup of fluent, somewhat more posterior aphasic speakers. He has considered the jargon of these patients to be the manifestation of a production deficit.

The diagnostic and treatment implications of word production anomia can be hypothesized. Benson has averred that patients whose naming deficit seems most purely motor are more responsive to such simple cues as the first sound or syllable of the target word than are patients anomic for other reasons. He has admitted, however, that some such speakers fail to respond to minimum cueing and sometimes even to maximum cueing. In our experience, patients whose naming deficits result from motor difficulties are easy to identify, especially once one has seen them for a session or two. Our experience teaches that they seldom, if ever, need specific naming treatment.

WORD SELECTION ANOMIA

For Benson, word selection or word dictionary anomia is the true anomia. The patient has difficulty evoking the name but comprehends it and can show knowledge of the word by gesturing, describing, writing, drawing, or by showing dismay at errors. One such patient from our clinical practice was trying to produce the name of a tight end for the Green Bay Packers. He could not produce the player's name, but stood up, walked to the

door of the office, started down the carpet, made a head fake, broke into the open, caught the pass, tucked it in, and rambled to the credenza. Benson has said such patients usually recognize the correct name but may not profit from being cued with the same behavior or responses they use as substitutes for the word they cannot think of. They may describe an item, for example, but not respond correctly to the clinician's description. They may gesture a target in an apparent effort to aid their own retrieval, but not profit from the clinician's gesture. These dissociations have been mentioned previously. They are repeated because their value as warnings to the clinician warrant it.

A popular line of research (Marshall, 1975, 1976; Marshall et al., 1980) has identified the behaviors accompanying word-finding difficulty as self-generated cues. The implication is that aphasic people use these behaviors to help themselves retrieve words. A common clinical suggestion is to reinforce the most powerful of these "cues" during treatment. Benson's profile of the typical word selection anomic person, however, suggests that some accompanying behaviors in some patients may simply be symptoms rather than strategies. Differentiating symptoms from strategies in individual aphasic people is a crucial step in treatment planning.

SEMANTIC ANOMIA

Patients with semantic anomia usually do not recognize the words they cannot produce. Benson has admitted that this form of anomia may differ only in severity from the previously described word selection anomia. His alternative suggestion, however, is that the two may differ fundamentally. They may differ in locus of lesion and they may differ in underlying neuropathophysiology. The damage in word selection anomia may be to processes crucial to accessing known words. The damage in semantic anomia may be to semantic fields. In the former, the word really is on the tip of the tongue. In the latter, nothing at all is sitting on the tongue. If they differ in these ways, they may differ in response to treatment as well.

LIMITED ANOMIAS

no fruit + veg names

Category specific, modality specific, and so-called disconnection anomias have been described. Hart, Berndt, and Caramazza (1985), for example, described the case of a patient with inordinate difficulty naming fruits and vegetables. It is arguable whether these limited deficits should be called aphasic, because aphasia traditionally is present across modalities. Our own position is that these limited anomias can be included with the aphasias as long as diagnostic testing confirms they are not the result of perceptual deficits.

The clinical significance of the limited anomias is contingent on one's clinical purposes. Probably such anomias do not often bring a patient to therapy. They may, however, be present in a patient referred for evaluation, and their discovery may be of diagnostic importance. If seen for treatment, they offer fertile ground for clinical experimentation. The clinician interested in finding out if impaired performance is helped by pairing it with less impaired performance would do well to treat such pure patients.

LOCALIZATION OF THE ANOMIAS

That naming deficits appear to be ubiquitous in aphasia has one potential implication for the localization of naming in the brain: wide areas of cortical and subcortical tissue may subserve the performance. But, because all naming deficits do not appear to be identical, it is probable that all nervous system areas do not make the same contribution to naming. Indeed, Benson (1979b) has said that site of dysfunction seems to be a significant influence on type of naming deficit. Goodglass, Klein, Carey, and Jones (1966) agreed about the possibility of localization for naming based on the "psychological character of different word categories" (p. 87). Buckingham (1979) also hypothesized that different types of words may have different localizations.

Benson's candidate for the primary naming area is the angular gyrus in the parietal lobe of the major (usually left) hemisphere. Producing a name is thought by Benson to result from "simultaneous synthesis of both simple and complex percepts from multiple sensory modalities, a process called intermodal association" (Benson, 1979b, p. 319). Benson has an explanation of what happens, for example, when one sees a picture of a cat. A flood of visual, acoustic, tactile, kinesthetic, olfactory, affective, and environmental associations are evoked (depending, presumably, on one's experience with cats). Benson has provided a series of figures depicting the connections of the angular gyrus to the primary sensory and other cortical areas and has suggested that these areas and these connections are necessary to development of naming. Benson has recognized, of course, that the neural bases of naming are more complex than can be portrayed by a diagram.

He has specifically hypothesized that cross-modal association and actual word selection are separate processes with separate neuroanatomic substrates. He has paired word selection with a "hypothetical word dictionary" (p. 324). By drawing upon his own extensive case material, he has said that pure anomia results from a lesion at the junction of the temporal and occipital lobes. He has been unwilling to say that the dictionary is stored in this region. He has said, however, "that entry into and use of a functionally discrete lexical repository is a significant portion of the task of word finding and that the temporal-occipital junction area of the dominant hemisphere appears essential for that task" (p. 324).

Buckingham (1979) has localized naming functions in the posterior superior temporoparietal region of the left hemisphere, an area he has said is important to retrieval. He has referenced neurophysiological evidence from Fedio and Van Buren (1975) in support of his position.

Other naming deficits may result from lesions outside the angular gyrus and temporal-occipital regions. Anterior lesions cause Benson's word production anomia and can be seen in Broca's or conduction aphasia. Difficulty naming colors is thought to result

Difficulty naming colors

from a posterior lesion that disconnects the right visual area from the left hemisphere language area. Geschwind (1967) reported on a specific anomia for objects presented to the left hand following a lesion to the corpus callosum. In addition, specific modality deficits may result from lesions to the relevant sensory analyzer regions so that a tactile anomia would result from a discrete parietal lesion, for example, and a visual anomia would result from an occipital lesion.

Other areas may also be crucial to naming. Ojemann (1975), for example, discussed the importance of subcortical structures, as did Knopman and colleagues (1984). These last authors have posited that naming depends on posterior, superior temporal-inferior parietal cortex and on insula-putamen areas of subcortex and that the naming problems resulting from lesions to these different areas are also different. Semantic paraphasic errors predominate in the first; phonologic paraphasic errors predominate in the second. Even the right hemisphere may contribute to the naming of at least some words, perhaps those associated with action, or those that may be easily visualized. And because words do not usually appear outside linguistic, cognitive, and affective contexts, wide areas of the left hemisphere, including the frontal lobes, are no doubt crucial to naming, especially in connected speech.

Problems localizing the anomias remain. Benson (1979b) has said that all the limited category anomias and their localization are controversial and await confirmation. Goodglass and Geschwind (1976) have complicated the issue even further. They observed that, except for the modality specific anomias, word finding difficulty may have little localizing significance. In support of this point, they observed that anomia can be symptomatic of tumors far from the language areas, "suggesting that word-finding is sensitive to raised intracranial pressure, without the necessity of a discrete structural lesion" (p. 404). They did add that when the anomia is isolated or pure the "lesion is almost always in the temporal or temporo-parietal area" (p. 404). Knopman and colleagues (1984) did not agree that

naming functions are not localizable. They did report, however, that naming dysfunction is not inevitable from either the temporal-parietal or insula-putamen areas identified in their research. They stated, "we found that naming in some patients resisted damage of regions that caused severe naming deficits in other patients" (p. 1469).

Treatment cannot await a neuroanatomic model of naming, nor does treatment need such a model. The foregoing section was merely a reminder to clinicians to look beyond the angular gyrus and to expect some naming deficits even when the speaker is not an "anomic" aphasic person.

ASSESSMENT

All the major aphasia examinations have at least one subtest for naming, usually confrontation naming, requiring that the patient provide specific names for specific objects. Some, like the Boston Diagnostic Aphasia Examination (BDAE) (Goodglass & Kaplan, 1972), sample naming of objects from a variety of categories—body parts, colors, and objects, for example. The Boston Naming Test (Kaplan et al., 1983) tests the aphasic person's ability to name 60 objects. Limited data from children and nonaphasic and aphasic adults are provided for these 60 items, thereby allowing the clinician to draw at least weak conclusions about an individual patient's performance. The Western Aphasia Battery (WAB) (Kertesz, 1982) also tests naming in detail.

Formal tests, especially those relying heavily upon picture naming, may not provide sufficient information for diagnosing the nature of the naming disturbance (Kohn & Goodglass, 1985) or for treatment planning. As a foundation for such planning, we select from the following: confrontation naming of pictured and real objects, naming in response to descriptions, naming in response to gestures, written compared to verbal naming, naming as part of cloze, naming in response to first sound or syllable cues, naming during process and picture description, naming in delayed imitation, and naming of opposites (boy and _____, night and _____). We also observe what a patient does when attempting to name and try to judge the effectiveness of these activities.

These data combined with the history and a total speech-language profile become the basis for decisions about whether and when to treat naming and about the appropriate methods. This chapter's bulk and separate status are not evidence that we always treat naming. We do not. On the other hand, when patients want to talk better and have difficulty providing specific names or their equivalents, we provide them with naming therapy.

GUIDELINES FOR STIMULUS SELECTION AND ORDERING

Busy clinicians have no time to judge the difficulty of all stimuli prior to each session. Many rely on their clinical experience for a general notion of item difficulty. These notions govern stimulus selection in much of aphasiology. For the treatment of naming, a considerable body of literature on stimulus characteristics that seem to influence the names aphasic people find easy and hard is also available. We have provided the following discussion of guidelines based on that literature for three groups of clinicians: those wanting to publish their treatments and in need of rigorous stimulus control, new clinicians in need of the literature's help while their own experience is accumulating, and seasoned clinicians trying to sort through the debris of a failed program for evidence about what went wrong.

INFLUENCE OF FREQUENCY

Rochford and Williams (1962, 1965) completed an extensive series of studies on the influence of word frequency. In the early study, 36 aphasic people named a series of pictured objects whose frequency of occurrence in written English (Thorndike & Lorge, 1944) had been determined. Each picture was exposed for one second. Some of the stimuli apparently presented problems for the subjects that had little to do with their specific naming deficits. For example, the subjects were unsure of what to call some stimuli where a part of the object rather than the whole object was to be named (patients have similar difficulties with some of the Boston Naming Test items [Kaplan et al., 1983]). The data were analyzed nonetheless and a significant interaction of frequency and correct naming was discovered, but only for the extremes—the very common and the very rare.

In an even more extensive series of studies, Rochford and Williams (1965) further studied the influence of frequency on aphasic naming. They first measured the influence of frequency on ability to name and found, as they had three years previously, that the two were significantly correlated. They next compared the ability of a group of aphasic people to name objects and body parts. They said, "It can be concluded that the visual and semantic context provided when naming body parts does not facilitate the word search and that this task offers further evidence for the correlation between word frequency and relative word finding difficulty" (p. 409). Not satisfied, they went on to measure the potency of compound words such as "hedgehog" in which the frequency of the two words was controlled. Common-common words were easiest, common-rare were next, and rare-common were hardest. The first two kinds of words were not significantly different but were both significantly easier than the third.

In another experiment with 11 aphasic people, they confirmed that frequency of occurrence also influenced the accuracy with which verbs could be named. Rochford and Williams won themselves a place in the universal reference list, and it appears that most researchers since their time have attempted realistic control of frequency of occurrence. Clinical research into treatment programs for naming also controls for it. Daily clinical activity probably does so only serendipitously. Clinicians know that good treatment can usually override all linguistic influences. Working clinicians merely compensate for rare stimuli by working harder. We mention frequency of occurrence in this clinical text nonetheless, because frequency may explain why we sometimes leave aphasia therapy so tired.

INFLUENCE OF OPERATIVITY

Gardner (1973) hypothesized that an object's operativity helps determine how easily its name is evoked. Objects with high operativity can be "operated upon" and therefore "known through a variety of actions and sensory modalities" (p. 213). An orange is high in operativity; a curb is low, for example. Gardner studied the influence of operativity on the naming of 11 anterior aphasic, 11 posterior aphasic, and 11 non-aphasic people. Stimuli were four pictures—the interior of a house, a city street, the body of a woman, and a country scene. These four pictures contained 72 target objects whose operativity and frequency were known. Each subject was shown the pictures and asked to name specific items as the experimenter pointed to them. Failure was followed by the opportunity to select the correct word from a series of four; the object's name, a semantic foil, a phonetic foil, and an unrelated word.

All aphasic people had naming difficulties, but little difficulty recognizing the correct word from the series of four. Items high in operativity were easier to name than ones low in operativity, and in this study, operativity had a more profound influence even than word frequency. This last finding is interesting because frequency is seldom dethroned by anything short of intense therapy. It is also noteworthy that in a later but similarly designed study (1974), Gardner reported that operativity and frequency made equal contributions to correct naming. He ended the 1973 report with some hypotheses about operative and figurative words and about naming.

Of figurative objects such as "curb" he said, "figurative elements depend primarily on associations within the visual modality" (p. 219). About naming in general, he said, "naming depends upon the capacity to arouse some subset of the actions or sensory experiences (schemes) normally involved in activity with the object...the aphasic patient may have greater difficulty (than normal) in initiating this process (arousing one or more schemes) or may need to activate more

schemes before producing the required name" (p. 219).

Gardner was disinterested in the treatment use of his data, and translation must be chary. We have three prosaic suggestions: clinicians might test the facilitating power of allowing patients to manipulate treatment items while attempting to name them, they might rely on multiple modality cueing, or they might want to use operativity as a way of understanding what an individual patient finds easy and hard.

INFLUENCE OF LARGE AND SMALL DRAWINGS, REAL OBJECTS, AND REDUNDANCY

Benton, Smith, and Lang (1972) tested the ability of 18 aphasic people to name real objects and large and small line drawings of the same objects. Objects were significantly easier for the aphasic patients to name; the size of the line drawings made no difference. They interpreted their data as showing that redundant stimuli are easier to name because they evoke a larger number of associations.

Bisiach (1966) used nine aphasic patients test for differences in the potency of realistic colored drawings, simple line drawings, and distorted line drawings. The distortion was created by drawing a set of slashed lines over the original drawings. Patients were required to name the pictures within 15 seconds. The aphasic subjects were more successful with the realistic drawings. Bisiach concluded that amount of information or redundancy in the stimulus influences naming within the visual modality. With regard to the nature of aphasic naming deficits, he stated, "Without denying the possibility that the structures responsible for the naming process may themselves be damaged, it is nevertheless apparent that in anomic subjects the language disturbance is at least partly conditioned by factors acting at the level of the mechanisms of interaction between the sensory analyzer and the verbal sphere" (p. 95).

Corlew and Nation (1975) tested a portion of the redundant stimuli idea by testing 14 aphasic people with life-size, realistically shaped and colored versus uncolored line drawings, and found no difference. Bisiach (1976) replied to Corlew and Nation, blaming a difference in subject selection for the differences between his and their studies. He may be right; it is difficult to know. But about something else he is absolutely accurate, at least in our view. He said researchers should continue to manipulate the physical characteristics of stimulus objects for what the results may say about naming. We agree; clinicians should continue manipulating also for what the results may say about treatment.

INFLUENCE OF ALTERED STIMULI

Faber and Aten (1979) measured the amount and correctness of speech elicited from aphasic speakers by intact and altered pictorial stimuli. Their instruction to 10 nonfluent and 3 fluent aphasic people was, "Tell me what you see." Two sets of stimuli, matched for frequency of occurrence, were used to elicit naming. The altered stimuli were such things as a broken pencil and a bent coat hanger. The aphasic people produced an equal number of correct names to both lists. The altered subjects, however, elicited a greater number of topically related words. This finding led the authors to suggest that the altered condition effect is due to the arousal of multiple associations surrounding the concept of the object" (p. 184).

Rochford and Williams (1962) measured the influence of "stylized" or "unconventional" pictorial representations. They compared aphasic people's ability to name stylized rare words—unicorn and rosary—with common words—bee and dog—having "unconventionalized pictures." The rare words were easier. Type of representation then has an influence.

Common reps = easier

INFLUENCE OF SINGLE AND COMPOSITE PICTURES

Williams and Canter (1981) compared the naming of 40 aphasic people (10 Broca's, 10 Wernicke's, 10 conduction, 10 amnesic [anomic]) when confronted with simple drawings of single objects and when the single objects were combined into groups of four and presented in a composite picture. The confrontation naming of single objects was completed in a traditional way. Names were elicited for the composite pictures by instructing each patient to describe the pictures. High and low frequency picturable nouns were tested. Errors were classified into 1 of 12 categories.

The Broca's aphasic people were significantly better in confrontation naming. The Wernicke's aphasic people were significantly better in context. No clear trend emerged for the conduction and anomic aphasic people, although individuals from both groups generally showed clear preferences. Overall, high frequency words were easier than low, a predictable finding. Delay, phonetic attempts, and substitution of related words were in the top four most frequent error types for all groups, but some of the less frequent error types such as neologisms helped to distinguish the groups.

These results have clinical utility. They suggest first that even Broca's aphasic people have word finding difficulties. Next, the authors reinforce the notion that "situational context" may influence naming, especially by those with Wernicke's aphasia. They add to their findings their prejudice that poor naming reflects impaired access and conclude that treatment should stimulate retrieval processes. Presumably, this might mean featuring context for Wernicke's and simple pictures for Broca's aphasic people. Myers and Linebaugh (1984) have written a cogent warning about the complexity of pictured stimuli with aphasic people that helps to flesh out the issue of stimulus complexity.

INFLUENCE OF CATEGORIES

A study that provides information both on stimulus selection and on the nature of word storage was completed by Goodglass and colleagues (1966). These authors studied 135 aphasic people (35 Broca's, 35 Wernicke's, 17 amnesic, and the rest unclassifiable). They compared the naming and comprehension of five semantic categories—objects, letters, numbers, actions, and colors.

Object naming was the hardest, and the comprehension of object and action names was the easiest. These authors observed that production and comprehension of the same lexical items may involve different processes, an issue that is beginning to receive experimental attention (Butterworth, Howard, & McLoughlin, 1984). The issue is important clinically. Butterworth and colleagues (1984) suggested that "practice in semantic word discrimination may improve the accuracy of word-finding more than therapy aimed specifically at output itself" (p. 425), at least for some patients.

Goodglass and colleagues (1966) also said that different semantic categories may be "experienced differently psychologically and produced through different processes" (p. 85). Clinicians have to ask if words from different categories can be taught with similar or identical methods—perhaps not. The case of actions and objects is especially interesting in this context, because of the possibility that the right hemisphere makes a greater contribution to the comprehension and use of verbs than to objects.

INFLUENCE OF FREQUENCY AND PICTURABILITY

Goodglass, Hyde, and Blumstein (1969) determined the relationship of frequency and picturability to the appearance of nouns in the speech of Broca's and Wernicke's aphasic people. The data were the nouns taken from transcribed interviews with 17 people with Broca's aphasia and 21 with fluent aphasia, this last group consisting of both Wernicke's and anomic aphasic people. They discovered that the fluent aphasic people used a high incidence of high frequency, nonpicturable nouns. They said such words may be conditioned by the more normal syntactic context that the fluent aphasic people are better able to create than are their more syntactically impaired Broca's aphasic peers. The nouns that the Wernicke's and anomic aphasic people produced were parts of more or less "cast-iron" phrases involving words such as "time," "way," and "day." They made the interesting obser-

vation that "the observed frequency effects are not the cause but a predictable result of the well-known difference between the speech pattern of the two types of aphasia" (p. 118).

INFLUENCE OF PHONEMIC CUEING

A number of researchers have confirmed phonemic cueing's potency. Li and Canter (1983) chose to see if phonemic cueing, in which the speaker is provided with the first sound or two of the target word, varied in its influence according to the type and severity of aphasia. Forty patients (10 Broca's, 10 Wernicke's, 10 conduction, and 10 anomic) served as subjects. Comprehension, naming, articulation, and responsiveness to cues were measured. The results showed that the Broca's aphasic patients were significantly more responsive than were the Wernicke's aphasic patients, who were the least responsive. Conduction and anomic aphasic people occupied an in-between position, closer to the Wernicke's patients. Mild and moderate patients, regardless of type, were more responsive to phonemic cueing than were severe patients. The findings compelled the authors to observe, "Clinically, it may be beneficial to reserve phonemic cueing for aphasic patients with mild to moderate naming difficulties and to use a general stimulation approach, such as Schuell's intensive auditory stimulation for those with severe anomia" (p. 102).

TIMING STIMULUS PRESENTATION

Clinicians have noted that the timing of stimulus presentations is sometimes as crucial as the stimuli themselves. It is easy to err by going too fast or too slow. Brookshire (1971) was among those to study this phenomenon. Specifically, he measured the effects of trial time (exposure time) and intertrial interval on naming. He first looked at naming in relation to the exposure time of stimuli to be named. Stimuli were exposed 3, 5, 10, 30, and a self-regulated number of seconds. Correct naming increased with amount of exposure but the steepest increase was between the three and five second intervals. Not much is gained by longer exposure. Of the self-paced trials, Brookshire stated, "Self-paced trials appear more efficient than machine-paced trials of comparable duration" (p. 295). In a second experiment, the stimuli were exposed for three seconds, but the intertrial interval, which was constant in the first experiment, was either 0, 5, 10, or 30 seconds. Naming was slightly better at the 30 second interval, with no significant differences for 0, 5, and 10. The improvement at 30 seconds, however, was not characteristic of all six experimental subjects. Brookshire concluded that the exposure time is more potent than the intertrial interval. He also said that if a patient is to be allowed a long time to name, the stimulus should remain in view the whole time. In another experiment, he discovered that a 30 second stimulus exposure interval was associated with better naming than a 10 second interval. In one additional experiment, he confirmed that the stress for a quick response can erode performance.

The clinical uses of his data are several: (1) patients may do better if allowed to regulate treatment's pace, (2) patients may do better if stress for quick answers is avoided, and (3) amount of exposure to stimuli may be more important than time between presentations. Because Brookshire repeated the stimulus presentation in these experiments he had data on how his six people did with repeated exposure to the same stimuli. They did not learn. He was quick to point out that the subjects did not receive knowledge of results, so his experiment is unlike typical therapy. He did say, however, that naming does not seem to improve with simple repeated attempts to name, an observation that clinicians devoted to stimulation should remember.

OTHER INFLUENCES

Other influences on naming are the modalities and cues presented in those modalities. Some researchers have compared modality influences either singly or in various combinations. Others have looked at single cues versus a series of cues within a single modality. Others have combined the two. Some of the studies were designed primarily for what they might reveal about aphasia. Others were designed primarily for what the results could teach about treatment. We admit that such a division is especially arbitrary, because concepts of the disorder and concepts of treatment influence one another, and most researchers, regardless of their main concern, speculate about their finding's contribution to understanding both aphasia and management. We will preserve the distinction for our convenience, but readers may sometimes have to disregard it for the same reason.

INFLUENCES OF THE MODALITY

Gardiner and Brookshire (1972) used eight aphasic people and a set of high frequency nouns to determine the influence on naming of auditory, visual, and combined auditory and visual stimulation. In the auditory condition, each subject repeated words uttered by the examiner. In one set of experiments, the visual condition required the patient to name pictured objects as they were flashed on the screen. In another set of experiments, the visual stimuli were written, single words. In the combined conditions, the experimenter named each item as it was presented visually so that the subject both saw and heard the name. In the tradition of research from Brookshire's laboratory, conditions were controlled against threats to validity.

The results have interesting therapeutic implications. Performance in the visual condition was always worse than in the combined and auditory conditions, and performance in the combined condition was always slightly better than in the auditory condition. Of the two visual conditions, picture naming was somewhat better than word reading. This study seems to confirm the traditional practice of combining modalities, although the difference in response adequacy one gets by having the patient imitate while looking at a picture of the thing to be imitated may not be worth the effort. The superiority of naming objects over reading words is more than a little surprising and alerts clinicians to test for stimulus differences. As another example of the importance of attention to individuals, one of their persons was better in the auditory than in the combined auditory-picture condition. Gardiner and Brookshire's analysis of the individual patient responses reinforces the need for protean clinicians.

Because the investigators used several presentations of the single and combined stimuli, they could also draw some conclusions about changes in performance with repeated presentation and about the order effects of certain kinds of stimulation. Their findings were (1) improvement was obvious in both visual and auditory conditions, (2) improvement was not prominent in the combined condition, (3) improvement tended to occur earlier in the auditory than in the visual condition, and to reach a somewhat higher level in the visual condition, (4) performance in the combined condition was strikingly impaired if preceded by the visual condition, and (5) combined stimulation seemed to facilitate performance in the unisensory conditions. What a wealth of clinical data.

One striking implication of this study that has not received the recognition it perhaps deserves is that preceding an easy task with a hard one may depress performance on the easy one. Gardiner and Brookshire hypothesized that this deficit is caused either by a build-up of "noise" or because the patients simply could not shift their attention from the visual during the combined condition. Regardless of the reason, the findings are instructive for clinicians as they prepare their daily clinical experiments—treatment. Starting hard may be ill-advised. The study also confirms the need for diagnostic testing to determine each patient's response tendencies. The authors concluded with this clinical tip, "It would appear that alternating the presentation of stimuli in combined and unisensory conditions would improve the patient's naming performance in one or both unisensory modalities" (p. 356).

TREATMENT OF NAMING

FACILITATION AND DIDACTICISM

The foregoing reviews confirm that aphasic naming problems can differ and that some differences may be predicted from the type of aphasia the patient has. At the extremes of what may be a continuum, naming may fail either because of impaired access to intact semantic networks, as in many patients with Broca's aphasia, or because the networks themselves are impaired, as in many patients with Wernicke's aphasia. At the extremes of a therapeutic continuum for remediating these deficits, clinicians can select a simple facilitation approach in which correct names are merely elicited usually by dint of the clinician's creative stimulus selection and cueing, or they can select a more didactic approach in which the patient's knowledge about words and how to evoke them with self-cueing are enhanced.

These ends of the treatment continuum—facilitation and didacticism—have accummulated an alarming amount of semantic baggage both from within and outside speech-language pathology. We wish we could find less heavily burdened terms, but we cannot. We wish we could lighten their load. We probably cannot do that either. We may shift it and maybe even repack it a little, however, by discussing how the two approaches appear clinically.

In simple facilitation, clinicians choose the stimuli—usually high frequency of occurrence—and manipulate the timing, order, form—usually objects, pictures, or written words—and mode of stimulus presentation—usually auditory, visual, or auditory-visual—so that the speaker's success is nearly guaranteed. The right combination is repeated so that each treated response is elicited several, even several hundred, times within and across sessions.

This Schuellian (Schuell et al., 1964) treatment at its best. Stimulate, stimulate, stimulate. Errors are seldom analyzed except by the clinician who follows up patient errors with restimulation. Cueing hierarchies are used like escalators to whisk the patient along toward improved naming. The clinician does most of the work. The patient mostly profits from that work.

Such treatment is especially appropriate for acutely aphasic persons who are receiving help from physiological recovery or who have not yet realized how aphasia has changed their worlds. It is also for chronic patients, especially as they are entering treatment for the first time or for the first time in a long time, because such facilitation can be non-threatening as well as helpful. A facilitation approach has the additional advantage of allowing clinicians to put much of the naming literature to practical use, because much of that literature describes what aphasic people find easy and hard. Presenting easy stimuli the patient can respond to correctly is the facilitation method's body and soul. Finally, a stimulation approach is consistent with the view that aphasic dysnomia results from impaired access to intact or nearly intact concepts or semantic organizations.

Didactic approaches differ slightly or substantially, depending on how far along the treatment continuum they are. Clinicians still select the stimuli (with appropriate help from the patient) and still manipulate timing, order, form, and mode of presentation. The emphasis, however, is less on the number of correct responses and more on teaching the patient self-cueing and how to cope with errors. Errors are analyzed by clinician and patient together for what each error might teach about how to avoid it next time or how to correct it once it has appeared. Hierarchies are used like ladders. The patient is not whisked along, but advances by dint of self-analysis and self-cueing. Clinician and patient work equally hard.

A didactic approach is most useful with chronically aphasic people who can contribute somewhat more to their own recovery than can the typical acutely aphasic person who is often sick, depressed, and cognitively, as well as linguistically, impaired. Some of the literature helps clinicians plan this kind of treatment, and that literature will be reviewed. Although clinicians who use a didactic approach need not believe that dysnomia results from impaired semantic networks (Seron, Deloche, Bastard, Chassin, Hermand, 1979), they often do.

Handled correctly, didactic approaches need not be traumatic for either recent or chronic aphasic persons. Nor need they remind them of going back to school or of popular publications that promise a more powerful vocabulary in five days. In our experience, didactic approaches have a greater

chance of helping anomic speakers regain stable word finding than does simple facilitation, especially if (1) those speakers have only mild or moderate aphasic residuals, (2) anomia is a major symptom, and (3) they want to improve and will work hard for that improvement. It can be argued that there are too few data on naming to allow such statements. We agree we have not proved our position. We cling to it, however, because it seems to us that one risks less with a didactic than with a facilitation approach. If teaching does not work, probably nothing will.

CUEING HIERARCHIES IN NAMING TREATMENT

Cueing hierarchies to improve naming abound because the systematic presentation of an orderly array of cues is at the heart of aphasia treatment, especially for impaired naming, regardless of whether the practitioner believes in facilitation or in didacticism. Some cues appear in more than one hierarchy, although not necessarily always in the same place. More different than the cues making up the several hierarchies to be described, however, are their origins. A few seem to have been intuitive. Many resulted from analyses of how aphasic people perform when required to produce specific names in response to a series of cues presented in some random or counterbalanced order. A few hierarchies were incorporated into treatment programs, and the efficacy of each program was then tested.

The last section of this chapter summarizes a variety of task continua because all are useful to naming treatment. Some of the programs are fully developed. These can be applied as their progenitors dictate. Others are incomplete or incompletely tested. These can either be taken as is and tested in the clinic, or they can be dismantled, reassemble, and then tested in the clinic. We have only one caveat: be cautious both in the reading and use of what follows.

A NINE STEP DIAGNOSTIC HIERARCHY

Brown (1972) organized nine cueing conditions into a hierarchy based on his assumption that there are several stages in the naming of an object. He said, "As an indication of the stage involved, one may rely on the ability of the anomic patient to respond to such cues as the following, arranged in a tentative ascending order of efficacy for classical anomic aphasia" (p. 28). Even though this hierarchy was not intended for treatment, at least in its present form, we begin with it because of its completeness. Clinicians can always strip it for parts.

Because some of the steps are not self-explanatory, the hierarchy is presented along with the author's example, the word "razor."

1. Responsive, using functional ("It is used for shaving") or descriptive ("It has a metal blade") statements
2. Embedding, in which a word is embedded in a sentence ("You use a _____ for shaving")
3. Synonyms and antonyms
4. Rhyming words
5. Spelling the word
6. Open-ended sentences where the target word is to go at the end of the sentence ("You shave with a _____")
7. Automatic completions ("A straight-edge_____")
8. Phonemic cues (/reI/ or /r/)
9. Repetition

The assumption is that repetition is most likely to elicit the name and functional and descriptive statements are least likely to do so. Brown admitted, however, that different patients may have different hierarchies. Clinicians can use the hierarchy diagnostically and therapeutically. The cues can be systematically compared for their influence on each patient's naming. The cues can then be ordered from most to least facilitating, and the patient can be moved systematically and successfully from the easiest step to the most difficult. Other cues can be added or substituted. Indeed, the clinician can use this set of cues in all imaginable ways. Depending on one's purpose, for example, it might be useful to start with the hardest and move to the easiest and back again.

A HIERARCHY OF SIX CUES

Pease and Goodglass (1978) studied six cues: (1) providing the first sound or sound combination, (2) providing a superordinate ("animal" to cue "dog," for example), (3) providing an environmental context or location for the target, (4) providing a rhyming word, (5) providing a statement of function, and (6) providing a sentence completion cue. They studied 20 aphasic people using 173 pictured items, sorted into one of the six cueing conditions, depending on which cue seemed most appropriate to each word. Frequency of occurrence across lists was apparently controlled. Statistical analysis revealed the statistically significant power to evoke words of supplying the first sound or sound combination. This cue occasionally worked even with severe patients who were unhelped by the other cues. Sentence completion was the next most powerful cue. Rhyme ranked third in Pease and Goodglass's study, but was not significantly better than superordinate, function, or location.

A clinical cueing hierarchy organized from most to least facilitating based on these data, but that ignores the lack of a statistically significant difference among rhyme and the last three cues would be:

Step One: First sound or sound combination
Step Two: Sentence completion
Step Three: Rhyme
Step Four: Superordinate, Function, Location

On the other hand, Pease and Goodglass's data could be ignored altogether and the six cues could be organized into a six step hierarchy by a bit of diagnostic testing with individual patients. Our own experience is that these cues (like all the cues mentioned in this chapter) work differently not only for different patients but for different words and for the same patients with different words and at different times in their treatments.

A HIERARCHY OF FOUR CUES

Love and Webb (1977) compared the influence on picture naming by 20 Broca's aphasic speakers of (1) imitation, (2) providing the initial sound or sound combination, (3) sentence completion, and (4) reading. Presentation of 30 pictures in the four stimulus conditions was randomized except that imitation was always presented last because the authors anticipated that it would be easiest. Imitation, as predicted, was the most potent, providing the initial sound or syllable was next, sentence completion and reading were in last place and not significantly different. Love and Webb reported that this hierarchy was generated by more severe patients and that no hierarchy emerged for the milder subgroup, probably because stimuli were too easy.

Love and Webb's hierarchy resembles both Brown's and Pease and Goodglass's, and begins to affirm one's belief in the lawfulness of aphasia, a lawfulness that can be counted on (more or less) in treatment. Their data also remind us that cueing hierarchies and severity of aphasia interact.

A HIERARCHY OF THREE CUES

Barton, Maruszewski, and Urrea (1969) measured the potency of confrontation naming, sentence completion, and naming to description. Subjects were 9 persons with Broca's aphasia, 9 with conduction aphasia, 7 with Wernicke's aphasia, and 11 with anomic aphasia. Their hierarchy from most to least powerful based on group data is (1) sentence completion, (2) confrontation naming, and (3) description. They pointed out that 16 patients (approximately 44 percent) did not follow the hierarchy and that five found description the most rather than the least facilitating. That last finding should make all clinicians leery of all generic hierarchies. That description was more likely to produce a correct response by some patients than was sentence completion seems to fly in the face of clinical sense. Diagnostic testing makes a good face guard.

COMBINING CUES

Weidner and Jinks (1983) used 24 nonfluent aphasic people placed into either a mild or a severe aphasia group to study the individual and combined potency of (1) printed words, (2) initial syllable, and (3) sentence completion. Stimuli were 100 commercially available pictures. Their experimental design required nine stimulus sets and was reasonably complex but allowed for the comparison of the three cueing conditions by themselves and in several combinations. Stimulus set A, for example, began with the printed word cue, which was then combined with sentence completion if the speaker was unable to name, and both were then combined with the initial syllable if the speaker was again unsuccessful. In contrast, stimulus set G required that the three cues be presented one after the other, first written word, then sentence completion, then presentation of initial syllable. Both procedures resemble what clinicians do in treatment, and this similarity to treatment is one of the study's attractive features.

The authors did not find a best hierarchy, a not unexpected finding. However, the authors did report that combining cues is more potent than presenting them singly or in succession. Apparently, a combination of two was as good, statistically, as a combination of three; although patient severity and other idiosyncratic variables no doubt influenced how individuals did. Written word cues were the most successful single cues for mildly aphasic people. Initial syllable cueing was least effective for both mild and severe groups, a somewhat surprising finding in light of how well initial sound cues usually fare in this kind of research. The severe group seemed to respond about equally to all cues, but their performance may have favored either sentence completion or written word cueing. The authors ended with a reasonable clinical suggestion; determine each speaker's cueing hierarchy.

A COMPARISON OF TWO HIERARCHIES

Goodglass and Stuss (1979) compared two hierarchies: (1) picture followed by phonemic cue, and (2) verbal description followed by phonemic cue. They tested 10 Broca's, 7 Wernicke's, and 6 anomic aphasic people. The examiner provided three characteristics of the object to be named in the verbal description condition. The other conditions were traditional ones. The authors measured latency and correctness of patient responses to determine the relative effectiveness of the two hierarchies. The Broca's aphasic people performed better than all the other groups on both hierarchies, and like the Wernicke's aphasic people, they did better than the anomic patients with the confrontation naming condition. The Broca's aphasic people were significantly better than the Wernicke's aphasic people in naming to description. The phonemic cues were especially successful for the Broca's aphasic people. For all patients, confrontation naming usually elicited a correct response at once or not at all (each subject had 30 seconds to name each target).

These data have a number of interesting clinical implications. They suggest that Broca's aphasic people may respond equally to a variety of cueing hierarchies. They support the conclusion from other studies that the naming difficulties of different types of aphasic people are different. They suggest that descriptions are weak cues for all patients, perhaps because descriptions require substantial understanding and memory.

CUEING HIERARCHIES USED IN TREATMENT

Previously reviewed hierarchies were not used therapeutically. In other words, they were not used to change behavior, they were merely used to elicit responses once or a few times. Clinicians recognize that once is inadequate and a few times may be only a little better if a patient is going to begin talking better outside the clinic as the result of systematic talking inside it. However, these hierarchies could be used clinically, and that is why they were presented. Some hierarchies whose therapeutic efforts have been studied have also been reported in the literature. Testing does not make such hierarchies better than those previously described. Indeed, many of the steps in both kinds are the same. The advantage of these next to be described are that directions for using the hierarchies as well as the hierarchies themselves are normally reported. The result is a more complete clinical package.

A HIERARCHY CREATED BY PATIENTS

Linebaugh and Lehner (1977) allowed a series of patients (number not recorded) to determine by their errors the relative potency of 10 cueing activities. The 10 were then organized into a hierarchy, and five patients were treated. The method of using the hierarchy resembles a common clinical practice. Treatment started at the top of the hierarchy, in this case, with confrontation naming and then proceeded down it, one cue at a time, until a correct name was elicited. Following a correct response, each patient was directed back up the hierarchy, only to reverse once again if the name failed to emerge in response to a given cue.

The hierarchy, from least to most powerful cue, is:

1. Confrontation naming
2. Direction by the clinician to have the patient state the function and then try to name
3. Direction by the clinician to have the patient demonstrate the function and then try to name
4. Statement of function by the clinician
5. Statement of function by the clinician accompanied by demonstration
6. Sentence completion provided by the clinician
7. Sentence completion plus silent posturing of the target word's first sound provided by the clinician
8. Sentence completion plus audible production of the target's first sound provided by the clinician
9. Sentence completion plus audible vocalization of the target word's first and second sounds by the clinician
10. Imitation

To study the hierarchy's potency, the authors assigned words of approximately equal frequency to treated and untreated groups. Treated words were moved up and down the hierarchy as previously described. According to Linebaugh and Lehner, more than one reversal was seldom necessary for the five patients. They are reported to have learned the treated lists, and the learning reportedly generalized to untreated words. Linebaugh and Lehner added without explanation that two patients "showed greater improvement on the generalization words" (p. 28) than on the treated ones. They said their program is consistent with two principles of treatment: (1) elicit a response with the weakest possible cues, and (2) systematically fade the cues. They observed that their hierarchy "facilitates the word retrieval process as a whole" (p. 28).

Their recipe for treatment is a good one. It need not be the entire therapeutic offering, but it can be an important portion. Because it is orderly, it can easily be modified to fit individual tastes. We like it especially because it is the first to include self-cueing. We seldom use a hierarchy that does not.

A THREE STEP TREATMENT HIERARCHY

Thompson and Kearns (1981) placed 40 written (not pictured) words into four lists. Lists A-1 and B-1 were semantically related, as were lists A-2 and B-2. These four lists were then put into a multiple baseline design, and each list was treated in turn by progress through a three step task continuum. The three steps were (1) sentence completion, (2) sentence completion plus cueing with the first sound or sound combination, and (3) sentence completion plus imitation. Progress from step to step, beginning with step one, the most difficult, depended on the patient's reaching a 90 percent criterion on the treated set of words.

Their aphasic speaker, a 64-year-old woman, was four years postonset of a left hemisphere stroke when the study began. Treatment was two or three times per week for 84 sessions. She benefited at least a little from the treatment. Treated words responded to the hierarchy and gains were maintained, but treatment effects did not generalize. We have included their study not only for its hierarchy, but because the treatment design can be a model for clinicians interested in clinical research. This report's other strength is its contribution to our thinking about what treatment does. Unlike most other authors quoted thus far, Thompson and Kearns did not believe

that their results confirm improvement in a "general retrieval process." If such were the case, they reasoned that generalization would have been expected. Instead, they seemed to suggest that something about the semantic fields or concepts was disrupted in their speaker. They were also quick to remind us that other hierarchies and other patients might have behaved differently. We cannot argue with their caveat. We can, however, reinforce their feeling about disturbed fields in aphasia. Many aphasic people, even if they are not globally aphasic, have them. Merely evoking words may not be therapeutic for such patients.

HIERARCHIES AND RAPID MOVEMENT

To improve naming, Basso (1978) used a variety of cueing hierarchies; rapid, repetitive stimulation; and quick movement up and down the appropriate hierarchy. Her general approach was to elicit automatic responses which were then moved toward increased "intentionality." The typical program begins with a step in which the patient is shown a picture which is to be pointed at and named. If the patient fails to respond, the clinician then supplies an open-ended sentence—and if need be—a phonemic cue, and asks the patient to try again. Basso said that a forceful production of the sentence creates a verbal environment that makes the patient's utterance nearly automatic.

Once the patient has begun to name (and it is assumed names will appear), the clinician has a choice of ways to make the task harder. Because treatment begins with a single picture, the patient can be faced with a greater number of choices from which the target is to be selected and named. According to Basso, the challenge can also be increased by having the patient supply the word as the completion to a nonfacilitating, open-ended sentence such as "This is a _____." Once a response emerges from any of these conditions, the clinician then asks for a repetition of the name after a delay. Next, the patient can be helped to create sentences with the target word. This seems like a giant clinical step to us, unless the sentence, like the name, is elicited first of all with maximum cues which are then faded. Another of her methods, although it is not clear where it appears in a given hierarchy, is for the clinician to help patients decide on a word by having them "look for the required word within the correct semantic sphere" (p. 12). If the target is "cat," a patient can be asked, "Is it a dog?" or "Is it a horse?" and so on. Basso's report was somewhat informal, so no data were provided, nor did she outline specific steps. Her thesis, however, is clear: Do what must be done to elicit a response, then help the speaker respond with ever increasing independence until the target words appear predictably in volitional, connected speech.

HIERARCHY FOR THE LANGUAGE MASTER

Keenan (1966) reported on a hierarchy to improve naming that used the Language Master (Bell & Howell, Co., Chicago, IL). As part of program development, he prepared two sets of words on Language Master cards. In Set I, which included nouns, verbs, and numbers, the patient saw on one side of the card the pictured target, one pictured foil, and the target's written name. When put through the machine, each Language Master card produced the target's name. The picture of the target and the printed name were represented on the reverse side of each Set I card. In Set II, the face of each card pictured the target and its written name. The name was again recorded on the magnetic recording strip. The written name was the only thing appearing on the back of the card.

The card sets were presented in a hierarchy of nine tasks. Because these tasks are a useful set of procedures, they are repeated here. The first three procedures use Set I; the others use Set II.

1. Patient listens to the recorded name, reads the name, and then points to the appropriate picture. To check the answer, the patient then turns the card around and imitates (or reads aloud) the spoken and printed words.
2. Patient points to the target without playing the card. He or she checks by looking at the card's back side and then plays the card and imitates the signal.
3. Patient listens to the name but the printed form is covered from view. He or she checks by exposing the written name, then plays the card and imitates the signal.
4. Patient looks at the target while the written name is covered, then plays the card and repeats the name, then writes the word and checks the answer by comparing with the name written on the card.
5. Patient looks at the target and printed word, then copies the word, then says the name, and finally checks the response by playing the card.
6. Patient looks at the back side of the card with the word covered, plays the card, writes the word, and then checks the written response.
7. Patient copies the word from the back side, speaks the word, and then plays the card to check the response.
8. Patient looks at the picture with the written word covered, writes the name, checks the answer, plays the card, and then repeats the spoken word.
9. Patient looks at the picture with the written name covered, says the name, then plays card to check the answer.

Keenan said a limited number of patients have made "satisfactory progress" with this and similar programs. It is unclear how the program is to be used. Strict use presumably requires the clinician to move through each of these steps. Keenan, if asked, would probably say that the program is to be fitted to the patient. If such custom designing is done, steps can be omitted, reordered, and even redesigned.

A CUEING HIERARCHY COMBINED WITH DRILL

Rosenbek and colleagues (1977) treated a 58-year-old anomic aphasic man who was aphasic secondary to a closed head injury, subdural hematoma, and subsequent surgery. The design was a withdrawal design in which the patient was alternately admitted to the hospital for a month of treatment (three times) and then released to return home without treatment for a month.

The authors combined a task continuum with traditional multimodality drill. The program shares some features with the Language Master program just reviewed. In step one, both a picture and written word were presented, and the patient named it or read it aloud. No effort was made to determine which the patient was doing. Correct naming was followed by drill in which the patient spelled the word orally, wrote the word, and then named it once again. If the patient failed to name in response to the picture and written cue, the clinician then spelled the word aloud and had the patient say the word that had just been spelled. This was an especially powerful cue for their speaker. If all that failed, the patient was given the word to imitate, although this cue was not mentioned in their report. In step two, the clinician showed the patient a picture of an object and simultaneously provided an open-ended sentence cue. If the name was not forthcoming, the clinician provided the first letter (but not the first sound). If it still did not appear, the clinician spelled the whole word. In step three, the clinician's job got simpler, and the patient's more difficult. The clinician merely showed a stimulus picture. The patient had to name the picture and then, if possible, create a sentence, preferably a function sentence, using the word. In step four, the clinician presented two or more related pictures, which the patient had already seen at previous steps, and the patient was required to generate one or more sentences about them.

Several kinds of cueing condition are included in steps one and two, and it is impossible to know how many repetitions of particular steps and cues were required for the patient to learn. It is reported, however, that no learning or generalization occurred until near the end of the second treatment month. When progress began, it occurred on both treated and untreated words and seems to have spread to other kinds of speech-language performance. "Seems to" because all changes occurred within the first year and spontaneous

improvement may have been occurring and adding its influence to that of the clinician. A pattern of degeneration during withdrawal that would have suggested clinician control over the naming response was not consistently demonstrated.

OTHER KINDS OF PROGRAMS

Not all programs are constructed around a kind of therapeutic Jacob's ladder, although an ordering of something—stimuli, amount of cueing, amount of independence—characterizes most programs not only for naming but for all symptoms of aphasia. The following programs feature hierarchies less and other principles—auditory stimulation, deblocking, priming, multimodality stimulation—more than did the programs just reviewed.

SCHUELLIAN TREATMENT: I

Helmich and Wipplinger (1975) studied the influence of Scheullian treatment on naming in one "neurologically stable" 54 year old person with mild aphasia and a prominent naming deficit. Treatment began eight weeks after a single cerebrovascular accident (CVA). Forty-five words from the Peabody Picture Vocabulary Test (PPVT) that the patient failed to identify on two administrations of the test were selected for treatment.

The 45 words were randomized into one of three conditions: no treatment, maximum treatment, and minimum treatment. The difference between maximum and minimum was only in the number of repetitions of the stimuli. The treatment comprised four steps: identification, contextual cue, differentiation, and tracing-copying. In identification, the patient was shown a picture while the clinician named it. In contextual cue, the patient saw a picture while the clinician used the word in a sentence. In differentiation, the target's picture was included in a display of four and the clinician pointed to the target and named it. In tracing-copying, an extremely busy step, the clinician first printed the word, then read it. Next, the patient copied the word and the clinician named it.

The program emphasized the stimulus rather than the response and patients were not to respond verbally until the four steps were completed. In the minimum condition, the four steps were presented once for each target. In the maximum condition, each of the four steps was presented four times. Maximum and minimum treatments were presented on alternate days during four weeks of treatment. Beginning on the second day, each session began with a confrontation naming test of the words treated in the previous day. At treatment's completion, and again two weeks later, all PPVT words were retested.

The authors reported that maximum and minimum stimulation improved naming equally. Untreated words apparently showed an unstable pattern of slight improvement. The authors concluded "application of a planned treatment program enhanced the naming skills" (p. 26) of their patient. They also said "that using a reduced amount of stimulus repetition maintains therapeutic effectiveness, yet results in a more economical use of therapy time" (p. 28). They admitted that small gains on untreated items could reflect either generalization or spontaneous recovery. Predictably, they favored the former. Unfortunately, their design prevented their being sanguine. They said, for example, that their patient was neurologically stable yet they reported, almost as an aside, that his hemiplegia improved during the treatment's course. Perhaps they meant by medically stable only that he could tolerate the treatment. And, although limbs and language can and do change independently, the motor system's change makes us wonder about physiological recovery, especially because this patient was studied only two months following his CVA. Two months is within the period of physiological recovery for many patients. Nonetheless, their study is useful as a sample of how two clinicians translated Schuell's suggestion (Schuell et al., 1964) for repeated, multimodality stimulation into a four phase treatment.

SCHUELLIAN TREATMENT: II

Wiegel-Crump and Koenigsknecht (1973) studied the influence of a Schuell-like stimulation program on the naming of four aphasic people. All four were at least three months postonset and had undergone only limited speech-language therapy. All had moderate to severe naming deficits. The authors noted they purposefully excluded mildly and profoundly involved speakers.

The researchers began with 150 picturable words from three frequency of occurrence distributions and from five superordinate categories: household items, clothing, food, living things, and action words. Confrontation naming and picture referent matching tasks were created. The 150 words were presented twice prior to treatment and words to be treated and those to be saved as generalization items were selected from the error responses. Food items went entirely untreated to serve as a measure of generalization across superordinate categories. Twenty treated and 20 untreated words equated for frequency of occurrence within each of the four treated superordinate categories were finally selected. To measure treatment and generalization effects, all 150 words were presented for confrontation naming and picture matching at the beginning of every sixth session.

Eighteen one-hour treatment sessions held two or three times a week constituted the treatment period. Treatment was based on Schuell's principles. Rate, rhythm, stress, and length of stimuli were adjusted "to provide maximum optimum stimulation" (p. 413). To further reinforce the treatment, each treated word was presented 10 times, then presented in 5 short sentences, then presented alone 10 more times. In addition to this auditory stimulation, each word was presented pictorially, and if a particular stimulus presentation failed to elicit a response, "auxiliary stimuli" such as gestures, associations, open-ended sentences, and word-initial speech sounds were also provided. As the authors said, "Clinical time was most profitably spent in stimulating and in eliciting language, not forcing the patient to respond" (p. 413).

The patients improved progressively as measured during the sixth, twelfth, and eighteenth sessions. Naming of treated items increased as did naming for untreated items within the same category. Even naming within the untreated food category improved. Latency of response decreased overall, but did so most for the treated items. Frequency of occurrence had no effect on the results. The pattern of improvement caused the authors to conclude, "This equivalence of progress across super-ordinate categories... indicated that the amnesic component is symptomatic of disturbance of lexical retrieval and does not represent an absolute loss of information from the lexical store" (p. 414). They also used the patient's pretreatment superiority in picture-referent matching over naming and the significant change in all responses after only six treatment sessions as further proof of an intact lexical store. Whether or not their findings contribute to the argument about naming deficits in aphasia is arguable. What is not arguable is their contribution to our confidence about the efficacy of naming treatments.

AN ICONOCLAST'S PROGRAM

Von Stockert (1978) said, "I do not believe in repetitive sensory stimulation as a good technique for alleviating word finding difficulties. I consider it to be frustrating both for the patient and the therapist to repeat such stimulations for twenty times as Schuell recommends" (p. 101). He believes that "because the normal connexions do not work we have to activate detour connexions" (p. 101). What is his goal? "We try to enrich and strengthen the associative field... in order to get a verbal response such as naming" (p. 102). Von Stockert's program involves sets of words and words in sentences which are sorted into semantically related and unrelated groups. He called this a combined "lexical semantic" and "syntactic structural" (p. 102) approach and said it is appropriate both to Broca's aphasic persons with their syntactic problems, on the one hand, and Wernicke's aphasic persons with their semantic problems, on the other. We will describe only the lexical program in this section, but interested readers may want to consult the complete essay.

In Von Stockert's program, the clinician selects a target word which appears against a red background and then surrounds it with five related and five unrelated pictures. The patient's task is to order the five related pictures under the target and set the unrelated pictures aside. Mistakes are pointed out and the patient is helped to correct them. Once a correct array is spread out on the table, the clinician names first the target and then the five related words, all the while pointing to each one in turn. Patients are not required to speak; neither are they punished for spontaneous attempts to name.

In the next step, the written names of the objects are used. The clinician takes the target's written name, reads it aloud, and then places it by the target. The clinician then gives the other word cards, one at a time, to the patient, with instructions to place each under the picture of the object each names. The clinician adds additional stimulation by reading each word card and pointing to the appropriate picture. The clinician urges self-correction and aids correction if the patient can not do it alone. When this procedure is complete, training in syntax begins.

This program is multimodal and tries to keep pressure off the verbal performance. Speech is not forced, nor even emphasized. If the patient begins to say the names at any point in the program, however, that speech is encouraged. Once a patient has begun to talk, repeats may be requested. Unfortunately, the author reported no data, but said that studies were underway. Doubtless, data are now available. As a procedure to be integrated with others, this one seems logical. Its difference from simple stimulation, however, should not be exaggerated. Schuell would probably have approved, probably used exercises similar to the ones described here, and would probably wonder what all the fuss was about.

SORRT

Logue and Dixon (1979) were among the very few to assign their naming program an acronym. SORRT stands for Semantic, Oppositional, and Rhyming Retrieval Training. The program begins with listening. In step one, the patient is faced with word pairs that are either rhyming words, synonyms, or antonyms. The patient has to indicate what each pair is. In step two, the patient makes similar judgments about paired visual stimuli. The target and four other stimuli are presented on a card, and the patient selects the antonym, synonym, and rhyme. In step three, the patient is required to produce the same antonyms, synonyms, and rhymes the clinician has previously provided auditorily or visually. In step four, the patient is to produce additional antonyms, synonyms, and rhymes. Their patients seem to improve. Additional conrolled data would be welcome.

A COMPUTER PROGRAM

Colby, Christinaz, Parkison, Graham, and Karpf (1981) have published a computer program for anomic aphasic patients. It is based on the tip-of-the-tongue phenomenon previously reviewed. To a greater degree than all other programs reviewed, this one requires the patient to supply information about the target word. They described the program this way: "The general approach is: 1) to store as a data-base a lexical-semantic memory which in content and relations approximates the patient's lexical memory, and 2) to heuristically search this memory using clues the patient supplies about the target word" (p. 275). Patients' abilities to read, write, and make associations are measured prior to the program's initiation, and the program requires that they have considerable facility with all three. Indeed, they say the "conceptual-semantic" system must be intact.

The computer displays 15 topic areas. The patient first chooses a topic area for the word he or she cannot find. He or she then is asked for the first letter, then the last, then for letters in the middle and then for associations (What word does this word go with?). According to the authors, two or three bits of such information are necessary to retrieval. This program may be but one of a score of soon to be available programs for improving naming. This one requires considerable integrity of the semantic field and of the ability to spell. Broca's aphasic people will probably be better with it than will anomic and Wernicke's aphasic people.

DEBLOCKING

According to Weigl (1968, 1970), "The phenomenon of deblocking in aphasia consists in the total or partial disappearance of disturbances of various verbal performances when the disturbed, i.e., 'blocked,' verbal reaction is preceded by an unblocked adequate response" (1970, p. 288). Weigl said the patient should be kept ignorant of both the target to be deblocked and the deblocking stimulus, a position that Canter (1973) would probably sympathize with, because "the process must to a certain degree develop 'automatically,' unconsciously" (1970, p. 288). When deblocking works, it does so because "the capacity for decoding, coding and recoding verbal information is not completely obliterated" (1968, p. 144). Being less in awe of knowledge's effect on aphasic speech than Weigl, we are not much concerned with the aphasic person's knowing what we are up to. With this one reservation, we subscribe to the deblocking notion.

Deblocking can be direct as when "the key word appears in the prestimulation phase" (1970, p. 289). To deblock the word "slipper," in response to a picture, for example, one patient first heard several words, including "slipper" prior to seeing the picture of a slipper, which was itself just one of many pictures shown to the patient. Apparently, the word was forthcoming. The fate of the other names is not recorded. Indirect elicitation can be accomplished by presenting a "corresponding generic noun, the synonym, a semantically proximate word (i.e., plate instead of cup), an antonymical noun (i.e., darkness instead of lightness)" (1970, p. 289). Indirect elicitation is not easy to demonstrate with "slipper." "Wife" is easier. To evoke it, one might precede a picture with words such as "woman," "marriage," and "husband." Deblocking can be accomplished with a series of semantically related words which may include the target (direct) or not (indirect). To deblock "onion," as an example of elicitation with a series of related words, Weigl offered these deblockers, "hot, tears, sharp, frying." Perhaps it is the translation that makes "hot" appear. To accomplish deblocking of some responses, Weigl suggested stimulating the target with a chain of "restimulators." For example, a word to be named might be preceded by reading the word, copying it, and hearing it. Weigl said he had evidence confirming that deblocking of certain responses for certain stimuli was found to require a specific, unchanging order in the chained stimuli. We do not doubt it. Nor do we doubt that a one link chain (merely seeing the word's written form, for example) is sometimes all that is necessary to deblock a name, although we recognize that a patient's ability to read a word aloud is not evidence that he or she knows or can use the word spontaneously. Longer chains might be more appropriate in a total treatment aimed at improving performance in several modalities.

Clinicians recognize the possibility that certain kinds of cues will make it less rather than more likely that a specific name will appear. Weigl admitted that deblocking can lead to a "deviation-phenomenon" in which a related word from the deblocking stimuli appears as a replacement for the target. In our experience, related words are potentially but not inevitably disruptive. Clinical experimentation will resolve the issue for individual patients. Some researchers have already begun collecting clinically useful data.

Podraza and Darley (1977) completed a deblocking study using 80 words and 5 patients. They looked at the relative potency of (A) "phonetic prestimulation" in which the target's first sound was combined with a neutral vowel prior to the patient's seeing a picture of the target, (B) open-ended sentences, (C) prestimulation with two semantically unrelated words so that the target was presented along with two dissimilar words (e.g., if the target is "bee," the patient might hear "live, bee, goat"), (D) prestimulation with three related words (e.g., "sting, honey, hive"), and (E) confrontation naming.

A, B, and C were significantly better at evoking correct names than D and E, but were not significantly different from each other, and E was significantly better than D. Once again, stimulating with the first sound and with open-ended sentences are proven to be powerful, although the supremacy of one over the other is not established. Nor are the two conditions significantly better than giving the patient the target as part of a series of three. Prestimulating with related words, which has a kind of heuristic appeal, was less facilitating than just seeing a picture of the target. Of treatment, they said that each patient may need a unique hierarchy. They also said, "The problem of facilitating word retrieval in aphasia can be viewed as one of stimulating the patient with cues that provide what for him is the temporarily unavailable information that is blocking complete recall" (pp. 677–679).

PRIMING WITH ENVIRONMENTAL SOUNDS

Mills (1977) studied the therapeutic effect on naming of environmental sounds. His purpose was to test the potency of environmental sound cues in a naming program. He wanted to discover if an object's characteristic sound could become a "retrieval cue" (p. 71). He prepared lists of 32 words both with and without characteristic environmental sounds. Sixteen of each type were combined to form List A and sixteen of each type were combined into List B. Both lists were similar in word frequency. Four aphasic patients, each of whom had suffered a single, left hemisphere cerebrovascular accident at least one month prior to the study, were treated. Two were undergoing traditional treatment at the time of this study, but treatment other than the experimental type reported was suspended for the duration of the investigation. Prior to treatment, Mills demonstrated with an environmental sound recognition task that all four subjects "had a cognitive representation of environmental sound within their systems" (p. 71).

Prior to treatment, each patient was asked to name the 64 items. Subsequently, the four received four training trials of approximately 12 minutes each, during which each of the 32 List A and List B words was drilled once. In the treatment trials a picture was presented on a screen and an appropriate environmental noise was presented simultaneously through earphones. Correct naming was rewarded by the illumination of a red light. Words with no associated environmental sound (16 in List A and 16 in List B) were merely presented on a screen while white noise was presented through the earphones. Correct responses were again rewarded with the red light. Naming without environmental sound cues or feedback was tested after the first four treatment trials, then four more treatments were provided, and progress was tested once again. Both response time and accuracy were measured.

His results are encouraging, for although the difference between drilled and nondrilled environmental sound words and drilled and nondrilled words without environmental sounds was not significantly different after four treatments, it was after eight. Drilled words with associated environmental sounds were most improved, and undrilled environmental sound words were next most improved. He said, "The decrease in the drilled ES function indicates that providing the environmental-sound-based practice resulted in a retrieval strategy which was internalized by the subjects. The improvement in the nondrilled ES items indicates that the strategy learned was generalized to a lesser extent to the items in the nondrilled ES list" (p. 74).

TEACHING PATIENTS TO GENERATE THEIR OWN CUES

We have mentioned frequently that patients may have to learn cues to retrieval. Most programs already described have emphasized the name rather than how the speaker is to elicit it independently. Linebaugh and Lehner's program (1977) contained the roots of a difference, as did an early report by Berman and Peelle (1967), which summarized methods for teaching aphasic patients to generate their own cues. Unfortunately, Berman and Peelle did not provide data, but then very few did in those days. Among the methods they said improved naming were to have the patient (1) write the first letter, (2) sound out the first letter, and (3) use a self-generated sentence completion. Berman and Peelle also emphasized using what they called

associative errors to help elicit correct responses. Their article is important despite the absence of data because it emphasized teaching patients to help themselves.

MULTIMODALITY DRILL AND SELF-CUEING

If the anomic speaker is not being swept along by physiological recovery or if it appears that physiological changes will be incomplete and if the patient is eager to improve, we recommend introducing a program to teach names which relies ultimately on self-cueing. The implication is not that the speaker has no idea about what he or she is to say; it is only that the words he or she uses are unstable. Some words may be recognized but never used, others may neither be recognized nor used, others may be recognized sometimes and used sometimes. In our experience, patients' naming difficulties are never just one thing. Nor is our program. What follows then is a wide trail rather than a set of steps.

PROCEDURES: GROUP ONE

Procedures from Group One are diagnostic and involve determining words with which an individual speaker has difficulty. This is done in four ways—by listening to controlled spontaneous speech, by analyzing the patient's wants and needs, by using specific naming tasks, and by introducing a variety of words into treatment to find out if the speaker recognizes the words and can use them correctly. All four processes go on continually and simultaneously.

Usually, the clinician can guess at categories of words the patient can be expected to need and has only to introduce appropriate topics to see how many such words the patient can produce, how reliably, and with what self-generated cues. For example, a craftsman or tinkerer would benefit from knowing the names for tools and materials; a sports enthusiast needs to know the names of positions, equipment, mascots, and maneuvers; a homemaker's life is made easier by having the names of food stuffs, appliances, quantities, and the like. It is reasonably easy to develop a list of words for drill after short periods of discussion about such topics. Such lists can be confirmed and expanded by special formal and informal tests requiring the patient to identify and name selected words.

What a patient does during attempts to name can also supply grist for treatment's mill. We watch our patients respond and we note the predictable occurrence of gesturing, the appearance of synonyms and phonemically related words, the use of descriptions and gestures, and those long pauses with eyes turned skyward. We note, where possible, which of these seem to help and which do not. We also ask patients, assuming they are mild enough to respond, what they are doing that helps. Some of the things patients do are symptoms of difficulty; some of the things they do are attempts at self-cueing. By noting what precedes correctness and by asking the right questions, the clinician can tell the difference.

We do not worry about the number of words selected for treatment nor about how many words a speaker drills at any one time. We are influenced by the demands of single-case design, especially of the multiple baseline design, however, so we select (or try to) an even number of words so they can be randomly assigned to one of several equally sized lists. An excellent model for this kind of clinical research approach to stimulus selection is a study by Thompson and Kearns (1981). Once a group of words has been selected, treatment can begin.

PROCEDURES: GROUP TWO

The aim is to expand and strengthen associations and give the patient systematic practice with word use. Patients are first of all reinforced for what they are already doing to help themselves. For example, if a patient attempts to gesture an object's use or draw its shape, we have the patient continue to do so concurrently with saying the appropriate word. Patients who use sentence completion or description are told to keep doing so and are helped to build the most powerful cloze contexts and descriptions for individual words. Together, patient and clinician experiment with a variety of cloze contexts and practice creating the most vivid descriptions possible. Patients who write the first letter or first few letters in the air or on paper are encouraged to continue doing so, and writing and spelling drills then become a significant part of their treatment. If visualization, as of a bench in the park, helps evoke the word "bench," for example, such visualizations are drilled. Data suggesting the effectiveness of visualization are beginning to appear (Thompson, Hall, & Sison, 1986). Clinician and patient create the most vivid scenes possible and then rehearse these. Regardless of the specific self-cue being practiced, the emphasis is on drill. It is not enough merely to recall the word, the strategies for its access are also practiced so that the whole cluster is expanded, strengthened, and made more predictable.

As a word's stability increases, or simultaneously with efforts to increase it, other forms of the target word are introduced. For example, if the target is "bench," clinician and patient can discuss park bench, work bench, bench strength, being benched, bench presses, and going before the bench. We do not usually rely on a list of related words such as chair, couch, and stool, however, because our experience has been that such words are more likely to compete with the target than to enhance its strength. We do occasionally teach antonyms simultaneously, especially if they can be associated with very different gestures or other cues. Push and pull, for example, can be taught together. In fairness to Weigl and others, it is even possible to take related words which often emerge as substitutes for intended words, and by reinforcing both the target and one or more related words simultaneously, help the speaker learn to separate them. If nothing else, the speaker might learn "I always say 'P.J.'s' when I mean 'shirt,' so I must be trying to say 'shirt' because I just said 'P.J.'s'." Obviously, such word finding procedures take time. If the patients agree they have the time to spend and want to, we forge ahead.

No two words need to receive the same treatment. Some words cannot be gestured, for example, and some words have only one or two frequently used meanings or associations. What does work with all targets, however, is systematic drill with knowledge of results and analysis of errors. In contrast to traditional elicitation in which the clinician primarily restimulates, in this treatment clinician and patient share responsibility. Nonetheless, the treatment has features in common with elicitation: a high number of repetitions; careful stimulus-response selection, ordering, and timing; and the goal of keeping the patient successful enough so that treatment does not become more painful than failed conversations.

PROCEDURES: GROUP THREE

Group Three procedures are an admixture of procedures to increase generalization across words and situations. Our hypothesis is that treatments to strengthen associations, including as they do specific procedures to enhance self-correction and cueing, are more likely to generalize than is simple elicitation. Self-cueing is especially important because it helps "mediate generalization." So, as part of Group Three procedures, we both expand the number of treated stimuli within specific categories and we increasingly emphasize independent cueing.

More importantly, we try to increase the number of environments in which target words are used. Type of language use is one such environment. Names that appear within treatment's rigidly controlled stimulus conditions are more likely to appear in less controlled ones if the less controlled ones are also introduced in treatment. To this end then, we use the usual array of controlled spontaneous speech tasks—question and answer, summary of read material, controlled conversation, and

so on. Generalization across people can be aided by providing a variety of clinicians (when possible) and other listeners. Generalization across environments is harder. Family can help. So can friends. Doing what is necessary to guarantee that the speaker has learned the cues and feels comfortable with them is probably the most salutary of all.

A SUMMARY OF NAMING'S PLACE IN APHASIA TREATMENT

In the introduction we differentiated impaired access to intact semantic networks from intact access to impaired semantic networks. We also discussed a treatment continuum with facilitation on one hand and didacticism on the other. We are unsure about both the reliability and the validity of these distinctions and about the relationship of certain notions about the nature of the naming deficit in aphasia and responses to certain kinds of treatment. We are more sure about another way of talking about treatment programs. We think they can be categorized according to the amount and variety of cueing they provide and according to the amount of self-cueing they require of the patient. These differences among programs can be judged and quantified. This classification of programs, although not independent of theoretical constructs about misnaming and its management, has the advantage of being able to exist independently of such constructs. Its independence does not threaten its two eventual contributions: (1) improved naming for aphasic men and women, and (2) treatment data in support of more adequate models of naming in aphasic, and perhaps even nonaphasic, people.

10

TREATING ASPECTS OF VERBAL EXPRESSION

Because we have created a separate chapter for naming, which is also part verbal expression, we added "aspects of" to the title of this chapter. This subdivision is convenient but artificial. We made it because clinicians often make a similar distinction in their clinical approach to aphasic patients. We also made the division because the literature on naming and verbal expression in aphasia is too vast for a single chapter and because semantics and syntax (the topic of a major portion of this chapter) can be dissociated after brain damage.

IMPORTANCE OF VERBAL EXPRESSION IN TREATMENT

Verbal expression is at the heart of even our earliest therapeutic efforts with all aphasic people. Therefore, we start treatment for all patients, regardless of severity, by determining what they can say. Even when speech appears impossible, we do not abandon it to work only on comprehension or communication in some other modality. Rather, we design a clinical experiment to determine if any oral language can be stimulated or relearned, if the stimulated or relearned language is retained, and if the stimulation or learning generalizes. We usually work simultaneously on the other modalities, especially auditory comprehension, but speech work predominates.

If oral language does not begin to appear after two or so sessions, we change tack. The usual change is to an increased amount of auditory stimulation (Chapter 7), something that Schuell and colleagues (1964) would probably have had us do from day one anyhow, and a decreased amount of treatment for oral expression. We also intensify stimulation in the other modalities by having patients begin to copy, gesture, or read. But even when verbal expression is slow to appear, work on it is not abandoned. Rather, Base-10s (LaPointe, 1977a) are created so that changes in oral language are detected and at least a modicum of time continues to be dedicated to eliciting verbal expression. Usually, such persistence is rewarded unless the patient is and remains globally aphasic or has a syndrome characterized by inability to speak volitionally beyond a word or two and the inability to learn improved verbal expression despite significant improvement both spontaneously and with treatment in reading, writing, and auditory comprehension.

INFLUENCES ON TREATMENT DECISIONS

Clinicians use a variety of criteria for making decisions about how much to work on verbal expression, about what stimuli and methods to use, and about what to work on in addition. We will discuss two: (1) type of aphasia, and (2) distribution, severity, and natural history of symptoms. Both guide clinical decisions about the other communication modalities as well. Their specific influence on treatment decisions about verbal expression is this section's concern.

TYPE OF APHASIA

As a patient begins to talk automatically and spontaneously or upon imitation, the type of aphasia (assuming it is classifiable at all) becomes clearer. As aphasia type becomes clearer, so do the clinician's treatment goals. This is especially true for the major aphasic forms: Broca's, Wernicke's, global, and anomic. The reason is that labels are accompanied by neurophysiologic, neuropsychologic, and neurolinguistic hypotheses about the language deficits. For example, it has been hypothesized (Caramazza & Berndt, 1978) that Broca's aphasia results from a syntactic deficit and Wernicke's aphasia from a semantic deficit. The specific influences on treatment planning of labels and the hypotheses accompanying them will be further developed in a subsequent section of this chapter.

Admittedly, there are pitfalls, and maybe even pratfalls, when treatment is governed by the clinician's diagnosis of aphasia type. One pitfall is that hypotheses about why aphasic speakers sound as they do are always changing. For example, the notion that Broca's aphasic people have impaired syntactic abilities has only fairly recently replaced the ancient notion that Broca's aphasic speakers talk so as to conserve energy (Berndt & Caramazza, 1980; Kean, 1977). Probably, present hypotheses will be supplanted by newer ones yet (Kean, 1985). Fortunately, treatments governed by a particular hypothesis can also provide data on the adequacy of that hypothesis so that clinicians need not worry about working with presently popular but ephemeral hypotheses. In addition, a method's adequacy is determined by the patient's response rather than by the durability of its theoretical underpinnings.

A second potential pitfall is that perhaps 50 percent (Goodglass & Kaplan, 1983b) of

aphasic people have aphasias that cannot be typed. Poeck (1983) said adequate testing and intuition reduce the number to 25 percent. That the aphasia of one patient in four cannot be typed could be a serious influence on aphasia treatment if it were not for the fact that treatment planning can proceed even in the absence of a label. A catalog of the distribution and severity of symptoms and the natural (untreated) and treated course of those symptoms can be equally effective in focusing treatment.

DISTRIBUTION, SEVERITY, AND COURSE OF SYMPTOMS

Type of aphasia and distribution, severity, and course of symptoms are not synonymous. Certain clusters of abnormalities, for example, can occur uniquely and therefore, not qualify as a type of aphasia. A portion of the symptoms associated with a particular syndrome or type of aphasia can occur alone or in combination with symptoms considered to be part of another syndrome. In addition, similar symptoms can exist in two patients for different reasons, as when both Wernicke's and conduction aphasic people have literal paraphasic errors, or when Broca's aphasic and transcortical motor aphasic people have a paucity of oral language. Finally, as evidence of the difference, clinicians recognize that slight variations in symptoms can signal the existence of a clinically significant subtype within a particular syndrome (Hier & Mohr, 1977).

The distribution and severity of symptoms influence treatment of verbal expression. When verbal expression is normal or more preserved than other kinds of performance, as it is in alexia with and without agraphia, it can be used to help reestablish impaired performance. Methods are discussed in Chapters 8 and 11. When it is severely impaired relative to others kinds of behavior, the clinician can combine work on it with work on these other types of performance. The result may be a facilitation of verbal expression. Even when such facilitation fails to occur, however, work on other kinds of performance gives patients motivation-sustaining success, because they are improving in areas in which they are already reasonably good.

How profiles of performance are likely to change spontaneously and with treatment also influence clinical activities. Our principle for acutely aphasic people or for chronically aphasic people who have gone untreated is to devote at least some early effort to performances that are likely to be slow to return. This means treating the verbal expression of all patients in whom it is disturbed, because recovery of verbal expression often lags behind recovery of others kinds of performance (Henri & Canter, 1975; Kenin & Swisher, 1972). However, we do not recommend a generic treatment of all patients, because patients have different profiles of impairment and courses of recovery, patterns that are sometimes predictable by knowing the patient's aphasic type, and sometimes not (Ludlow, 1977).

ASSESSMENT

Whether one considers aphasia a clinical problem or a communication problem affects one's assessment, especially of verbal expression. We believe aphasia is both. So we assess how patients talk in response to a variety of controlled tasks, and we judge how they speak both in and outside (when possible) the clinic when no, or few, test restraints are imposed.

SPECIFIC TASKS

The reasons for using specific tasks in assessment include (1) classification, (2) treatment planning, and (3) progress testing. Most tasks contribute, albeit unequally, to all three. Because many of the best assessment tasks are included as parts of standardized tests and because standardized tests were extensively discussed in Chapter 4, this section will be brief.

IMITATION

Imitative tasks are especially important to classification and can be useful to treatment planning, but only if imitation and spontaneous speaking are compared. All major aphasia examinations include imitation tasks.

The Porch Index of Communicative Ability (PICA) (Porch, 1981) tests it briefly, however, so that PICA data usually have to be supplemented by other measures or informal tests. The Boston Diagnostic Aphasia Examination (BDAE) (Goodglass & Kaplan, 1983a) includes imitation of both high and low frequency of occurrence sentences and so is a better tool for testing imitation than many other measures. Our Standard Speech Sample (see Chapter 4) tests monosyllabic word, polysyllabic word, and sentence imitation. It also contains a section requiring patients to imitate three sentences or utterances of whatever length and structure they have previously used spontaneously in picture description. Procedures for this task are not rigidly structured. Clinicians are allowed to use more than three sentences, to ask for the imitation of correct and incorrect utterances, and even paraphrased ones.

Despite threats to reliability and validity, we believe informal measures of imitation can be important, especially to treatment planning. This is not to imply that one always uses imitation in aphasia treatment. We do not. Because imitation can be such a powerful cue, however, we do test almost every patient's ability to do it. On the other hand, we infrequently use imitative tasks to measure improvement, except with severe patients. Our reason is that we almost never judge a method's efficacy or a patient's progress by changes in imitation, choosing instead to measure spontaneous speech.

PICTURE DESCRIPTION

We always try to elicit one or more picture descriptions. We begin with the so-called Cookie Theft picture from the BDAE. We supplement it with unpublished pictures, depending on our needs. Picture descriptions are relatively easy to control and, therefore, make good test material in time-series designs (McReynolds & Kearns, 1983). They are also potentially rich sources of data about one aspect of a patient's spontaneous speech. Picture description probably does not predict social communication. It does provide information on how a patient can respond to one kind of structure and to the availability of cues of the sort provided by a picture.

The instructions are critical. Aphasic people (and probably nonaphasic ones as well) sometimes turn picture description into a naming task. "There's a _____" or "I see a _____." So, we ask them to tell us about what is happening, about what might have happened before, about what is likely to happen next, and about why something has happened. Of course, the direction "Tell me what you see" is all right too, again depending on one's purpose.

PROCESS DESCRIPTION

Clinicians anxious to elicit speech while simultaneously controlling their patient's output can have them describe processes: "How do you change a tire, get from Wisconsin to Arizona, make sweet bread enchiladas?" In our experience, this task is different from picture description. It probably stresses cognitive, including memory and ordering, processes more than does picture description. We use both when we want to track the treated or untreated course of a patient's aphasia. Ulatowska's group (Ulatowska, Doyel, Freedman-Stern, Macaluso-Haynes, & North, 1983) has described the procedure and how to interpret and score it.

STORY RETELLING

Ulatowska and her colleagues (Ulatowska, Freedman-Stern, Doyel, Macaluso-Haynes, & North, 1983; Ulatowska, North, & Macaluso-Haynes, 1981) have also structured story-retelling and picture-story sequences to elicit verbal expression. The method requires the aphasic person to retell a story previously presented by the clinician. The authors have also developed a method for analyzing aphasic performance.

Some formal tests have similar activities. For example, the unpublished Mayo Procedures for Language Evaluation based on the Minnesota Multiphasic Test for the Differential Diagnosis of Aphasia (MTDDA) (Schuell, 1965a) has one such task. The patient, after

having heard the clinician read it, retells the story of Marshall and Sutter's finding gold at the bottom of a California ditch.

TESTS OF FUNCTIONAL COMMUNICATION

Patients, as clinicians know, and as Davis and Wilcox (1985) demonstrated, may talk during a task differently from the way they talk during natural conversation. Natural conversation, however, is difficult to measure. Tests of functional communication such as the Functional Communication Profile (FCP) (Sarno, 1969) and the test of Communicative Abilities In Daily Living (CADL) (Holland, 1980a) are structured measures of functional abilities, including those of verbal expression. The FCP is an interview test; the CADL attempts to simulate extraclinic communication in the clinic. Both have been described in Chapter 4. They are mentioned here because they bridge a gap between the usual assessment procedures and naturalistic observation.

THE INTERVIEW

If a clinician has 10 minutes to evaluate a patient, five of those should probably be spent in the interview. A clever interviewer can find out how much patients can communicate, how they handle failure, and whether they have strategies for helping themselves. If family or caretakers are present, the clinician can identify the way patients and loved ones communicate with each other, what they do when communication fails, and—most important to prognosis—how important communication seems to be to all their lives.

ANALYSIS OF VERBAL EXPRESSION

Analysis of verbal expression can become a consuming passion. Methods abound. One that has achieved a substantial amount of fame was developed by Yorkston and Beukelman (1980). Their measure requires the clinician to record patients' picture descriptions and then count content units per unit time. Ulatowska and colleagues developed guidelines for evaluating responses to both story-retelling (1983) and process description (1981). Prins, Snow, and Wagenaar (1978) have also reported an elaborate scheme for codifying aphasic verbal expression. Others have developed systems for pragmatic assessment. Prutting and Kirchner's (1983) checklist of verbal and nonverbal behaviors is remarkably complete. More limited systems of codifying both nonverbal and verbal activities are also available (Davis & Wilcox, 1985). Holland (1983) has even outlined a system for describing how the aphasic patient does while going through the day with the clinician in tow. Davis and Wilcox (1985) have reviewed all these approaches.

Most such analyses are costly and time-consuming even when done with computer help. Our history of harried poverty has influenced our own activity. We do not rely on fine-grained transcription or computer analysis. We usually listen to a variety of samples and try to summarize them by selecting representative, trenchant examples of behaviors. We sometimes score certain dimensions such as relevance on a seven-point, equal-appearing intervals scale. Mostly, however, we rely on impression, unless we are preparing the patient's case for publication. For publication, we use one or more of the published methods previously noted.

GUIDELINES FOR STIMULUS SELECTION AND ORDERING

In our view, clinicians who have decided to improve verbal expression can (1) expand the complexity and length of what the patient says, (2) expand the patient's single word and short phrase repertoire, or (3) do both. Guidelines for choosing the stimuli can be garnered from the literature, although more guidelines seem to be available for the Broca's aphasic person than for any other.

EXPANDING COMPLEXITY AND LENGTH

If one's goal is to expand complexity and length, any number of clinicians have provided guidelines for stimulus selection. In her discussion of treatment for Broca's aphasic people, Horner (1983) suggested beginning with holophrastic utterances including expletives and nominatives followed by linked productions such as "the" + noun. Next, she recommended basic sentence types of the sort N + V + O, with care not to overemphasize the nominatives. She then added adjectives and introduced verb tense in the order: present progressive, regular past, and future.

Gleason, Goodglass, Green, Ackerman, and Hyde (1975) studied eight Broca's aphasic people and discovered a pattern of difficulty with syntactic structures. Their ordering of the relative difficulty of 14 syntactic structures is important because it provides specific suggestions about what might be good early, middle, and late stimuli when the clinician's goal is to expand complexity and length.

The four easiest structures, with the authors' example of each type, were:

1. Imperative intransitive such as "Sit down."
2. Imperative transitive such as "Drink your milk."
3. Number plus noun such as "Twelve cups."
4. Adjective plus noun such as "A funny story."

No statistically significant differences in difficulty were observed among these four sentence types.

Six structures of moderate dificulty that again did not differ significantly from each other consisted of:

1. WH-questions such as "Where did you put my shoes?"
2. Declarative transitive such as "The dog chases the cat."
3. Declarative intransitive such as "The baby cries."
4. Comparative such as "She was taller."
5. Passive such as "The man was killed by the train."
6. Yes-no questions such as "Did you call me?"

A final group of four constructions was significantly more difficult than all the others, although individual constructions in this group were not significantly different from each other. These were:

1. Direct plus indirect object such as "She gives her friend the dollar."
2. Embedded sentences such as "She wanted them to be quiet."
3. Adjective plus adjective plus noun such as "A small red car."
4. Future such as "He will work."

EXPANDING THE REPERTOIRE OF BRIEF UTTERANCES

Guidelines for selecting single word utterances are developed for naming in Chapter 9; those will not be repeated. Previously unmentioned guidelines will be outlined here. Blau (1983) has contributed questions to guide selection of a lexicon for children who cannot talk that is inclusive and sane enough to guide most of stimulus selection for a variety of aphasic patients. A paraphrased version of her list is presented in Table 10-1. Clinicians may want to consider this list when selecting stimuli for teaching or when certain stimuli have failed for no readily apparent reason.

TABLE 10-1.
Questions to Guide Selection of Single Word and Short Utterance Stimuli for Aphasic People.

Which vocabulary items might the aphasic person consider important?

Which vocabulary items do the primary caregivers stress as important?

Which vocabulary items refer to routine events experienced by the aphasic person?

Which items reflect preferences or dislikes for objects, actions, or people in the environment?

Which words reflect basic bodily needs and internal/emotional states?

Which communicative functions and semantic notions are currently being expressed by the aphasic speaker through speech and which through idiosyncratic signal systems?

Which lexical items does the clinician intuitively feel might have functional value for the aphasic speaker?

Adapted from Blau, 1983.

GENERAL TREATMENT PROGRAMS

Some methods are specific to certain aphasia types. Some methods are general and applicable to a variety of patients, whether or not they can be typed. Two of the latter will be described in the next section. Their integration into more type-specific programs will be discussed in a section when programs for specific groups and individuals are being presented.

PROMOTING APHASICS' COMMUNICATIVE EFFECTIVENESS (PACE)

Davis and Wilcox (1981) developed PACE. They described it as a treatment "that incorporates components of face-to-face conversation" (p. 169) into aphasia therapeutics. PACE's procedures are related, at least in part, to their assumptions about the language deficit in aphasia. One of their assumptions is that aphasic people retain competence to deal with at least some of the requirements of face to face conversation. These include such things as the ability to take turns and to signal when it is the communication partner's turn to send rather than receive a message. The method and its underpinnings have received a book-length treatment (Davis & Wilcox, 1985).

The method's core is for clinician and patient to take turns selecting cards from a pile placed face down on the table between them and to communicate the contents of each card by any means available—speaking, gesturing, writing, drawing. The most frequently used stimuli are pictured objects, actions, and stories. Topics, themes, or general ideas can also be written out and presented on cards.

REQUIREMENTS AND PROCEDURES

EXCHANGING NEW INFORMATION. The program's first requirement is that clinician and patient exchange new information. This requirement necessitates introducing some new stimuli every session or so. The authors admitted that newness is hard to achieve across several sessions because both clinician and patient come to know the stimulus set. Indeed, if patients do not, they are writing their own prognostic statements. To approximate the goal of newness, however, clinicians can select a large stimulus set and assemble each session's stimuli in some quasi-random fashion. Also, new stimuli can be added at intervals, and variations of each general stimulus type—animals, foods, celestial bodies, cars—can be used. This principle of requiring newness is one of the program's best features, at least in our opinion. Aphasic people are normal in many ways. They wonder at therapies requiring them to provide information they know the listener already has. About the only time such a peculiar arrangement occurs outside the clinic is during examination time.

TURN TAKING. The method requires that clinician and patient take turns being "sender" and "receiver." Although taking turns is not always a characteristic of extraclinic communication, as anyone who has endured an evening with a bore knows, it is better, at least for some patients at some times in their therapy, than a method requiring them to be receivers for most of each session. Turn taking becomes both reception and production training for the aphasic person, and it allows the clinician to model responses in a variety of modalities.

FREE CHOICE. The authors emphasized that patients are free to choose how they will communicate. The clinician provides pencil and paper, and perhaps even written or pictured items. Patients can write, draw, or select a pictured or written representation of each response item. These modes of communication then join speaking and gesturing in an array of options, used either singly or in combination, to communicate each idea. Leading the patient by demonstrating certain modes or combinations when it is the clinician's turn as sender is allowed, and often necessary. We use it. Our experience is that many patients try to talk and they respond to the listener's quizzical, uncomprehending looks with more talk rather than with attempts to communicate in some

other way. As a result, we often gesture, write, or point to pictures as a reminder that the patient can do the same thing. Explanations about why we are doing so when the patient knows full well that we can talk are advisable. We also follow the authors' recommendation to encourage speech at least part of the time, so that therapy is not silent.

NATURAL FEEDBACK. Providing the patient with appropriate, natural feedback is another of the program's better features. If the patient communicates an idea,however linguistically abnormal, the clinician acknowledges the message. As part of that acknowledgment, the clinician might say "I got it. You mean _____." If the clinician is unsure, the response can be something like "Um, I'm not sure. Did you say _____?" Included in this kind of statement may be a cue that will help the patient improve the next attempt. One of Davis and Wilcox's examples has the clinician responding to a patient's vague shaving gesture to communicate "razor" by saying "Do you mean shaving?" If the communication fails despite these initial cues, the clinician can ask more questions and try to lead the patient to a different mode or perhaps a different written, drawn, spoken, or gestured message. The authors were adamant that communication rather than accuracy be the goal and recommended that the clinician take a turn once the patient has communicated an idea.

The authors included a number of variations on their program to bolster their assertion that rigid principles can be broken for individual patients. These variations are important. We all need reminders that programs are not exquisite instruments that are destroyed by tinkering. Mostly, programs are pieces and parts to be assembled to fit individual goals and patients.

TESTING THE METHOD

Davis and Wilcox are interested in evaluating their method, so they have encouraged data collection. Table 10-2 shows one of their scoring systems for measuring how a patient does.

TABLE 10-2.
Example of a Communicative Rating Scale for Scoring a Patient's Sending Behavior.

Score	Condition
4	Message conveyed on first attempt.
3	Message conveyed after general feedback (e.g., "I'm not sure what you mean, can you tell me more?") indicates a lack of understanding.
2	Message conveyed after specific question feedback (e.g., "Are you talking about your son? Did he come to visit?")
1	Message is not completely understood by the receiver.
0	Receiver has no idea as to the nature of the message.

From Davis and Wilcox, 1981, p. 188. Reprinted with permission.

They reported two studies comparing PACE with what they called "directive unidirectional treatment" (p. 189). In both studies, it was reported that PACE was superior to the other treatment. Additional data have been slow to arrive, a tardiness that does not reflect on the method itself. One can only hope that the method works so well clinicians feel little need for data. Probably other forces explain the phenomenon, however.

GESTURAL REORGANIZATION

Gestural reorganization's goal is to improve speech by pairing meaningful gestures with spoken words and phrases. This program has not been as completely structured as PACE. It does have a conceptual framework, a general procedure, and the beginnings of experimental validation (Wertz, LaPointe, & Rosenbek, 1984), however.

CONCEPTUAL FRAMEWORK

Luria's (1970) concept of intersystemic reorganization is the program's basis. Luria believed that one kind of performance could be improved by pairing it with another kind of performance. One of his examples was of improving ball squeezing by teaching the squeezer to precede each squeeze with an eye blink. He used this somewhat unusual

example merely to illustrate the concept of pairing two kinds of performance. Behavior, according to Luria, can also be improved by using a unique form of sensory input to guide it. This, too, is intersystemic reorganization. One of Luria's examples was to have a Parkinsons patient walk by making sure that each step landed on one of a series of taped strips previously placed at appropriate intervals. He documented that both the eye blinking of the first example and the taped strips of the second are associated with better performance of the activity with which they are paired.

Our assumption is that verbal expression can be improved by the appropriate pairing of performances or with the systematic use of unique sensory inputs. Speech, for example, can be combined with meaningful gestures. Visual input, in the form of reading or some other visual signal, can be used to guide the articulators. Intersystemic reorganization may be the reason why improvement of oral expression occurs during either condition. Another hypothesis for the therapeutic effects of simultaneous gesturing and talking is that the gestural representation of meaning is more likely to be available to an aphasic talker than the verbal representation, although the data supporting this hypothesis are meager (Cicone, Wapner, Foldi, Zurif, & Gardner, 1979; Duffy & Duffy, 1981). The gestural performance, therefore, "deblocks" (Weigl, 1968) the verbal. Reading may also be a deblocker of speech. An even simpler hypothesis for the palliative effects of both gesture and reading is that memory for an utterance is enhanced by representing that meaning in more than one way.

A METHOD

The gestural program to be described needs rigorous testing. We use it in our clinic at regular intervals, but that use is not a test. Programs almost surely work for their progenitors. Whether they work for others is the issue. We offer the following as much for clinical experimentation as for clinical management. The much needed experimentation with gestures in aphasia has already begun (Kearns, Simmons, & Sisterhen, 1982; Tonkovich & Loverso, 1982).

STEP ONE

Our program's first step is to select a system of gestures. Our favorite is AMERIND (Skelly, 1979), because those gestures have been used with adult neurological patients, and because the meaning of many of the gestures is obvious or quickly taught to the user and significant others.

More important than the specific gestural system one employs with aphasic people, however, is that one uses emblems rather than illustrators. The terms *emblem* and *illustrator* are Ekman and Friesen's (1972). Emblems are meaningful gestures capable of standing for or replacing words and phrases. Cupping one's hand behind one's ear is an easily recognized gesture meaning "speak up," "I can't hear," "louder," or "turn it up." The index finger quickly drawn horizontally across the neck at approximately the larynx's level means "stop," "quit," or some equivalent.

Emblems can be paired with verbal expression to (1) increase the patient's overall communication, and perhaps (2) increase the amount of verbal expression, even after the gestures have been withdrawn. Illustrators, on the other hand, are timing or pacing gestures. They are appropriate for use with patients having a variety of neuromotor disorders such as apraxia of speech (Wertz, LaPointe, & Rosenbek, 1984) and dysarthria (Rosenbek & LaPointe, 1985).

Step one then, is to pick a system of emblems that may, in practice, be a combination of several systems, perhaps even supplemented by one or more idiosyncratic gestures invented by the patient or patient and clinician. The second activity in step one is to tell the patient what the gestural program requires and what it is to accomplish. Without such education and the patient's subsequent commitment, further steps will falter or be too shuffling to be efficient.

STEP TWO

Step two, the learning of the gestures, actually includes several substeps. Training usually begins with a recognition-comprehension drill which either documents that an individual recognizes and understands each gesture or that enhances such recognition and comprehension if they are impaired. Improved recognition or comprehension may require that patients match the clinician's gestures with gestures of their own, with pictured gestures and, for variety, even match pictures of gestures. If the patient requires considerable training in recognition or comprehension, treatment is likely to be protracted and gains are likely to be minimal. Improvement in speech as a result of learning the gestures is especially unlikely under such conditions. Most patients, however, unless they are globally or severely aphasic, will recognize and comprehend the gestures, or quickly learn the ones they do not immediately process. Once predictable recognition and comprehension are established for even a few gestures, treatment can advance.

Skelly (1979) has developed an elaborate set of procedures for moving beyond recognition and comprehension. Our own procedure is to begin teaching patients to perform the gestures they already comprehend. Some patients need merely to imitate. For these patients, the method is systematic practice of groups of 20 or so gestures until they can be produced reliably.

It is insufficient to have patients learn only predictable reproduction of the gestures, however (Coelho & Duffy, 1985). They need to use them spontaneously and communicatively as well. This expanded use may require several activities, beginning with practice in using the gestures as responses to questions such as "How do you show you're thirsty?" "What do you do if you can't hear?" When gestures can be used to answer questions, training can continue until the patient begins using the gestures spontaneously. If the clinician is not concerned about spontaneous use, however, treatment can move on as soon as the patient can quickly and accurately use each of the gestures in all situations the clinician can create in the clinic.

STEP THREE

Gestures and speaking are combined in step three. Early procedures vary radically from patient to patient, but almost always include the clinician's total or near-total control. The exception is for the patient who spontaneously accompanies gesturing with speech. These patients, when they appear, usually move quickly to other treatments not requiring a gestural accompaniment, so they will not be discussed further here.

Total clinician control means providing both the gestural and verbal models. During the patient's attempted replication, the clinician can simultaneously model both or only the most difficult response. Such modeling often is more crucial for the verbal part of the response than for the gestural, as gestural training has already occurred in step two. Sometimes, however, gesturing deteriorates at the beginning of step three. If so, simultaneous cueing can be near-total as when the clinician molds the patient's hand(s), and provides clear, unequivocal auditory, visual, and sometimes even tactile cues to the utterance. If even further clinician control is necessary, the clinician can initially separate the gestural and verbal by having the patient practice each separately. They can then be recombined.

The goal of step three is to strengthen the verbal so that it occurs ever more frequently without a gestural accompaniment. This means systematically eliciting fewer gestures and more verbal expression. If the patient cannot fade the gestural accompaniment, the pairing can continue, and the clinician can expand the number of gestured-spoken responses. This means selecting useful stimuli and practicing them until they are functional outside the clinic. If the gestures can be faded, clinician and patient can move to other methods, such as PACE, for expanding verbal utterances.

TREATMENTS FOR TYPES OF APHASIA

Different treatments for different types of aphasia are especially appropriate for verbal expression because typing of aphasia—at least during the time of this book's creation—is, or should be, based largely on the character of such expression. Therefore, this chapter features type-specific treatments more so than the other treatment chapters. What follows are summaries of our clinical practice with a variety of types. If we have not had success with a particular type, we do not discuss its specific treatment.

BROCA'S APHASIA

Once a clinician has decided to treat a Broca's aphasic person's verbal expression, the next decision is whether to (1) add to the repertoire of agrammatic responses, or (2) expand the complexity and/or length of utterances. No extant data support a choice of one over the other. In the absence of data, our general rules are to begin by expanding utterance length and complexity for the acute Broca's patient and to expand the chronic patient's repertoire of agrammatic utterances.

This rule is based on our experience, and statement of it is admission, not recommendation. Our experience is first, that acutely aphasic patients, unless they are globally aphasic and have massive brain damage, are likely to regain some portion of their previously normal utterances. We try to hasten that process. Experience, not surprisingly, has also taught us that chronic aphasic people are less likely to regain normal communication. This experience, paired with our belief that a greater number of agrammatic utterances communicates more than a lesser number of grammatic ones, leads us to try expanding the number of agrammatic utterances made by chronic Broca's aphasic people.

We do not apply this rule universally, however. If a patient wants more complex or longer utterances and seems to be capable of learning them, we respond to that want and ability, regardless of how long the aphasia has existed. Fortunately, clinicians never need to make a choice arbitrarily or even on the basis of duration of aphasia. Treatment done according to the guidelines of an alternating treatments design (McReynolds & Kearns, 1983) allows comparisons of both approaches. If one is superior, it is pursued and the other abandoned.

EXPANDING THE REPERTOIRE

Expanding the repertoire, as used here, means making agrammatic persons better talkers by teaching them a greater number of agrammatic utterances. The emphasis is on communication rather than correctness. We do not fear that an increasing number of agrammatic utterances will inhibit the return of more complex utterances. Beyn and Shokhor-Trotskaya (1966) do fear it. Nor do we worry about the gaps that continue to exist in the communication of even that person who knows every noun and verb in the language.

PROCEDURES: GROUP ONE

Patients with Broca's aphasia may be as impulsive as those with Wernicke's aphasia, probably because impulsivity is a frequent accompaniment of brain damage. Training for impulsive Broca's aphasic people begins with efforts to get them to wait until they understand what they are to do. Usually a few words and a gesture or two from the clinician followed by some practice with having to wait are sufficient. More frequent than impulsivity, however, and a greater therapeutic challenge with Broca's aphasic people, is their reluctance to respond. They are more likely than their fluent peers to defer to any available informant. Or failing that, they make only one or a few efforts to comply and then withdraw or otherwise signal surrender at the first sign of communication difficulty.

Nothing so prosaic as a simple wave of the hand or a bit of encouragement increases the responsiveness of most such speakers, especially if they are chronically aphasic. More frequently we have to take a number of more or less simultaneous steps. One is to win the speaker's trust and let it be known that being wrong is better than not trying. Leading each patient to some quick successes is also helpful, so we are careful to begin treatment by eliciting words and "cast-iron" phrases that we have heard them use during previous diagnostic sessions. Eliciting such words and phrases with imitation, imitation after a delay, and questions and answers may make these utterances more stable, and their speaker more confident.

Ludlow's (1977) advice about inhibiting stereotyped utterances also guides our early activities. We encourage patients to be wrong, but we discourage their use of stereotyped, invariant utterances. In other words, we encourage them to be wrong with élan and variety. Alajouanine (1956) observed that a measure of each patient's improvement is the ability to inhibit verbal stereotypes. During Group One procedures we try to hasten improvement by encouraging inhibition, a procedure helped immensely by having something else to say. That brings us to Group Two Procedures.

PROCEDURES: GROUP TWO

The first Group Two procedure is to select stimuli to be treated. We use Blau's (1983) guidelines as previously described with emphasis on those nominatives and verbs that are most useful for each person. Our stimulus selection is influenced as well by those authors (Horner & Fedor, 1983; Myers, 1980; West, 1978) who have hypothesized the right hemisphere's contribution to recovery from aphasia. We use a variety of dynamic rather than static, pictured items, and we are careful to drill verbs as well as nouns. We also use adjectives, if they seem important, and a variety of more or less "cast-iron" phrases: "I hope not," "Oh, my goodness," "You bet your life," and so on.

Once a corpus of utterances has been selected, treatment can advance. Some Broca's aphasic people can learn words by merely drilling them in the way students have been learning new vocabulary for decades. The essence of such training is systematic practice and knowledge of results. Because the aphasic learner is not merely a normal learner with a brain lesion, because aphasic language is not merely a reduced supply of normal language, and because imitation is different from purposive communication, such repetition is insufficient for most Broca's speakers. We have come to rely on a limited number of embarrassingly common alternatives to simple imitation.

The ubiquitous question and answer drill is our favorite. This method's essence is to have a patient imitate responses until they are stable and then use those same responses in answer to a series of appropriate questions. For example, if that patient has learned the word "quit," the clinician asks "What do you say when you've had enough of this?" The best materials for such drills come from the patient's own extraclinic activities. As but one example—although probably none are needed—one of our patients had flown to Las Vegas with his wife so that she could attend a sales meeting. Questions like "How'd you get there?" and "What'd you do?" prompted answers like "Fly" and "Craps." When other essential words such as "blackjack," "debt," "room service," and "nest egg" were unavailable, we provided and then drilled them.

Question and answer drill may be insufficient to help some Broca's aphasic speakers learn a larger repertoire, however. In such cases, the clinician may have to be more creative in stimulus selection and in preparing the therapeutic environment. It may help, for example, to represent some nouns, verbs, and adjectives in written form, with pictures, or as objects. These too can be practiced in as realistic a dialogue as two people can assume when they both know—as they should—that the immediate goal of their interaction is not communication but communication therapy. To make the written or pictured representation even more powerful, the clinician can have the patient repeat appropriate responses in the presence of those representations before beginning the question-answer dialogue.

Most patients seem to expect that they will talk as well outside the clinic as inside it. Most clinicians know better, and so try to involve spouses and caregivers in management from the very first. We begin by getting important other people to help with stimulus selection. We have them observe treatment, and we do treatment with them present. We give them things to do when we feel that a family relationship is strong enough to be a teacher-learner relationship as well.

Despite the most careful attention to stimuli, realistic drill, and family involvement, some patients may not learn. Others may learn treated stimuli during a session but give no evidence of retention or generalization. One interpretation of these failures is that some patients cannot learn even an expanded repertoire of agrammatic utterances if the treatment is exclusively or predominantly auditory-vocal activity. Procedures from Group Three may be more suited to this group.

PROCEDURES: GROUP THREE

Procedures in Group Three involve combining the modalities—pointing, gesturing, drawing, writing, and reading. This is not to say that we have every patient use everything, however. Our experience has been that Broca's aphasic speakers have a variety of ideas they can say and other ideas they are better able to represent in other modalities. This experience influences our treatment. We are less likely to merely combine modalities in an effort to teach a particular utterance than we are to find out which modality each patient has the greatest facility with for each utterance. As patterns emerge, we try to strengthen them. For example, Broca's patients are often able to use their fingers to portray numbers or to write out numbers that they cannot say at all or cannot say easily. We encourage their reliance on the method they do best. Similarly, patients, especially if encouraged to do so, often use meaningful gestures to represent ideas they cannot easily say. We reinforce these gestures just as we do using fingers and writing to portray numbers. The majority of patients can also draw. If they can, we encourage it. An integrated method for combining all these modalities is PACE (Davis & Wilcox, 1981, 1985), which was discussed earlier. PACE is the nonpariel Group Three technique.

Sometimes we do not use PACE, however, especially if we want to systematically combine modalities, perhaps with the hopes of using the stronger performance to aid the weaker one. Our alternatives to PACE are all variants (and some mutations) of multimodality treatment. The common goal of each variant is to combine modalities. Gestural reorganization, in which meaningful gestures are combined with speech, the specific steps of which were also described earlier, is an example of one such variant. Another possibility is to combine speaking and writing. This may work for the patient who can spontaneously write single words or who quickly relearns how words are to be written.

The method for combining speaking and writing is traditional. Step one is to guarantee that the patient's writing of some limited number of words is efficient and accurate. Words that the patient needs for communication, if they are initially inefficiently or incorrectly written, are practiced until they are consistently correct. When they are, treatment takes step two.

In step two, drill begins in earnest. Each word is either written and then said or said and then written. The relative amounts of writing and speaking vary, but generally, the weaker ability—in this example, speaking—is elicited more frequently. If writing a word correctly does not deblock its spoken equivalent, slightly different procedures can occur at step two. The clinician might, for example, say the word, have the patient write it, then say it again, and have the patient imitate the verbal model once or several more times. The clinician can also reinforce the association of the written and spoken forms by having the patient write each word, read each word aloud, and then say each one only after the written form has been faded.

The boundary between steps two and three is not rigidly drawn. The difference that does exist, however, is that in step three the verbal responses occur in the absence of most of the cues that were previously necessary to elicit them. A patient's failure to reach step three is evidence that (1) another modality, such as gesturing, needs to be combined with speaking, or (2) that efforts to improve verbal expression should be abandoned, and treatment should return to the approach of helping the patient communicate each idea with the modality best suited to it. PACE is again the method of choice.

EXPANDING COMPLEXITY OR LENGTH

Broca's aphasic people, especially acutely aphasic ones, can sometimes learn to expand the syntactic complexity or length of their utterances. Sentence complexity and length are not synonymous. Short sentences can be more complex than longer ones. Both complexity and length can be considered in stimulus selection and treatment, but efforts to separate them totally are probably not worth the effort, at least on most clinical days. One published program primarily for expanding complexity and one unpublished program primarily for expanding length will be described.

SYNTAX STIMULATION PROGRAM

Helm-Estabrooks, Fitzpatrick, and Barresi's (1981) Syntax Stimulation Program (SSP) expanded as the Helm Elicited Language Program for Syntax Stimulation (HELPSS) (Helm-Estabrooks & Ramsberger, 1986) is a complete package for increasing the Broca's aphasic patient's utterance complexity. It includes concepts, rationale for stimulus selection, description of specific stimuli, and methods for achieving experimental control.

STIMULI. Stimuli are multiple examples of eight sentence constructions. The order, with imperative intransitive utterances such as "Wake up" first and yes-no questions last, is based on data (Gleason et al., 1975; Goodglass, Gleason, Bernholtz, & Hyde, 1972) already described in detail in this chapter's stimulus selection portion.

THE METHOD. The program has two levels. Level A requires the clinician to provide the patient with a short dialogue that includes the target utterance. Standard dialogues have been created for each example of each construction. Each utterance is demonstrated in a simple, straight-line drawing. The patient hears the dialogue, sees the picture, then responds. In the authors' example of a Level A treatment, the clinician is to say, "My friend is oversleeping, so I tell him wake up. What do I tell him?" The patient is to say, "Wake up." After the patient responds correctly to 90 percent of the exemplars during two trials, treatment advances to level B, which requires the patient to complete the utterance. Their example is "My friend is oversleeping so I say _____." The patient is to complete the sentence with "Wake up." Treatment advances to the next sentence type when the patient gets 90 percent of the exemplars correct during two trials. A 90 percent correct criterion is used for moving from one level to another and from one sentence type to another.

THE RESULTS. The program was successful for their patient. It took him 22 30-minute daily sessions to meet criterion on the first five sentence types. The next three types were more difficult and required 21 sessions. Fortunately, the patient did more than merely use the sentence types during treatment. His performance on the expressive and receptive portion of the Northwestern Syntax Screening Test (Lee, 1969) improved and the gap between expressive and receptive scores on that test narrowed, primarily because of improved scores in expression. Generalization also spread to picture description and to conversation. Physiological recovery and friendly support were probably not influences, because treatment began three years after this 35 year old, right handed man's stroke and after nine months of another kind of language therapy.

Helm-Estabrooks, Fitzpatrick, and Barresi were not ingenuous. They recognized that generalization was limited for their patient as it often is for all patients. Limited generalization is their rationale for reminding clinicans to choose treatment stimuli with care. The patient may learn only what is trained. A rule is, train what is useful and relatively easy.

Salvatore, Trunzo, Holtzapple, and Graham (1983) studied seven patients, four with Broca's aphasia, to see if the hierarchy of sentence types suggested for the SSP was appropriate to their seven patients. It was not, even for the four Broca's patients. They suggested establishing a hierarchy for each patient, and they provided the method for doing it. These authors are standing on their colleagues' shoulders, not on their backsides. Their data do not move us to abandon the SSP, but to refine it to fit the individual patient.

A PROGRAM OF CHANGING CRITERIA

We developed a program to increase the amount and quality, including length, of the aphasic patient's spoken language. It begins by reinforcing one to two word utterances, then three to five word utterances, then six to eight word utterances, then nine or more word utterances. The heart of the program is a series of questions and answers using pictures as stimuli. The pictures are to guarantee that both patient and clinician know the subject and have a representation of it readily available. If the patient fails to answer a question about any given picture, a series of increasingly more powerful cues is provided. A correct response, once it appears, is systematically drilled. A patient with only moderate aphasia, or even moderately severe aphasia, would not necessarily start with one to two word utterances. Where one starts depends on what the patient can do predictably and functionally. Criteria can also be collapsed so that an individual begins with one to five word utterances, for example, and different criteria can be established for different kinds of utterances. Other modifications will be highlighted after the original program is described.

STIMULI. The stimuli are a series of realistic action pictures. Any number can be used. We use multiple of 5 up to 100, but more or less are appropriate. Our stimuli were selected from commercially available language stimulation card sets. They were selected because they portrayed human activities. Examples include a boy and girl playing with a dog, a woman dusting a bookshelf, a family eating a holiday meal, a man shoveling snow, a man and woman sawing wood. Judging the appropriateness of each picture to provide realistic, natural material for each of the 10 questions is important prior to using the pictures in treatment. Aphasic people have enough difficulty talking naturally, they should not (and usually cannot) be forced to talk unnaturally.

PROGRAM LEVELS. The program is organized into four criterion levels. At each level the patient is required to make a longer response. In Criterion I, the patient is urged to make a one or two word response describing each of a series of pictures. Three to five words are required at Criterion II. Six to eight words are required at Criterion III. Nine or more words are required at Criterion IV. Progress from one criterion to another—even from the first to the second—is not necessary for the patient or the program to be considered a success. Progress is stopped at whatever level the patient can accomplish and the number of treatment stimuli is expanded. Longer responses than are required at each criterion are not punished, but reinforced. The clinician may even set different criteria for different questions or pictures.

THE QUESTIONS. Responses about the pictures are elicited by a series of 10 questions. Quite arbitrarily we designed the program so that two randomly selected questions are asked about each picture. The 10 questions are listed in Table 10-3.

THE METHOD: CRITERION I. At Criterion I, each of a series of pictures is placed between patient and clinician, one at a time. The clinician instructs the patient to look at the picture, listen to the clinician's question about the picture, and then answer the question using only one or two words. The wording of these directions is tailored to the patient's understanding. After giving the directions, the clinician then asks the first of two questions, quasi-randomly selected from the list of 10,

TABLE 10-3.
Questions for the Changing Criteria Program.

1. How many people, animals, objects (as appropriate) do you see?
2. What is/are the person(s) wearing?
3. What is/are the person(s) holding?
4. What color are the clothes, sky, objects (as appropriate)?
5. What is around the neck, waist, wrist (as appropriate)?
6. How old is the person, animal, object (as appropriate)?
7. Where is the person, animal, object (as appropriate)?
8. What time is it?
9. What are they (add appropriate verb)?
10. What are they doing?

while simultaneously pointing to a relevant part of the picture. If the patient fails to respond or responds incorrectly, the clinician goes to the first cue, which is to provide the patient with a cloze structure so that the patient has only to fill in the blank with one or two words. If the patient again fails to respond or responds incorrectly, the clinician provides the answer and one foil. The patient then makes a choice. If the patient is still unsuccessful, the answer is provided and the patient imitates. If the patient is still unsuccessful, the clinician resorts to any traditional, remaining technique to elicit the response. If the patient still cannot respond, the clinician changes questions or pictures. If those changes do not help, the program is replaced.

Once a response is elicited, it can be drilled one or more times. Drill means the patient practices the correct response in a variety of modalities and as part of a question and answer dialogue. The number of times a response is drilled, if it is drilled at all, depends on how perseverative the patient is and how stable the response is, and is left to the clinician's judgment.

When possible and appropriate, a session at Criterion I, and at the other levels as well, involves at least two different questions about each of five pictures. A longer session or subsequent sessions can be easily created by adding more pictures or by randomly or quasi-randomly selecting more questions to be used with each picture.

Progress from one criterion to another is not dependent on rigid criteria. During our early development of the program we did not advance until a patient could make adequate responses to all the questions for each of 20 cards at two consecutive sessions. This guideline can be softened. One option is to get appropriate answers to a smaller number (15, 10, 5) of cards, another is to use fewer questions.

THE METHOD: CRITERION II. At Criterion II, the patient is told to make longer responses to each question. The goal is three to five words, and the same questions and pictures are used as at Criterion I. If the patient answers an individual question incorrectly, the clinician provides a cloze or cloze-like cue. If the patient is still incorrect or if no appropriate cloze cue can be created, two appropriately long choices, one correct and one incorrect, are provided and the patient is to say the correct one. If a correct response fails to appear, the clinician provides the appropriate one and has the patient imitate. If a correct response still fails to appear, the clinician tries to elicit the response with other, traditional methods. If the patient is still incorrect, and depending on the type of error(s) being made, the clinician can return to Criterion I, can introduce a new picture or a new card, or can abandon the program.

If the correct response appears, it is drilled using a repetition of the appropriate question, written cues, delay, and the other accoutrements of traditional behavioral treatment. As at all other criteria, the clinician can manipulate each of the patient's responses during the drill. A three word response can be shaped into a four or five word response, for example. Imitation is avoided, except as a last resort, and cues are faded before moving on to the next level.

THE METHOD: CRITERION III. Activity at Criterion III is similar to that at Criterion II except that the patient is requested to make a longer response. The target is six to eight words. Other potential differences are that some pictures and some questions may not appropriately elicit longer utterances, so these pictures and questions are deleted. The clinician should avoid requiring artificial responses merely to satisfy a goal for length of utterance. To do so, as several patients have shown us, is to thwart patient progress. Other pictures or questions can be substituted. Cues in response to errors are the same as at previous criteria. Failure at this level prompts a return to Criterion II.

THE METHOD: CRITERION IV. Criterion IV requires spontaneous descriptions of the same set of pictures in response to the same set of questions, with substitutions and addi-

tions as appropriate. The goal is sentences of nine or more words or several consecutive sentences without intervention from the clinician. Requirements about length and number of sentences are influenced by common sense. Two adequate seven word sentences are not rejected nor is the patient forced to create unnatural utterances or to make trivial observations to meet an arbitrary length requirement. Cues are provided in response to failure just as at other criterion levels.

Failure at this conversational or spontaneous level prompts a return to Criterion III. Failure to reach this criterion does not mean that the patient or the program has failed.

Because the changing criterion program is reasonably complex, an extended example has been included. This example may help interested clinicians more comfortably judge and even use this program.

THE METHOD: AN EXTENDED EXAMPLE USING A PICTURE OF A MAN AND WOMAN MAKING COFFEE AND QUESTION 10, "WHAT ARE THEY DOING?"

Criterion I. Instructions: I'm going to ask you a question about this picture. Keep your answer short. Use only one or two words.

Procedure 1. Clinician shows the picture and asks some form of "What are they doing?" If response is correct, it can be drilled. Drill means using other modalities such as reading, and using questions and answers, repetition, and supportive instructions to elicit the correct answer 2 to 10 (or so) times. If response is incorrect or if the patient fails to respond, and if a simple repetition of the instructions and/or question is insufficient, clinician moves to *Procedure 2*. If response is correct but drill seems inappropriate, a new picture or question can be introduced.

Procedure 2. Clinician shows the picture and provides the patient with a cloze cue. The cue's wording is left to the clinician, as is the amount of information the patient is to supply. Examples are: "They are making _____," "They have a coffee pot, they are making _____," and "They have a coffee pot, they are _____ _____." If response is correct, clinician returns to *Procedure 1* and drills or not as appropriate. If response is incorrect or if patient fails to respond, clinician moves to *Procedure 3*.

Procedure 3. Clinician shows the picture and provides the patient with a multiple choice cue. The cue's wording is left to the clinician. Examples of multiple choice cues are "Are they making coffee or tea?" and "Are they making coffee or brewing tea?" If response is correct, clinician returns to *Procedures 1* and *2* and drills or not as appropriate. If response is incorrect or if patient fails to respond, clinician moves to *Procedure 4*.

Procedure 4. Clinician shows the picture and provides a correct response. An example is for the clinician to say, "Say what I do, 'Making coffee'." Patient is urged to imitate the model. If response is correct, clinician returns to *Procedures 1, 2,* and *3,* and drills or not as appropriate. If response is incorrect or if patient does not respond, clinician moves to *Procedure 5*.

Procedure 5. Clinician shows the picture and then tries any and all cues for eliciting a correct response. These may include, but are not limited to, written, gestured, and real object cues and systematic attempts to elicit an imitated response. If response is correct, clinician returns to *Procedures 1, 2, 3,* and *4* and drills or not as appropriate. If response is incorrect or if patient does not respond, clinician moves to another picture or to another question.

Criterion II. Instructions: I'm going to ask you a question about this picture. Make your answer a little bit longer than before (if patient has already completed *Criterion I*). Make it three, four, or five words (if patient is beginning the program at *Criterion II* or if the first instruction seems inadequate).

Procedure 1. Clinician shows the picture and asks some form of "What are they doing?" If response is correct but short, clinician reinforces the response and asks the patient to "Make it longer," "Say more," or some equivalent. If response is correct, it can be drilled. If it remains too short, is incorrect, or if the patient fails to respond, and if a simple repetition of the instructions and/or questions is insufficient, clinician moves to *Procedure 2*.

If response is correct but drill seems inappropriate, a new picture or question can be introduced.

Procedure 2. Clinician shows the picture and provides the patient with a cloze or cloze-like cue. The difference between the two is that in the cloze, the patient has merely to finish the utterance. In the cloze-like cue, the clinician provides information which the patient can then turn into a response. The cue's wording is left to the clinician, as is the amount of information the patient is to supply. An example of a cloze cue is "They got out the pot and coffee so they could _____ _____ _____." If response is correct, clinician returns to *Procedure 1* and drills or not as appropriate. If response is incorrect or if patient fails to respond, clinician moves to *Procedure 3*.

Procedure 3. Clinician shows the picture and provides the patient with a multiple choice cue. The cue's wording is left to the clinician. Examples of multiple choice cues are "Would you say, 'They are making coffee' or 'They are brewing tea'?" If response is correct, clinician returns to *Procedures 1* and *2* and drills or not as appropriate. If response is incorrect, or if patient fails to respond, clinician moves to *Procedure 4*.

Procedure 4. Clinician shows the picture and provides a correct response. An example is for the clinician to say, "Say what I do, 'They are making coffee'." Patient is urged to imitate the model. If response is correct, clinician returns to *Procedures 1, 2,* and *3* and drills or not as appropriate. If response is incorrect or if patient does not respond, clinician moves to *Procedure 5*.

Procedure 5. Clinician shows the picture and then tries any and all cues for eliciting a correct response as at *Criterion I*. If response is correct, clinician returns to *Procedures 1, 2, 3,* and *4* and drills or not as appropriate. If response is incorrect or if patient does not respond, clinician moves to another picture, another question, or the previous criterion.

Criterion III. Instructions: I'm going to ask you a question about this picture. Make your answer a bit longer than before (if patient has already completed *Criterion II*). Make it six, seven, or eight words (if patient is beginning the program at *Criterion III* or if the first instruction seems inadequate. Modeling a correct answer may help).

Procedure 1. Clinician shows the picture and

asks some form of "What are they doing?" If response is correct but short, clinician reinforces the response and asks the patient to "Make it longer," "Say more," or some equivalent. If response is correct, it can be drilled. If it remains too short, is incorrect, or if the patient fails to respond, and if a simple repetition of the instructions and/or questions is insufficient, clinician moves to *Procedure 2*. If response is correct but drill seems inappropriate, a new picture or question can be introduced.

Procedure 2. Clinician shows the picture and provides the patient with a cloze or cloze-like cue. The cue's wording is left to the clinician, as is the amount of information the patient is to supply. An example of a cloze-like cue is "The man and woman have the coffee pot out. What are they doing?" If response is correct but short, clinician reinforces the response and asks the patient to "Make it longer," "Say more," or some equivalent. The length requirement need not be held to slavishly. If response is correct, clinician returns to *Procedure 1* and drills or not as appropriate. If a correct, short response is all that can be elicited, it too can be drilled or the patient can be systematically helped to expand it by the clinician's skillful providing of cues. If response is incorrect, or if patient fails to respond, clinician moves to *Procedure 3*.

Procedure 3. Clinician shows the picture and provides the patient with a multiple choice cue. The cue's wording is left to the clinician. Examples of multiple choice cues are "Would you say 'The man and woman are making coffee' or 'The man and woman are brewing tea'?" or "Would you say, 'The boy and girl are making coffee' or 'The man and woman are making coffee'?" If response is correct, clinician returns to *Procedures 1* and *2* and drills or not as appropriate. If response is incorrect, or if patient fails to respond, clinician moves to *Procedure 4*.

Procedure 4. Clinician shows the picture and provides a correct response. An example is for the clinician to say, "Say what I do, 'The man and woman are making coffee'." Patient is urged to imitate the model. If response is correct, clinician returns to *Procedures 1, 2,* and *3* and drills or not as appropriate. If response is incorrect or if patient does not respond, clinician moves to *Procedure 5*.

Procedure 5. Clinician shows the picture and then tries any and all cues for eliciting a correct response as at previous criteria. If response is correct, clinician returns to *Procedures 1, 2, 3,* and *4* and drills or not as appropriate. If response is incorrect or if patient does not respond, clinician moves to *Procedure 5*.

Procedure 5. Clinician shows the picture and then tries any and all cues for eliciting a correct response as at previous criteria. If response is correct, clinician returns to *Procedures 1, 2, 3,* and *4* and drills or not as appropriate. If response is incorrect or if patient does not respond, clinician moves to another picture, another question, or a previous criterion.

Criterion IV. Instructions: I'm going to ask you a question about this picture. Make your answer even longer and more complete. Make it nine or more words. Try to use more than one sentence (these instructions are determined by common sense and the patient's competence).

Procedures: The procedures are similar to those previously described. The object is to help the patient make adequate responses yet retain all possible independence.

The program's object is not merely to teach the patient a set of two, three, or more word responses. It is to teach a set of strategies for communicating. It helps patients focus on details, monitor themselves, use time creatively, and do all the other things that successful communication requires. Patients need not move through all the criteria. Even stable and generalized performance of Criterion I ability may be sufficient for severe patients. Collapsing the criteria so that the patient's goal is one to five and six or more words is also a sane modification in response to the individual patient.

WERNICKE'S APHASIA

Martin (1981a), in his evaluation of Wepman's treatment (Wepman, 1972), sprinkled a liberal amount of his own view throughout the essay. Martin said,

The fluent aphasic's particular behavioral characteristics, his lack of strong inhibitory skills, as well as his difficulties with auditory comprehension and inter- and intrapersonal monitoring all militate against the automatic use of the structured task initially for either comprehension or expression. (p. 150)

He recommended that treatment begin with the clinician's learning to understand the patient's communication. In other words, the clinician rather than the patient changes. Once the clinician has learned to listen, the next step is to teach others how to understand, or so said Martin. In our experience, this step is usually unnecessary because families nearly always understand more than clinicians. A more crucial contribution to families is reassurance that they are not hurting the patient or retarding progress by responding to the jargon. They know how to understand; they need reassurance that it is all right, that the patient may even benefit.

Our own view, and doubtless, Martin shares it—at least in part—is that enhanced communication is always the goal with aphasic patients, but that the speaker as well as the listener must change. Helping the Wernicke's aphasic speaker reduce distractibility and impulsivity is the usual first step. In our view, this reduction is more likely if the clinician imposes structure on the patient's communication and on the environment in which that communication takes place. The amount of that structure depends on the patient's duration of aphasia and needs. Chronic patients are often better able to respond to structure than are acute ones. Patients with a strong need to communicate usually respond better than those who value other things more than they value communication.

PROCEDURES:GROUP ONE

The aim of procedures for Group One is creation of a therapeutic structure. First, the patient learns to wait. This means instructing, encouraging, and—if necessary—gently but firmly forcing each patient to be silent until a message has been delivered. We usually begin with a terse explanation about the necessity for listening and not talking. To test the explanation's effectiveness, we make a series of short statements, usually about ourselves. We avoid greetings and familiar or emotional topics because they are likely to ignite a patient response.

Not surprisingly, Wernicke's aphasic patients sometimes begin talking during our explanation of why they should not. Even when they are able to be quiet for the explanation, they seldom can resist responding to our first treatment utterance. To counter this impulsivity, we keep our explanations short, keep our statements during drill banal or arcane, force each patient to attend to us, and even inhibit their speaking by laying our hands on theirs and by signaling them in other ways about their need to simply listen. Some clinicians even touch them on the face, have them clench their teeth, or hold a "bite block" between their teeth. The bite block is only appropriate in well-established, trusting clinical relationships because the bite block is unnatural and invasive. If a patient accepts the block, and if it obviously helps comprehension and perhaps even speaking, its use can be brief because most patients learn those things that are obviously palliative. When they do, the bite block can be replaced by gentle reminders and an occasional touch.

When the patient can listen to explanations and general statements, we move to a series of yes-no questions to which we and the patient know the answers. "Is your name _____?" "Do you live in _____?" "Is your child a _____?" The patient has only to answer with the spoken equivalent of "yes" or "no." We inhibit any tendency on the patient's part to respond before the question is complete. We also try to use a variety of questions so that the answers are less predictable. We try to avoid questions to which "maybe" is the answer. We supply bountiful prompts about why listening is crucial and we help patients identify those times when rules of listening have been violated. Sometimes we even elicit nodded rather than spoken answers: "Merely shake your head. Don't talk."

Patients who have waited as requested, but who then give incorrect answers often try to correct those answers with explanations, sometimes of excruciating length. We agree with them that answers need to be correct as well as appropriately delayed. Then we get them to let us continue controlling the situation by allowing us to repeat the question so that they can answer correctly. When they have learned to wait and to make short, yes-no responses we continue to drill, but with a minimum of explanation. Like other patients, those with Wernicke's aphasia often get into a groove once they make a few correct responses and fully understand the task. Clinician explanations may only jar the stylus unnecessarily. This kind of treatment need not last a long time, and indeed, may take only a few minutes at the beginning of each session before treatment advances to procedures from Group Two.

PROCEDURES: GROUP TWO

Group Two procedures help the patient move from yes-no to a variety of other short, intelligible utterances. Most patients, regardless of severity, make short, intelligible, stereotyped responses. Questions to elicit these repeatedly and predictably are a good Group Two procedure. We use high frequency of occurrence questions about the weather, hospital food, family, and other appropriate topics. Unless patients understand why certain questions are used repeatedly they may decide to begin embellishing the answers, if for no other reason than to add some variety to treatment. Often unintelligibility is embellishment's companion, so we are careful to explain every therapy activity in short, matter of fact sentences and to discourage embellishment.

As a further step, the clinician can ask questions that allow patients to make a series of related statements about a series of related quetions. A dialogue might go like this: "What is your name?" "Was that your father's name?" "No?" "Then what was his name?" "Who were you named after?" "What did you name your first child?" And so on. The reader can supply thousands of other examples from experience. The point is to try for a kind of chaining of short responses. Such chaining makes the treatment dialogue somewhat realistic without causing the clinician to lose control.

Another procedure is to use multiple choice questions and supply the patient with one answer and one or more foils: "In the Northern Hemisphere, does a toilet bowl's water swirl clockwise or counterclockwise?" This procedure can also be inserted as a cue in the chaining approach described previously. These multiple choice questions require that the clinician know a good deal about each patient's and the world's history. Such knowledge allows quick intervention when the patient begins to embellish unintelligibly, a result often of the patient's trying to talk about something he or she knows too little about or has forgotten the particulars of. Questions to avoid are those the patient may be unsure of and those that are emotionally laden. Questions about illness are usually inappropriate and should be probed gingerly and abandoned quickly if they elicit confusion, confabulation, or circumlocution.

The clinician should continually remind the patient of the treatment's rationale and hold tightly to rigid criteria of acceptability or intelligibility. Rigid criteria are even more crucial as the clinician expands the stimuli because fluent patients relish telling the whole story—a story that is likely to be unintelligible if the patient, rather than the clinician, is in control.

When limited, intelligible answers to easy questions begin to occur frequently, the clinician can advance to questions requiring longer answers. "How long can you refrigerate fresh squirrel meat?" "How do you feel about allowing 18 year old people to drink?" "What will you do when you leave the hospital?" If a patient's speech deteriorates, the clinician has choices. Unintelligible answers can be interrupted and another topic introduced. Or, if the clinician has at least some idea of what the patient has said—such knowledge being likely as the clinician is still a dominant influence on topics at this stage of therapy—the patient can be stopped and the clinician can help refocus the patient on the same topic. Refocus can come from picking up on a word or two and turning these into a question the patient can then confirm. "Did you say something about your best friend's being a beer can collector?" If the clinician's query is confirmed, the patient can be urged to repeat the answer. If nothing has been intelligible, the old game of "20 Questions" may save the conversation. If 20 Questions fails, the clinician can always repeat the original question after a pause. If that fails, clinician and patient may have to begin again with a new question and answer. Or, they may need to kick back, sit quietly, and have a sip of lemonade.

When a speaker is responding correctly to a variety of questions, the task can be made even harder. A good transition from predominantly clinician controlled to clinician and patient controlled therapy is to have the patient ask a question similar to the one just asked by the clinician. This is close enough to imitation to make success likely, yet it also resembles much of conversation: "Oh hi! How are you?" "Fine, how are you?" "Good, still living where you were?" "Yes, how about you?" and so on.

We do not believe that each session needs to use different questions. We repeat some of the same material time and time again. Such repetition is not antipragmatic: consider the social rituals upon arriving at work each morning. Nor do we believe that a session needs to feature only one activity with the expectation that more difficult activities will be used in the next session. Instead, we suggest moving back and forth among questions of mild, moderate, and extreme difficulty so long as the patient is as successful and independent as possible.

Nothing in these suggestions is inconsistent with an emphasis on communication or on pragmatics, because the goal is always to help the speaker produce something that the largest possible number of people can understand. We recommend using no more clinical control than that goal requires.

PROCEDURES: GROUP THREE

Once the patient is making the best possible approximation of good responses within the rigid restraints of Group Two activities ("best possible" being a clinical judgment based on samples across several sessions), restraints can be loosened. Both topic selection and clinician control can be altered. Often, of course, these two changes are really one change. As topics become more general,

or important, or familiar to the patient, the clinician's control over treatment almost inevitably weakens. Almost, but not quite. Clinical diligence is mandatory and a return to previous instructions and activities may be necessary, at least for short periods. The topics themselves may even help retain constraints. Shared experiences, a news item, a television show, a particularly memorable moment in hospital ward living can provide discussion material. The clinician can and should encourage the speaker to evaluate each response and can let the patient know in a variety of ways that unacceptable aphasia has invaded an utterance.

If the patient continues to improve, the clinician needs to make sure that clinical progress is being transferred to the outside. Family or other caretakers need to know what kind of responses the patient is capable of, how to elicit them, and how to respond when communication fails or is less than optimal. Observing therapy (if possible), a family or caregiver's conference, even a letter packed with specific details are all ways of educating these other people. When they and the patient feel secure, treatment can end.

Treatment need not advance to Procedure Three kinds of activities. Some patients remain too severe to do more than a bit of these. Discussion, usually short, of everyday affairs may be as far as they can advance. So be it. Treatment of verbal expression can stop there. All Wernicke's aphasic people, even severe ones, are excellent communicators. Many of them draw, write, and gesture. They do not come to treatment to communicate, they come to communicate better. The family can be helped to lead the patient toward these short periods of more effective conversation by using the methods from Procedures One and Two. They can also learn to accept and encourage communication in other modes. Clinical treatment can end.

GLOBAL APHASIA

Globally aphasic people deserve treatment, and that treatment can be worth everyone's time (Collins, 1983, 1986). Verbal expression may not be a realistic long-term goal for such persons, but short-term attempts to establish or expand it are a legitimate therapeutic activity for both acute and chronic globally aphasic people.

Attempts to train verbal expression, even if they are unsuccessful, accomplish several goals. The patient's response to the treatment can (1) help confirm the diagnosis, (2) help confirm the prognosis, (3) help establish long-term treatment goals, and (4) perhaps help improve the patient's nonspoken communication.

PROCEDURES: GROUP ONE

Confirming the diagnosis is crucial because globally aphasic patients usually recover less and may recover later (Sarno & Levita, 1981) than most other aphasic types. To know the diagnosis then is to have important prognostic and treatment planning data. Confirming the diagnosis requires different kinds of information, depending on each professional's definition and description of global aphasia. For us, globally aphasic persons retain a significant amount of cognitive ability, but reveal themselves by their profound linguistic involvement and persisting inability to associate speech movements with the meaning of those movements. Formal testing will usually establish the amount of aphasic deficit. Procedures in Group One establish the patient's ability to associate movements (usually speech movements) and the meaning of those movements.

Step one in determining a patient's ability to associate movement and meaning is to elicit serial productions, imitated words and phrases, or automatic, meaningful responses about health, the environment, the food, or any other appropriate topic. If utterances of any sort can be elicited, step two is to have the patient indicate the meaning of what has been uttered. How such confirmation is achieved is determined by what has been said. Numbers can be confirmed by a show of fingers or by pointing appropriately. Words and phrases can be gestured, written, pointed to, matched, selected as objects, consistently comprehended, and even repeated predictably.

Experienced clinicians recognize, however, that patients may know what they have uttered but still be unable to use any clinician-conceived mode or activity to confirm that knowledge. In these cases, the continued, appropriate use of utterances may be the best evidence for understanding. Usually, however, assiduous testing will confirm knowledge when such knowledge exists. Patients match names of people with photographs indicate with their fingers the number of children they have, and in a variety of other ways show that they know. If they cannot do any of these things despite considerable training, a likely hypothesis is that they are globally aphasic.

We realize the matter may be more complicated than we have portrayed it. Globally aphasic people eventually begin understanding some portion of what is said to them, understanding that is enhanced by routine or predictability and by liberal visual cues. They also regain the ability and willingness to garden, window shop, and draw to an inside straight, and even read the obituaries if they did these things before. These abilities confirm that meaning, in some sense, is preserved or regained, and that it is inaccurate to say that meaning is lost in global aphasia. Having worked with globally aphasic people for decades, however, we are not convinced that global aphasia is solely a performance deficit. Rather, it seems a mix of impaired competence and performance with the performance deficit being greatest for verbal expression.

Diagnostic treatment can establish, perhaps better than any other method, the profundity of the coexisting competence deficit. The more profound that deficit, the more firm is the diagnosis of global aphasia, the more bleak is the prospect for oral language, and the more likely it is that treatment will focus on enhancing whatever residual abilities the patient has and on counseling both patients and families about making the best possible use of, and adjustment to, what remains.

If the globally aphasic person shows evidence of the ability to associate movements and meanings, that information promises, but does not guarantee, evolution into either apraxia of speech or Broca's aphasia. Evolution to Broca's aphasia is more likely the longer postonset the patient is, because evolution from total or near total speechlessness to apraxia of speech usually happens rapidly (Mohr et al., 1978). These different courses, however, are of greater importance to prognosis and long-term treatment planning than they are to immediate treatment planning. The reason is that acute, severe apraxia of speech and severe aphasia are managed similarly in the early stages, because the common clinical emphasis is on communication—on helping the patient learn to communicate something meaningful. Selected activities to enhance such communication are at the heart of Group Two procedures.

PROCEDURES: GROUP TWO

Our goal with patients who seem to be associating movements and meanings is to establish at least a small repertoire of useful spoken or spoken and gestured responses. Stimuli can be nearly anything, including recurring utterances (Helm-Estabrooks & Barresi, 1980), but usually consist of at least one greeting; the words yes and no, or some synonyms; a proper name or two; a variety of single words to express needs; and even one or more phrases, especially if such phrases appear in the patient's more spontaneous untreated repertoire.

We usually begin treatment with imitation alone or with imitation supplemented by gesture and by reading. Portions of a published task continuum (Rosenbek, Lemme, Ahern, Harris, & Wertz, 1973) may be useful here. In that task continuum, a response is first established with immediate imitation, then imitation after a delay, then the patient produces each response several times consecutively without intervention from the clinician. If the patient makes an error, the clinician can restimulate immediately or advise the patient briefly (aphasic people wither under a verbal barrage, even a well-intentioned one) and then restimulate. If a correct response is still not forthcoming, a new stimulus can be introduced. At all steps, the clinician is careful to provide clear auditory and visual models. The amount of delay between what the clinician says and the patient's imitation can be varied, as can the number of the patient's consecutive repetitions and the number and spacing of practice utterances overall.

Imitated responses are not volitional purposive ones, however, so clinicians need to plan one or more activities to help patients begin using each utterance purposively. It is tempting to be facile about such carryover activities, because so few data confirming their efficacy are extant. In practice, however, it usually suffices to have a patient practice each utterance in response to questions and in a variety of situations resembling "real life." Group treatment and the careful education and structuring of each patient's environment outside the clinic are helpful as well.

FLORANCE AND DEAL'S PROGRAM

Eliciting responses from severely aphasic people with simple imitation is often difficult, especially if they are globally aphasic. Multiple cues to help the patient understand what is to be said can be helpful. Gestures, objects, and written stimuli are the most logical additional cues. Florance and Deal (1977) have published a protocol for what they call "nonverbal" patients that combines features of multiple cues and planned carryover activities. The program is outlined in Table 10-4.

This program resulted from five years' experience and is carefully organized. Procedures for testing and scoring and criteria for moving between levels are specified. Sentence stimuli were used with the 15 patients on whom Florance and Deal reported data. Any stimuli could be used, however, and the interested reader may wish to consult the original article for more details.

Methods described thus far have been for patients in whom the union of speech and meaning has been previously confirmed or for those in whom that union can only be discovered by structured, protracted treatment. If, during such treatment, a patient repeats adequately, but cannot use a response in any other context, a breakdown in the realtionship of meaning to speech movements can be hypothesized. If the patient has great difficulty

TABLE 10-4.
Florance and Deal's Program for the Nonverbal Patient.

STEP I. Training Target Sentences

Part A: Auditory, visual and graphic stimuli—production of target sentence (TS) with simultaneous auditory and visual cues.

Part B: Auditory stimulus—production of TS with visual cues only.

Part C: Auditory stimulus—production of TS without cues.

Part D: Graphic stimulus—independent production of TS.

STEP II. Pseudoconversational Procedure

Part A: Stimulus: Pre-established question
Response: Trained TS

Part B: Stimulus: Pre-established question
Response: Any appropriate response

STEP III. Generalization

Conversational sample utilizing training content topic, training and related responses. Stimulation of novel utterances.

From Florance and Deal, 1977. Reprinted with permission.

using the response in all other modalities as well, the data strongly suggest a coexisting competence deficit and the presence of global aphasia. When a diagnosis of global aphasia has been confirmed, the clinician has to make choices. In our experience the continued drill of verbal expression is not one of the choices. Procedures in Group Three, on the other hand, may be appropriate.

PROCEDURES: GROUP THREE

Helm-Estabrooks, Fitzpatrick, and Barresi (1982) have developed a program called Visual Action Therapy (VAT) for globally aphasic people. They say the program may prepare the globally aphasic patient for more traditional treatment of verbal expression.

This program, like others with which Helm-Estabrooks is associated, combines concepts and procedures. The program relies primarily on gestural responses by the patient and visual input from the clinician; no one speaks. The patient is taught to gesture the function of eight objects as a result of progress-

ing systematically through a three stage program of 24 steps, 12 at stage one and six at each of the other two stages. As originally published, the program begins with tracing, advances through the matching of objects and pictures, and moves on to the imitation of gestures with objects or pictures of the objects present. It ends with the patient's being able to gesture each object's function even though the object is no longer present. Neither clinician nor patient talks during the treatment. Patients are helped to understand what is required of them by observing gestures from the clinician.

The authors reported that VAT training of globally aphasic patients was accompanied by significant changes in gesture and auditory comprehension as measured on the PICA (Porch, 1981). They also reported a trend toward improvement on the PICA reading subtests. Along with other researchers (Gardner et al., 1976; Glass et al., 1973), these authors hypothesized that VAT "may reintegrate some of the conceptual systems necessary for linguistic performance" (p. 388). A discussion of modularity and this program's effect appears in Chapter 1.

If an individual patient responds as Helm-Estabrooks and colleagues' patients did, it is recommended that VAT be followed by traditional therapy emphasizing auditory comprehension and speaking. Unfortunately, the profession has no data on what the specifics of that treatment should be. Our experience—although limited—is that a patient may do best with a continuation of a gestural program either alone or in combination with speech. In other words, nothing is sacred about VAT's eight items. Sixteen items, or 40, or some other number can be taught, especially if learning appears to be more efficient as more items are introduced and if speech, such as naming, begins to appear as the program continues. An alternative to expanding on VAT-type stimulation is a return to the imitative and multimodality programs already described. Yet another alternative is to concentrate on auditory comprehension (Chapter 7) or writing (Chapter 11) as alternative/augmentative modes of communication.

PROCEDURES: GROUP FOUR

If the globally aphasic person moves into the Broca's range, methods from that section will be appropriate. If not, protracted treatment of any sort is inappropriate because it seems to us that abandoning such patients to treatment is an injustice. Neither is it fair merely to end treatment; the end must be prepared for.

Preparation for an end to treatment can begin with the most complete cataloguing of remaining abilities possible. Globally aphasic people can win at cards but cannot rub it in. They can select items for purchase even when they cannot read the warranty. They can indicate assent about a child's education even when they cannot defend their reasons. They can vote even when they cannot campaign for their favorite. And so on.

When the catalogue is complete, portions of it that the family may not be aware of or secure with can be discussed with them. Once families are educated and reassured, they become even better clinicians than they were naturally at the time of the patient's insult. All that remains—usually—is to give families freedom to call anytime they have questions or feel the need for reevaluation.

TRANSCORTICAL MOTOR APHASIA

Transcortical motor aphasia (TCMA) is relatively rare, but the pattern of deficit lends itself to logical treatment approaches. Although some authors (Alexander & Schmidt, 1980) have recommended against therapy because symptoms disappear so rapidly, others (Benson, 1979a) have reported persisting symptoms. Presence or absence of recovery, however, is not the issue. A variety of medical conditions improve spontaneously, but such recovery is hardly an argument against their treatment. The keys to treatment are to discover what the patient can do despite the total or near total deficit in spontaneous speech and to manipulate selectively those strengths to enhance the return of volitional-purposive verbal expression. Depending on severity, the patient with TCMA is able to imitate a variety of utterances and may be able to understand, name, and read aloud with reasonable facility. These abilities can sometimes be structured so that they aid speech's return.

PROCEDURES: GROUP ONE

The first cluster of Group One procedures comprise a program developed and tested by Lentz, Shubitowski, Rosenbek, and McNeil (1983). The program relies on imitation and naming to improve spontaneous speaking and was completed within the constraints of the multiple baseline design (McReynolds & Kearns, 1983). The patient for whom the program was developed was 64 years old. Two weeks prior to treatment's initiation, he had a left, anterior cerebral artery stroke resulting in severe TCMA.

Step one was to have the patient list, either verbally or in writing, the most important nouns and verbs suggested by each of a series of pictures. His relatively preserved ability to name verbally and in writing despite an inability to create spontaneous sentences made this first step logical. When he could not retrieve appropriate nouns or verbs, the clinician would point out important objects and cue him with descriptions, cloze-type sentences, and in a variety of other ways. He nearly always responded to such cues with a greater variety of words. If a crucial word did not appear, the clinician would provide it, but only as a last resort. When he had produced or been supplied with a list of three or more relevant words, he was asked to start a sentence with one of them and then try to expand it into a phrase by using one or more of the other words. For example, about a picture showing a plane in flight, he provided the words "plane" and "fly." His response to the request for a sentence was, "Plane is flying."

He was told at the beginning of treatment that long, complex, complete, even grammatical utterances were not required. He was merely to say as much as he could. He was subsequently rewarded for any attempt. The best attempts were discussed and drilled. Imitation was used to help him correct or expand the ones that were too incomplete to be effective communication.

Despite being in a period of physiological recovery and improving as a result, the data from the multiple baseline design suggest that treatment contributed to his change. To get these data, 20 pictures were randomly assigned to one of four treatment groups. Reliable seven point, equal-appearing intervals scoring systems for judging both grammatical completeness and relevance of responses were used to measure baseline, acquisition, retention, and generalization of responses. Treatment was initiated with each group in turn. Baseline performance for all groups was variable and was being influenced by physiologic recovery. The data on grammatical completeness appear in Figure 10-1. Treatment effects are not striking. Treatment's influence on relevance is more obvious and compelling, as shown in Figure 10-2.

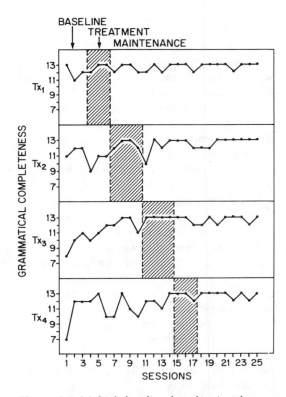

Figure 10-1. Multiple baseline data showing changes in the grammatical completeness of a transcortical motor aphasic person's responses during a treatment program to improve picture description.

PROCEDURES: GROUP TWO

If reading is somewhat preserved, reading aloud can also be therapeutic for the person with TCMA. We have used two variations. The first is to have the patient begin each session with more or less uninterrupted reading followed by controlled speaking. The clinician selects the reading material from published treatment material or from other sources such as the newspaper, according to the patient's ability to read. Such extended reading sometimes deblocks verbal expression, and drill following the reading can be closely, barely, or not at all related to ideas just read, depending on how generalized the deblocking effect is.

The patient's performance after a period of reading will advise the clinician about how similar reading and subsequent talking must be. If reading deblocks only a limited number of related utterances, we emphasize our second Group Two procedure, which is to have the patient improve the ability to say a limited number of responses by first reading them carefully aloud.

Regardless of whether the patient reads

a lot for general priming of verbal expression or only a phrase or two for specific priming, the reading itself will usually be an incomplete treatment. The patient may be able to say a few general things after having read for a few minutes or—and this is more likely—may be able to produce a few utterances after reading them aloud several times. However, the facilitating or deblocking effect may not endure or will not spread to unread material. To make it spread or generalize requires systematic extension of control. Such control comes easiest—at least in our experience—from more focused reading. The procedure begins with the reading of appropriately complex stimuli. When such stimuli are read correctly, they are then to be used more pragmatically as answers to questions. If the transfer from aloud reading to question-answer is difficult, a step involving imitation

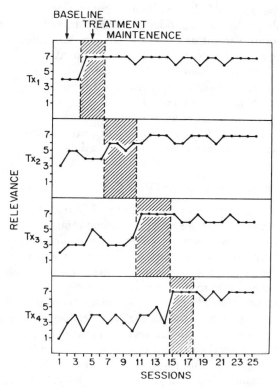

Figure 10-2. Multiple baseline data showing changes in the relevance of the same transcortical motor aphasic person's responses during a program to improve picture description.

can be interposed between the two. If the clinician is very prepared, read responses can also be used to describe pictured stimuli. This of course requires having the same object, theme, situation, or idea represented both in pictures and in writing.

Control can be increased further by the progressive fading of reading and the increased use of more pragmatic activities. Usually, patients with TCMA are being swept along by physiological recovery even as they are receiving this treatment. The result is that more planning is likely to go on in the earlier stages than in later ones.

OTHER APHASIC PEOPLE

Thus far we have not specifically discussed conduction and transcortical sensory aphasic (TCSA) people and those aphasic speakers who cannot be classified. We have not treated enough TCSA people to know how to do it. We have treated several people with conduction aphasia, but we have no data confirming our success. That is different from saying we have not helped them. We may have; we just cannot confirm it. Other people think they have also and have published favorite methods (Simmons, 1983).

Our problem with the conduction aphasic person is the same as our problem with the unclassifiable person. We are unsure of the reasons—beyond brain damage, which is of scant help in treatment planning—why they perform as they do. One solution—for us, if not for them—is to fall back on two general principles; two principles that often lead to a single therapeutic approach. The first is that it is good therapy to provide the aphasic speaker with a simulus that elicits a successful response. The second is that beginning with performances the patient is capable of, either alone or in combination with a performance that is not so intact, is worth carefully controlled trial.

PROCEDURES: GROUP ONE

Group One procedures are to identify the patient's strengths, unless that has already been done, and then to begin facilitation by directing the therapy at those strengths. Patients who can copy or write, copy or write. Patients who can comprehend, listen. But because listening is enhanced by having to act, some kind of action needs to be part of all listening drills. That action need not be talking, however. It can be nodding, pointing, matching, looking, reading, counting, or gesturing. In fact, we seldom ask patients to respond verbally in the kind of treatment being described here, preferring instead to let speech remain in the background. If speech emerges from that background and if it is adequate, or useful, or better than silence, so much the better. Even if the speech, when it does appear, is very good, we do not force it or move it to the foreground. Rather, we are content to treat only the strengths, and reinforcing strengths becomes treatment's only goal. If speech begins to appear from the background, our failure to shift our full attention to it will not result in its shrinking back into the background. Oral expression emerges from some patients only if it is allowed to do so on its own.

At other times, the clinician may want to coax speech as well as some other performance from patients. The least invasive way of doing this, and the one we begin with, is to talk ourselves while simultaneously helping patients with some other activity. We will, for example, simply say each word as we are working with it in another modality such as writing. We might even talk about the word being represented. For example, we often say the word, or describe its function, or make a personal comment about it. If the word is "coffee," we might volunteer that we only drink decaffeinated, or instant, or fresh ground, or that we are trying to cut back or whatever. The danger is in talking too much and destroying the patients' performance of even the nonspeaking activity. On the other hand, if patients observe that they also drink decaffeinated, we might simply congratulate them on their good taste and if they say they are cutting back, we compliment their good sense. If experience has confirmed that one response is not likely to be followed by another, we suppress the desire to continue the conversation and return instead to the specific task at hand. If experience has confirmed that more than one response is likely, we give them every chance to appear.

If speech begins occurring at predictable intervals, a greater emphasis on it may be appropriate. That greater emphasis may take the form of more direct attempts to elicit speech or the predictable repetition of previously correct responses. The appearance of more speech usually means patients are regaining sufficient language to use it a variety of ways. Speech that happens only at irregular intervals is usually speech that will remain distressingly unpredictable.

Subsequent treatment can take one of three forms, depending on whether verbal expression begins to improve. If it does not, the clinician can continue emphasizing other modes of communication and then discharge the patient when sufficient competence in these alternative modes has been achieved. A minor variant of this approach is to schedule periodic follow-up so that treatment can be resumed if verbal expression begins to appear spontaneously and if resources to support the treatment are available. If verbal expression—regardless of how limited—emerges, the clinician has a different option, an option summarized under Group Two Procedures.

PROCEDURES: GROUP TWO

Group Two procedures require that patients begin speaking in accompaniment to their other activity. The main difference between Group One and Group Two procedures is that speech is moved from the background to the foreground in Group Two. In other words, patients are made to realize that speaking is part of the drill. Performance in nonspeaking modalities becomes cues to aid the retrieval of verbal expressive items. The program at this point can be described as reorganization and the methods have been described previously.

These procedures are common in speech pathology because one or aphasiology's enduring shibboleths is that weaker modalities are to be combined with stronger ones. Group Two procedures, therefore, are provided as grist for several experimental mills. Our general approach is to begin with the reorganizer (called either the deblocker or the facilitator by others). The reorganizer, as described here, is a nonverbal response and can be written, gestured, heard, or read. It can be presented one or more times. The subsequent verbal response can occur simultaneously with the reorganizer or right after it. Once elicited, the verbal can be repeated once or several times, with or without the accompanying reorganizer. If the patient progresses, the reorganizer may be presented less frequently, until it is finally unnecessary.

If the patient's progress stops and the reorganizer is necessary to elicit all or most verbal responses, the clinician is faced with the dilemma of deciding what to do. If resources are available and if the patient agrees, the reorganization can continue with experimental rigor to see if the patient eventually begins to learn improved, independent verbal expression. Two other options are possible, again depending on resources and the patient's (and clinician's) attitude. Treatment can return to an emphasis on the reorganizer or can be halted. This latter decision causes anguish, but it is simply the case that some patients cannot improve. These men and women are not well served by protracted treatment.

CONCLUSION

Probably the majority of lay people judge patient progress by changes in verbal expression. Certainly, most patients gauge their own improvement by how well they are talking. We serve our profession and our patients by improving verbal expression. Fortunately, except in global aphasia, it usually can be improved, and even in global aphasia, treatment of verbal expression is justified.

And when does tratment of verbal expression stop? The question admits to no single answer. When verbal expression is normal, however, is not one of the possibilities, because brain damage makes normal impossible. The realistic answers are (1) when the money runs out and no free services are available, (2) when the patient wants to quit, (3) when change is no longer occurring, (4) when the speaker is functional. Better speaking is the best popular test of a treatment's effectiveness. Knowing when to quit is the best professional test of a clinician's competence.

11

TREATING APHASIC
WRITING DEFICITS

The second R, "ritin," appeared independently in distant parts of the world at different times, and it ranks among humans' highest intellectual achievements (Tzeng & Wang, 1983). Its emergence was probably necessitated by primitive societies' transition from hunting to agriculture and a subsequent need to keep records (Wang, 1982). Ten thousand year old clay tokens found along the Iran-Iraq border contain marks and perforations that indicate a simple system of recordkeeping. Amazing!

But, not all are impressed with this ancient art of placing marks on a surface begun 10 millennia or so ago. Today, some write very little; others write not at all. Conversely, one of us is so enamored with the art he cannot refrain from rewriting the fifth draft before it leaves the secretary's typewriter! One person's abstinence is another's addiction. Nevertheless, all, regardless of inclination, will find the ability to write disrupted after becoming aphasic. This chapter is about that disruption and our attempts to mend it. We will discuss how writing goes awry following brain damage, how one determines what is wrong, whether this can be changed, and if it can, how we go about it.

APHASIA, AGRAPHIA,
AND APHASIC AGRAPHIA

Our recurring refrain implies aphasia is a general language disorder that disrupts all language modalities. Writing, being one of these, takes its lumps.

Marcé (1856) was the first to describe a writing disturbance following brain damage, but Benedikt (1865) gave us the term *agraphia* and suggested it was a symptom of aphasia. Earlier Trousseau (1864) and later Dejerine (1891) observed and described writing deficits in aphasic patients. Jackson (1866) linked writing impairment in aphasia to similar deficits seen in speech and reading. And Exner's (1881) attempts to localize writing in the brain left his name as a landmark in the left hemisphere.

Controversy abounds, as it always does when something is submerged below the surface of comprehension, about the presence of agraphia in patients who are not aphasic. "Pure" agraphia (Hecaen, Angelergues, & Douzens, 1963) implies the presence of a writing deficit in the absence of other language deficits. Lecours (1966) suggested Lee Harvey Oswald suffered a pure or "isolated" agraphia that coexisted with preserved spoken language, reading, and above average intelligence. Benson (1979a) also listed agraphias that are not necessarily aphasic and, apparently, result from focal lesions.

Certainly, nonaphasic writing disturbances may follow neurologic damage. Dementia erodes writing (Bayles, 1984), as does acute confusional states (Chedru & Geschwind, 1972) and right hemisphere brain damage (Myers, 1984). But, can one be aphasic without being agraphic? Geschwind (1973) has argued one cannot. The reported cases of aphasia without writing disturbance, he believed, result from insufficient evaluation. Geschwind claimed some aspect of writing will always be disrupted if aphasia is present. We agree. The converse, "pure" or "isolated" agraphia without coexisting aphasia, dementia, or confusion, must be rare, because we seldom see it. We leave its description and explanation to those who do.

CLASSIFICATION AND APPRAISAL OF APHASIC WRITING

Appraising writing has an advantage not found in appraising other aphasic deficits—auditory comprehension, reading, and oral-expressive language. In writing, immediate tracks are left. One may deny, "I didn't say that" or ask, "What did I say?" But writing leaves a trace. It confronts us after the fact, and it is there for analysis.

How we look for an aphasic person's writing problems is guided by the requirements of the formal tests, discussed in Chapter 4, and informal exploration we devise. All of the standardized measures—Minnesota Test for Differential Diagnosis of Aphasia (MTDDA) (Schuell, 1965a), Porch Index of Communicative Ability (PICA) (Porch, 1967), Boston Diagnostic Aphasia Examination (Goodglass & Kaplan, 1983a), and Western Aphasia Battery (Kertesz, 1982)—contain subtests that require the taker to write, copy, and draw. The latter two tests do not use writing performance to determine the presence of aphasia or to rate its severity, but they do permit collecting a sample of the patient's writing. Even the "functional" measures—Communicative Abilities In Daily Living (CADL) (Holland, 1980a) and Functional Communication Profile (FCP) (Sarno, 1969)—consider an aphasic person's ability to put marks on paper. Our informal probes range from observing whether the patient elects to use pen and paper if they are present to whether and how he or she edits what has been written.

The formal and informal measures confirm Geschwind's (1973a) contention that all aphasic people have difficulty writing. Some have problems resulting from using a nonpreferred hand necessitated by the presence of right hemiplegia. Others have minor twists and turns in their spelling and syntax that would go undetected if we did not know they had suffered a left hemisphere CVA. And, in some, writing is completely devastated. Aphasic writing deficits, therefore, are relative to the aphasic person and the person he or she was before becoming aphasic. Those who wrote premorbidly will probably want to and try to postonset. Those who did not probably will not. We encourage the former and we respect the latter. Aphasic people, no matter how severe, can and should be permitted to make choices.

What we see when we appraise writing resembles what others have observed. Individual letters are omitted, substituted, distorted, added, and reversed; words are omitted or substituted and their order may be altered; syntax is fractured by word omissions or rearrangement; and punctuation is absent or incorrect (Darley, 1982). When the marks are intelligible, we can classify them into Benson's (1979a) four error types: defects in the mechanics of handwriting (orthography), defects in syntax, defects in semantic content, and defects in spelling.

We, like Weisenberg and McBride (1935), observe that aphasic writing frequently resembles aphasic oral expression. Broca's aphasic patients reveal agrammatism in both speech and writing. Wernicke's aphasic patients speak and write with some preservation of syntax. Although a rare case (Assal, Buttet, & Jolivet, 1981) may display a dissociation between oral expression and writing, for example, the fluent speech seen in Wernicke's aphasia and agrammatic writing found in Broca's aphasia, the differences between aphasic speech and writing, usually, are more in quantity than in quality. Goodglass and Hunter's (1970) observation that the length of grammatical strings in speech usually exceeds those in writing is, we believe, generally correct. Thus, although there are rare exceptions, Lord Brain's (1961) suggestion that written language is the most fragile of language skills appears true. Porch (1967) demonstrated that written performance in a large sample of aphasic patients was poorer than verbal or gestural performance.

Most of all, we see a wide range of severity. As shown in Figure 11-1, the global aphasic patient may put pen to paper and leave a series of insoluble tracks. The mildly anomic

patient may communicate his or her intent, but the presence of aphasia can be detected. Keenan (1971) reported that writing was the most sensitive indicator of aphasia in mildly involved patients.

CLASSIFICATION

Some have attempted to classify aphasic writing. And, like the attempts to classify aphasia, this has generated controversy. Schuell and colleagues (1964) observed writing deficits in all five of their MTDDA prognostic groups, supporting the belief that aphasia is a general language deficit crossing all modalities. Goodglass (1981) has listed specific writing deficits for the aphasic types that can be classified with the Boston Diagnostic Aphasia Examination. These are summarized in Table 11-1.

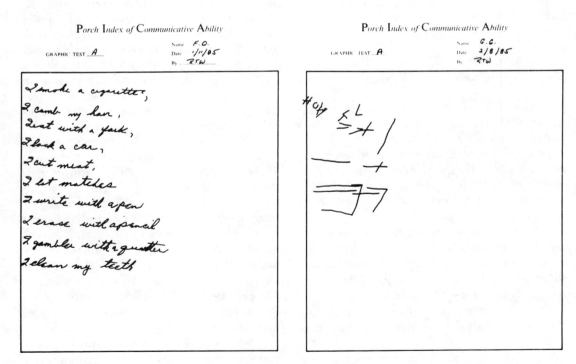

Figure 11-1. The range in the severity of aphasic writing deficits is demonstrated by two patients' performance on PICA Subtest A, writing the function of objects. G. G. was classified as global aphasic on the Western Aphasia Battery and performed at the 9th Overall percentile on the PICA. F. O. was classified as anomic aphasic on the Western Aphasia Battery and performed at the 90th Overall percentile on the PICA. G. G. wrote with his nonpreferred left hand, and F. O. wrote with his preferred right hand. Reprinted with permission from Consulting Psychologists Press, Inc., 577 College Avenue, Palo Alto, CA 94306.

TABLE 11-1.
Writing Deficits Characteristic of Different Types of Aphasia.

Type	Writing Deficits
Global	The patient may be able to copy and to write his or her name. All other writing is totally agraphic.
Broca's	Letter formation, recall of spelling, and sentence formation are similar in severity to oral expression. Agrammatism in writing usually resembles agrammatism in oral expression.
Mixed nonfluent	Writing ranges in severity from complete agraphia to incorrect spelling in grammatically defective simple sentences.
Transcortical motor	Writing is similar in severity and the types of errors to that seen in the writing of Broca's aphasic patients.
Wernicke's	Writing deficits range from total agraphia to written paraphasias, semantic substitutions, and garbled syntax. Agrammatism rarely appears in the writing of Wernicke's aphasic patients.
Transcortical sensory	Writing is usually severely impaired.
Conduction	Writing deficits vary, but are usually present. Spelling and grammatical errors are seen, but syntax is not agrammatic.
Anomic	If the lesion involves the angular gyrus, writing is impaired. If it does not, anomic patients write as well as they speak.

Adapted from Goodglass (1981).

Before becoming too enamored with a belief that aphasic writing can be classified, we remind ourselves that Goodglass (1981) cautioned only 40 to 60 percent of aphasic patients can be classified usefully and reliably. The same, we assume, is true of these patients' writing. Probably fewer would be classified if classification were based solely on writing. The descriptions listed in Table 11-1 indicate two signs, severity and syntax. Globally aphasic patients display more severe writing deficits than other types, and there is a range of severity within each type. And, writing deficits appear to separate into a fluent and nonfluent dichotomy. Written agrammatism is more likely to be present in the writing of Broca's, mixed nonfluent, and transcortical motor patients than it is in the writing of Wernicke's, transcortical sensory, conduction, and anomic patients. Beyond severity and syntax, writing deficits vary as much or more within a type of aphasia as they do among types of aphasia. Thus, we agree with Benson's (1979b) observation, "The variations of

writing disorders that can follow brain damage combined with marked premorbid individual variations have defied demonstration of exact clinical-anatomical correlations of agraphia" (p. 37).

APPRAISAL

Regardless of what the literature tells us or what we have seen previously, neither refutes what a single patient does when plowing through our appraisal tasks. What a patient tells us about his or her writing deficits guides what we may or may not be able to do about improving these. This is what we want to know.

Our appraisal of writing usually begins during the first few minutes we spend with a patient. We place a pad of paper and a pencil on the table when we sit to chat about what happened to the patient and why he or she happens to be where he or she is. We use these, and we watch to see whether the patient does. Those who do are probably telling us something that makes them different from those who do not. Attempting to write or draw information that will not come verbally implies, we think, that person is willing to use all of the resources at his or her disposal to make some music. Those who are right hemiplegic and spontaneously pick up a pencil with their nonpreferred left hand and try to put it to use make us smile. Those who show no awareness that tools other than their tongues are available worry us. For these, we do not request attempts to write at this time, but we are not above a few clandestine forays. For example, we may say "My name is. . ." and we say it and write it. This is followed by "And your name is. . ." and we wait and watch to see what is done. For the most part, this initial meeting is conversation, not correspondence. The paper and pencil ploy is to establish their presence and to indicate, surreptitiously, they are available for use should the patient choose. And, we keep them present except when the rigidities of a standardized test banish them.

STANDARDIZED MEASURES

Formal appraisal of writing comes during the administration of a general language measure, the PICA, BDAE, or WAB. We are after a sample of written syntax, word-finding, writing to dictation, and drawing. Each of the standardized measures provides what we seek. We administer one or more of these, depending on the time we have to invest in appraisal and how quickly we are able to learn what a patient is trying to tell us.

The PICA provides six writing tasks, and five of these require responses to the same stimuli. This permits a look at consistency in response to the same stimuli across a variety of tasks. In addition, the PICA indicates the influence of stimulus conditions on the patient's written responses. For example, some things we believe may help actually hinder. PICA Subtest B requires the patient to write the names of objects. Subtest C involves writing the names after they are spoken, and Subtest D requires writing the names after they are spelled. We expect performance to be better on C and D than it is on B. For most

aphasic patients, it is. But, for a few, it is worse, indicating that auditory assistance erodes performance. We always look not only at what patients do, but also at how what we do influences what they do.

In addition, the PICA's multidimensional scoring system provides a quantifiable code that describes written performance. This permits establishing treatment targets, for example, selecting a frequent behavior (i.e., related responses) for movement up the scale (i.e., to cued or repeated responses). Further, each written subtest can be converted to a mean score and a percentile. And, all subtests can be combined to obtain a Graphic Modality mean or percentile. These are compared with verbal and gestural performance to determine how writing relates to other aphasic deficits. Finally, PICA written performance provides a baseline for detecting subsequent change. Comparison of writing subtest scores obtained early postonset or pretreatment with those collected later or after treatment permits detecting improvement or the lack of it.

Figure 11-2 shows a PICA Modality Response Summary for E. S., a 66 year old man who became aphasic subsequent to suffering a left hemisphere frontal-parietal infarct about two weeks before we met. He wrote with his nonpreferred left hand because dense right hemiplegia required him to do so, and he did not write very well. Comparison of performance among Graphic subtests indicated, with one exception, what is usually seen in an aphasic person's writing; poorer performance on more difficult tasks and better performance on easier ones. The exception was a dip on Subtest E, copying words. He omitted some letters in some words, and he produced some illegible letters in others. He was either trying to tell us something, or he was being careless. We made a note to find out which. What he did tell us was that his writing, though incorrect, was in the ballpark. His related responses communicated and might be used to supplement what would not come in speech. In addition, we had a baseline, 60th percentile Graphic performance; an indication of severity; a sufficient sample to focus some treatment; information that E. S. wanted to

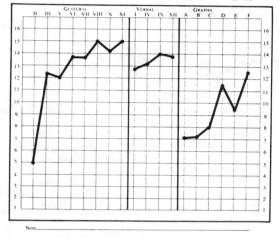

Published by
CONSULTING PSYCHOLOGISTS PRESS
577 College Avenue   Palo Alto, California

Figure 11-2. PICA Modality Response Summary showing a comparison of gestural, verbal, and graphic performance for E. S. at two months postonset. Reprinted with permission from Consulting Psychologists Press, Inc., 577 College Avenue, Palo Alto, CA 94306.

write and would try to do so with his non-preferred left hand; and support to justify our diagnosis that E. S. was aphasic. Thus, putting him through the PICA Graphic subtests satisfied the purposes of appraisal.

The BDAE and WAB sample similar written performance. Both provide some things we want to know that are not appraised by the PICA. For example, both contain the most useful and important task we can administer, writing one's name. In addition, both provide a range of subtests from serial writing, the alphabet and numbers, to written picture description. Within this range are some useful modality comparisons. For example, writing words to dictation is compared with oral spelling of the same words and constructing these from anagrams. Determining

modality strengths may indicate which can be used to improve another in subsequent treatment. Finally, both the BDAE and the WAB contain drawing tasks. These are found in the Spatial and Computational supplement to the BDAE and the Constructional, Visuo-spatial and Calculation section of the WAB. Obtaining a sample of a patient's ability to convey information by drawing reminds us that not everything we put on paper to communicate need be lexical. An aphasic patient's picture may not be worth a thousand words, but it may provide the one word that cannot be said or written. Scores derived from the BDAE writing measures are expressed as subtest totals, and these can be converted into percentiles. WAB scores are subtest totals and, eventually, are combined with reading performance and provide a part of the WAB Cortical Quotient (CQ).

Figure 11-3 shows E. S.'s written description of the WAB picture. Those with no previous exposure to this family picnic scene by the lake could probably interpret his productions as, "The boy is reading a book. The girl is pouring a drink. They are listening to the radio." "The guy is flying a kite" may be a bit more difficult. Nevertheless, most of E. S.'s writing communicated. It also indicated he wrote slowly, and he did not write profusely.

Figure 11-4 shows how E. S. produced the WAB drawing stimuli. All were done from verbal commands; no pictorial examples were used. Although his performance would not win a prize at the local art fair, except for the cube and house, E. S. produced reasonable facsimiles of the stimuli. He could, therefore, supplement what he said and wrote with drawing.

Other standardized language tests sample aphasic patients' writing, for example, the MTDDA. We do not prescribe administration of a specific test. We do advocate appraising writing with one of them. Any of those mentioned will satisfy the purposes of appraisal—make a diagnosis, state a prognosis, determine severity, and focus treatment.

A useful scale for describing the severity of aphasic writing was developed by Schuell

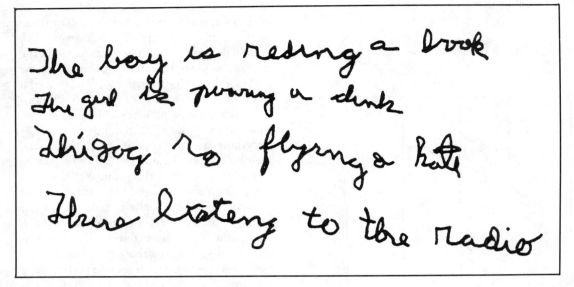

Figure 11-3. E. S.'s written description of the WAB picnic scene picture at two months postonset.

(1965a). As shown in Table 11-2, a patient's writing can be described on an eight point scale ranging from "No observable impairment" to "No functional writing." This can be used to describe a patient's writing to family members and those in other medical or rehabilitation disciplines, and it can be used to measure change.

INFORMAL MEASURES

In order to seek additional information about a patient's ability to write, we use informal measures. These look for performance not sampled by the standardized tests. Typically, we want to know how our patients write what most people write, if they can communicate by drawing, if their performance improves if we provide anagrams, and if they can profit from the pictures and letters on a communication board.

We want to know how our patients write what most people write. Cursive exposition of the function of 10 common objects may tell us something about a patient's ability to write, but few do this outside the confines of a treatment room. Most of us write our name, our address, our phone number, and other bio-graphical information. We write checks and notes to ourselves and others, we fill out forms, we make lists, and we write cards and letters. We do some writing to dictation, especially during a telephone call, and we do some copying of information we may need later. These are the things we write, and, probably, these are the things our patients wrote before becoming aphasic. So, we find out what they can do now. We have them fill out a form, write a check, make a list, take a phone message and write it down, copy an address or phone number, and write a note at the bottom of a greeting card. What we request is tempered by the patient's severity and willingness to take pen in hand. What we observe, frequently, amazes us. Sometimes, when patients are asked to write what people write and not what patients write, they write more like people.

We have heard an aphasic patient say "doodle" when he meant fork, but we have never seen an aphasic patient doodle. For most aphasic patients, pencils are foreign, and they are taken up only after a request from a therapist to write. Few of us ask our patients to draw outside the dictates of a standardized test. Clinicians who have asked their patients

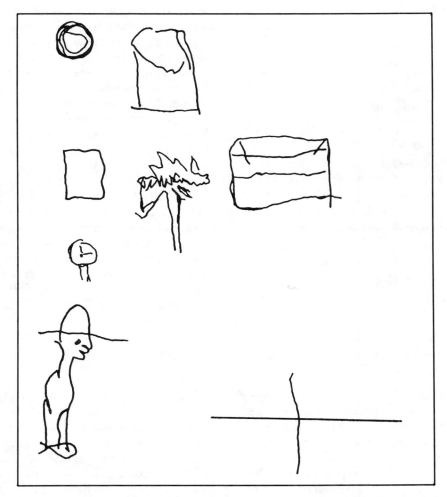

Figure 11-4. Responses on the WAB drawing stimuli by E. S. at two months postonset. Productions show attempts to produce a circle, cube, square, tree, house, clock, person, and line bisection.

to draw have something to tell the rest of us. Gardner and Winner (1981) observed many professional artists retained their premorbid artistic talent after becoming aphasic. Hatfield and Zangwill (1974) found several aphasic patients who could communicate with their drawings but not with words. Lyon (1984) has demonstrated that some patients can draw when they cannot talk or write and that these patients' communication through drawing can be improved by treatment. So, we have begun to appraise our patients' ability to communicate by drawing. The tasks include copying shapes and line drawings, an auditory request to draw an object without a model, draw an action (e.g., running), or an emotion (e.g., sadness), and answer a question with a drawing (e.g., Who is Bob Hope?). In some patients, drawing conveys what will not come verbally or in writing. In others, drawing indicates no more semantic or syntactic inventory than is present in speech or writing. But, that is what we want to know.

Sometimes, a leg up will get one on the way to the top. A few aphasic patients who cannot get letters going can get going if you give them the letters. That is why we keep a box of anagrams around and why we explore

TABLE 11-2.
Schuell's Scale for Quantifying Aphasic Patients' Writing.

Level	Description
0	No information
1	No observable impairment
2	Can write an acceptable letter with only minimal errors
3	Spontaneous writing is present with mild impairment of spelling and formulation
4	Can write short, easy sentences spontaneously and to dictation
5	Spelling vocabulary of 100 or more words; can write some phrases and sentences
6	Can write name and a few words to dictation
7	No functional writing

Adapted from Schuell (1965a).

a patient's ability to use them. Anagram tasks on the BDAE and WAB can be supplemented with more useful stimuli. These range from selecting letters to form one's name, address, and the names of family members to arranging letters to match a printed stimulus. Typically, we provide the necessary letters, in a random array, to produce what is requested, plus two extra letters. For more severely aphasic patients, we provide only the letters needed. Those who have difficulty arranging letters to produce a spoken word are probed with dictated spelling of the word, one letter at a time. We look for errors in selecting letters and in sequencing letters, and we look for a patient's ability to recognize errors and his or her ability to repair errors he or she makes.

Finally, we determine patients' ability to use another means of graphic communication, a communication board. These come in a variety of sizes and contain a range of content. The communication board shown in Figure 11-5 is representative. The front contains pictorial stimuli that can be used to express basic needs. The back contains an alphabet and space to add additional stimuli. The board is covered with plastic to permit writing on it with a grease pencil and easy erasure. We begin by orienting a patient to the board. He or she is asked to point to pictures we name or identify by function. Similarly, use of the alphabet is determined by having the patient point to letters we name. Those who can identify pictures and letters are pushed to see if they can communicate with the board. We ask "How would you show someone you are hungry?" or "you want to shave" and so on. Use of the alphabet is determined by asking a patient to spell his or her name, the names of family members, or spell out one word answers to questions. Those who can use the communication board to supplement what they can say, gesture, write, and draw take it with them and are encouraged to use it until improvement makes it obsolete. We encourage patient, staff, and family to keep the board present and to keep it active.

SUMMARY

Formal and informal appraisal of writing tells us what a patient can do and what he or she is willing to do. Not all who can write, draw, and use a communication board are willing to. Some who are willing cannot. For the unwilling and the unable, treatment for writing is placed on hold until interest or ability surfaces. Most attempts to command interest in the reluctant or success in the chronically unsuccessful are internecine. For those who want to write and who show some potential for being able to write, the appraisal methods discussed should have identified what is wrong and how some writing may be resurrected.

PROGNOSIS

Knowing what is wrong with writing and having a hunch about how to improve it does not guarantee improvement will follow. One wants to know a patient's prognosis for improving writing. And, like our ability to predict change in any other modality, our precision in giving writing a prognosis is underwhelming. Nevertheless, we try.

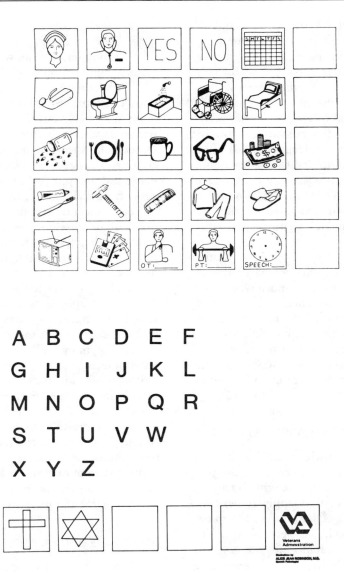

Figure 11-5. Front and back sides of a communication board used to supplement communication in other modalities.

Experience and the literature tell us writing will improve in some, but not all, aphasic patients. For example, Butfield and Zangwill (1946) reported improved writing in 72 percent of their treated patients, and Basso, Capitani, and Zanobio (1982) observed 56 percent of their treated patients made gains in writing. However, writing usually improves less than auditory comprehension, reading, and oral expression (Basso et al., 1979). A rare patient (Anderson & Ulatowska, 1977) may differ and show more gains in writing than in oral expression.

Treating writing deficits increases the probability of improvement. Fifty-six percent of Basso, Capitani, and Zanobio's (1982) treated patients displayed improved writing, and only 28 percent of their untreated patients improved. Similarly, Wertz, Collins, and colleagues (1981) found writing improved significantly more in patients who received writing treatment than in patients whose treatment did not include writing therapy.

Like change in the other modalities, most of the improvement in writing occurs within the first three months postonset. However, Wertz, Collins, and colleagues (1981) found treated patients continued to display significant improvement in writing at 6, 9, and 12 months postonset. And Haskin's (1976) patient displayed marked improvement during five months of treatment begun at 10 years postonset.

Thus, some aphasic patients' writing improves, especially if they receive treatment. Predicting whether and how much writing will improve in a specific patient is difficult and not very precise. We employ the tools we use to predict overall change in aphasia discussed in Chapter 4, but here we will focus on those signs that apply specifically to writing and the results of brief bouts of prognostic writing treatment.

PROGNOSTIC SIGNS FOR WRITING

General prognostic variables have a negative or a positive influence on the probability of improvement. The same is true for prognostic variables that apply to writing. Four specific indicants have surfaced from our experience, and each has been observed by others. These are premorbid literacy, the patient's desire to write, the presence of a dissociation between speech and writing, and the status of a patient's phonologic and lexical-semantic writing ability.

PREMORBID LITERACY

There are some whose strengths were not meant to be educated in schools. These range from those who spent only "three winters" in the classroom to those who obtained a high school diploma by simply putting in their time. Damage in the left hemisphere does not convert the premorbidly illiterate person into a reader and a writer. Those who could not

write before becoming aphasic will not do so after. They tell us, if they are able, and those who cannot reject requests to write on our formal appraisal measures.

Unfortunately, years of education are a poor indicant of premorbid writing ability. Some who never lasted a semester in school wrote flawlessly before becoming aphasic. Others who spent the mandatory 12 years in class never mastered literate writing. So, information about premorbid writing skill must come from the patient, his or her family, or a friend, not a transcript. Moreover, literacy in all of us is seldom present or absent. It resides in degrees. Thus, one must probe the patient, family, or friend to find out how much the patient wrote and how well.

Inability or reduced ability to write before the onset of aphasia is a negative prognostic sign. Holtzapple (1972) has documented that writing does not change in premorbidly illiterate or marginally literate patients. Her results indicate ability to copy shows gains, but writing does not budge. Our experience is similar. In fact, these patients are reluctant to work on writing or even participate in writing's appraisal. We honor their wishes, admire their wisdom, and focus our efforts on other modalities. For those who are willing, we may attempt to resurrect legible production of their signature, but the future for writing is not bright for the premorbid nonwriter.

WILLINGNESS TO WRITE

Some who could write before becoming aphasic will not attempt to write after. Why? Premorbid ability to write does not mean one did. Writing in most aphasic persons is disrupted more than performance in other modalities. Writing for most, aphasic and nonaphasic, is the least frequent and most inefficient means of communication. And, if hemiplegia renders the premorbidly preferred right hand useless, some are reluctant to cross the bridge to left-handed writing even though they could. The patient may use any or all of these reasons to reject any work on writing. One gentleman told us "I don't want to hand write. I want to talk teeth." His wish was honored.

Patients who do not want to write because they wrote little before becoming aphasic, who feel their writing deficits are beyond repair, who cannot or will not use their left hand to write if right hemiplegia dictates they must, or who prefer to concentrate on oral expression and eschew written communication have a poor prognosis for improving writing. Conversely, those who wrote before becoming aphasic and seek to after, who believe writing deficits can be mended, who try and find they can use their left hand if the preferred right hand is nonfunctional, and who are willing to divide treatment's time between both oral and written expression have a brighter prognosis for improving writing. We have treated both kinds of patients, and the former are more numerous than the latter.

DISSOCIATION BETWEEN SPEECH AND WRITING

One of aphasia treatment's cherished beliefs is to emphasize the patient's strengths. This is done to maximize communication in the strong modality and to use it to boost performance in weaker modalities. Although untested, many treat this belief as truth. Its application in treating aphasic writing is frequently moot, because written expression is usually not the strongest modality. Most patients listen, read, gesture, and speak better than they write. A few, however, display better writing than speech.

Hier and Mohr (1977) reported a patient who revealed a dissociation between oral expression and writing. The latter was less impaired than the former. Shubitowski, Lentz, Rosenbek, and McNeil (1983) found a similar patient, and during a treatment trial, they demonstrated improved writing with little change in speech. This dissociation, better writing than speech, appears prognostic. Those who write better than they talk may be telling us their writing will improve more than those who display the expected poorer writing than speech or those who show equal impairment in both.

PHONOLOGIC AND LEXICAL-SEMANTIC ABILITY

Hatfield (1983, 1985) has postulated two routes in converting words to print, phonologic and lexical-semantic. Impairment of one, the other, or both of these may occur in aphasia. Phonologic dysgraphia is an impaired ability to convert phonemes into graphemes but reasonably preserved lexical-semantic ability. Surface dysgraphia is the reverse; impaired lexical-semantic ability with reasonably preserved phonologic to graphemic conversion. Deep dysgraphia results when both abilities, phonologic and lexical-semantic, are impaired.

The prognostic implications of Hatfield's classification lie in the presence or absence of a strength that can be exploited in treatment. Those with phonologic or lexical-semantic dysgraphia have a preserved ability. Those with deep dysgraphia have no preserved ability. Prognosis for improved writing, we speculate, is better for the former than for the latter.

SUMMARY

Prognostic signs that apply specifically to writing are few. Those listed here indicate the patient who could write before becoming aphasic, who wants to write after onset, whose writing is superior to oral expression, and who has relatively preserved phonologic or lexical-semantic ability has a more favorable prognosis for improving writing than the premorbidly illiterate patient who has no desire to write after onset, whose oral expression is better than writing, and who has impaired phonologic and lexical-semantic skills. Of course, neither patient exists, because prognostic signs do not simply exist; they coexist. In combination, they render most statements about a patient's future effete. Thus, we look elsewhere for evidence to predict change in the aphasic person's ability to write.

PROGNOSTIC TREATMENT

The four prognostic indicants listed in Chapter 4—ability to learn, retention, generalization, and willingness to practice—

can be examined to predict potential for improving writing. This, of course, requires investing time and effort. The methods involve developing brief, single-subject prognostic treatment designs.

ABILITY TO LEARN

H. M. was severely aphasic at two years postonset when he returned to the hospital for prostate surgery. Dense right hemiplegia rendered his premorbidly preferred hand useless. Appraisal revealed nonexistent writing ability and marked impairment in copying. Nevertheless, he was fond of pencil and paper, indicated by his frequent unsuccessful attempts to use them. His overall management included attacks on auditory comprehension, reading, and oral-expressive deficits. Along with these, we constructed a single subject design to determine whether practice would improve his ability to copy. Ten stimuli composed of biographic information—name, address, wife's name, etc.—were produced in large type on worksheets. These were baselined in three sessions, followed by 10 days of homework which required him to copy each stimulus five times a night. Repair of errors was done each day during a few minutes of his treatment session for other deficits. In addition, a daily criterion run was done to see if H. M. was learning. Figure 11-6 shows he was willing and he was able. The PICA scoring system indicated improvement across the 10 days. H. M. learned, and other writing tasks became a part of his treatment.

RETENTION

W. B.'s wife went to work after he became aphasic. He was home alone, and he had sufficient oral expressive language to handle telephone calls. But, his writing was not adequate to take messages for his wife and teenage daughters. A writing to dictation task that employed a telephone message form, shown in Figure 11-7, was employed. Ten stimuli, each containing the name of the person called, the name of the caller, a brief message, and the caller's telephone number, were selected,

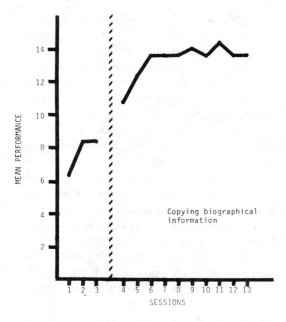

Figure 11-6. Prognostic treatment for H. M. indicating ability to learn. Ability to copy 10 biographic stimuli was baselined in 3 sessions, practiced as homework, and tested in 10 sessions. Performance is shown as the mean of 10 productions scored with the PICA multidimensional scoring system.

drilled in daily treatment, and assessed in a daily criterion run. Figure 11-8 shows W. B.'s ability to take telephone messages improved during treatment, and he retained his ability during withdrawal, after writing treatment had moved on to other targets. W. B. learned, and he retained. Both indicate a positive prognosis for improving writing. He continued to have difficulty with messages to his younger daughter about punk rock records and concerts. W. B. preferred the classics.

GENERALIZATION

C. W.'s auditory comprehension, reading, and oral-expressive language rebounded quite nicely during the first nine months after the occurrence of a left hemisphere CVA. But his ability to write lagged, and this 70 year old Annapolis graduate whose IQ topped 150 wanted to write. So, we set up a multiple baseline design to see whether intensive drill

TO: _____

FROM: _____

TELEPHONE NUMBER: _____

MESSAGE: _____

_____

_____

_____

Figure 11-7. Telephone message form used to evaluate W. B.'s ability to learn and retain.

would improve writing the names of objects and whether there would be generalization to untreated stimuli, writing the function of the objects. Figure 11-9 shows that the treatment worked; written confrontation naming improved. In addition, there was a gradual but

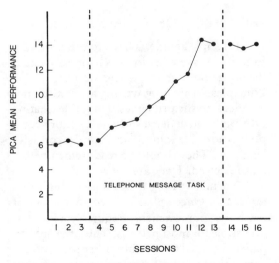

Figure 11-8. Results of telephone message task to evaluate W. B.'s ability to learn and retain. Message writing performance improved during 10 treatment sessions and remained improved after treatment on this task had stopped.

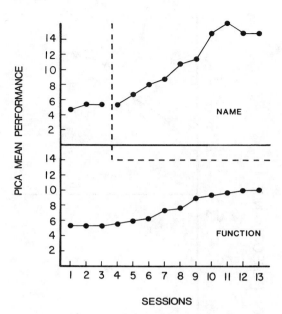

Figure 11-9. C. W.'s generalization in a multiple baseline design showing performance in writing the names of objects, treated, and writing the functions of objects, untreated.

definite generalization to the untreated stimuli. Writing function also improved. Because neither patient nor clinician has time to take on all of the words in treatment, we hope for generalization from treated stimuli to untreated stimuli. Without it we are doomed. For C. W., generalization occurred, and prognosis smiled.

WILLINGNESS TO PRACTICE

Improving writing requires the aphasic patient to practice, and it requires him or her to want to practice. Both are difficult. There are better ways to spend an evening than copying and completing. Nevertheless, we want patients to be willing. If they are, prognosis is good. C. W., our example for generalization, was, and he displayed this by destroying a single-subject design. Figure 11-10 shows what he did to our plans to treat one set of words beginning with "F" while continuing to baseline two additional sets, "M" and "R," in a multiple baseline design. We were looking for generalization from treated words

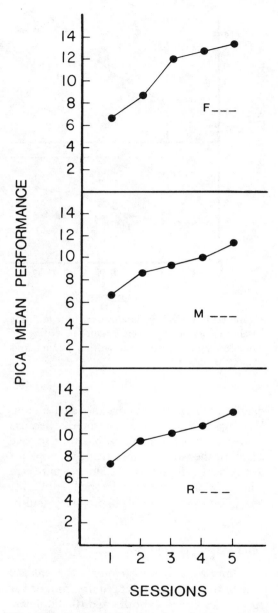

PICA MEAN PERFORMANCE

SESSIONS

Figure 11-10. Ascending baselines for three sets of words showing the results of C. W.'s willingness to practice between sessions.

to untreated words. C. W.'s tenacity and willingness to practice never got us out of baseline. He left us after the first baseline condition to tell his wife what he had deduced. Writing treatment was now turning to practice with words beginning with "F," "M," and "R." At

his insistence, they spent the afternoon and evening practicing. The results of this were evident during the next baseline session. Subsequent afternoons and evenings spent in the same activity, without our knowledge, made our baseline look like Mount St. Helens. It erupted! After five similar sessions, we inquired. C. W. told us how he was spending his time out of our sight. He was willing to practice, and he did.

TREATMENT

After the patient's writing deficits have been determined by appraisal, after the patient indicates a willingness to write, and after determining prognosis for improving writing is favorable, one focuses, administers, and evaluates treatment. We begin by listing some principles that guide treatment. Next, we consider the stimuli to be employed and how these should be controlled. Then, we decide whether time should be devoted to the mechanics of writing. And, finally, we select methods appropriate for the patient. These include traditional treatment, writing programs, and computer assistance.

PRINCIPLES FOR TREATING WRITING

Principles guide. They are the things up front that make what follows happen, unsnarl the snags, and get us where we want to go. Principles for treating writing are similar, not identical, to the principles that guide treating other aphasic deficits, those in auditory comprehension, reading, and oral-expressive language. They should be read, remembered, and reviewed. Here are a few.

Normal writing is not a goal. Improved writing is. Once aphasic, normality is out of reach. But improvement, frequently a lot of it, is possible for most patients. Thus, the aphasic patient is urged to keep his or her focus on the gains. We look back to see how far we have come. However, we do not look back beyond onset and seek the way we were.

Writing as compensation for impaired speaking is acceptable and encouraged. This includes drawing. Pencil and paper may help tongues along, and writing and drawing combined with speech and gesture may communicate what none alone will. Therefore, although we may practice writing in isolation, we encourage its use as part of total communication.

Writing treatment is structured. It involves careful selection of stimuli, exact specification of responses, constant analysis of performance, a knowledge of results, systematic repetition, and good humor. Structure does not mean rigidity, because writing treatment, like all treatment, is dynamic. It may follow a hierarchy, but it should not be forced to. Steps are ordered as hypotheses, and they are reordered when a hypothesis is refuted. The goal is getting there, not following a specific route. The potency of techniques is measured by whether a patient writes better within and across treatment sessions, not by our assumption that what we do should work.

Writing treatment leads the aphasic patient toward becoming his or her own editor. Initially, the burden for providing a knowledge of results may rest with the clinician. But gradually the load is shifted and shared. We ask patients to read what they have written, and if it is not right, we prod them to recognize their errors, to correct, and to revise.

Periodic reevaluation of progress is crucial. Improvement is identified and applauded. Persisting deficits are noted and attacked. The measures for reevaluation may be formal or informal and, usually, are both.

Writing treatment acknowledges what kind of writer and what kind of person a patient was before becoming aphasic. Clinicians who treat all aphasic people the same are not clinicians. "I never hand wrote!" one patient told us. Another resented our stealing any time from writing therapy to mend other deficits. We honored the desires of both.

Writing deficits have not read Goodglass and Kaplan (1983b) or Kertesz (1979). Prediction of how writing is disrupted is possible, but it does not take preference over what the patient across the table displays or needs. A writing treatment package for Broca's, or Wernicke's, or any other type of aphasia does not exist. Too much difference in each individual patient's history prevents treating any as a member of a group.

Similarly, no single set of tasks will improve writing deficits, and neither will a strong clinical preference. The goal is to communicate on paper; not to win a Palmer penmanship prize or construct the essay with the fewest run-on sentences. Conversely, striving only for the "functional" or "pragmatic" may move writing no further than filling a page with perfectly formed and joined ovals. Specific tasks need to be drilled on the way to the primary goal, turning writing into communication. The clinician who knows this explains it to the patient and promotes acceptance of time spent on seemingly nonfunctional practice.

Writing stimuli must be appropriate and adequate. They cause something to happen. Initially, what happens may be valuable only for analysis and planning the next step. Ultimately, what happens should communicate. An inappropriate or inadequate stimulus evokes nothing. The patient sits watching the absence of his or her pen's influence on paper. Select stimuli carefully and be ready to revise stimulus selection.

Similarly, concentrate on antecedent rather than consequent events. Planning correctly—stimulus and task selection—increases the probability of getting it right. All of the "nice jobs" or "good goings" must await a successful response. And, if the patient knows the response is successful, the reinforcements are not necessary. Writing correctly is its own reward. So, we concentrate on doing what we can to ensure a successful response, and the time to do that is prior to the patient putting pen to paper.

Exploit strengths, but beware of dissociation. Some preserved abilities, for example, auditory comprehension, may assist some patients in improving their writing. Hearing it may help write it. But, this must be demonstrated. We avoid using the good to make the bad worse.

Finally, generalization is promoted by preparation. We check generalization with multiple baseline designs and pre- and posttreatment testing. We seek it with repetition, training a large number of useful stimuli, teaching self-generated cues, making the patient his or her own editor, involving family and friends in treatment, and extending treatment beyond the clinic with appropriate assignments. We urge the patient to use treated writing behavior other than on demand.

These are the principles. We urge clinicians to have some and to use them long enough to determine whether they are appropriate. But, it is not a clinical sin to abandon a principle when a patient's performance indicates it should be.

STIMULUS SELECTION

R. H.'s writings had gone up in smoke, and on the page, he viewed the ashes. Could he kindle what may be left? He could not, the way he was going about it, because he was using the wrong fuel. R. H.'s attempt was a letter to his sister explaining where he was and what had happened to put him there. Our evaluation indicated he had difficulty copying words and no intelligible writing beyond that. He attempted to prepare something for the afternoon post, and he failed. His letter to his sister had the effect of a pancake dropped from a height of two inches. R. H. did not know what we did about the need for appropriate stimulus selection. His residual language would not push a pen through "cerebral vascular accident." In fact, it could not master "stroke." Our knowing what he did not is why he came to us and why we were able to help.

One of our principles is careful attention to stimulus selection. Another is to concentrate on antecedent events. Treatment stimuli are a large part of the antecedent event, and they must be selected and ordered carefully to ensure the consequent event, writing, has the highest probability of being successful.

We know, of course, that stimuli and responses are not separated in time and that methods influence both. But, we also know the most buoyant method will not keep a written response afloat if both are burdened by leaden—too long, too complex, not meaningful—stimuli. So, we take time here to discuss how we select and order stimuli for treating writing. Specifically, we will consider stimulus modalities and their combinations and stimulus content—length, complexity, and meaningfulness. We know we cannot prescribe for all patients, but we know there are means for finding out what is best for individual patients.

STIMULUS MODALITIES

Writing treatment stimuli are, like most treatment stimuli, presented in the visual, auditory, or tactile-kinesthetic modalities. Frequently, two or more of these are combined if, and only if, combining modalities helps. So, we are cautious about multimodality stimulation, and we use it only when the patient demonstrates combining modalities improves performance.

VISUAL. Visual stimulation is inseparable from writing treatment. It may be present initially, as a printed letter or word to be copied. It is always there as a consequent event: the patient's response. Most sections on writing in the aphasia treatment workbooks (Keith, 1980; Ross & Spenser, 1981) contain a number of treatment tasks that utilize visual stimuli—copying, separating compound words into two or more words, unscrambling letters to form a word, filling in the blanks in a printed sentence, etc. The assumption is that visual stimuli are good stimuli for treating writing. There is little evidence to support this. Nevertheless, most writing treatment contains a lot of visual stimuli, perhaps because visual stimuli permit some graphic effort by even the most severely involved patient. Many who cannot write can, at least, copy. That is the task of choice when the clinician harbors hope that copying will give way to something more functional.

Porch (1967) has demonstrated that copying is the most preserved of writing abilities in most aphasic patients. We agree, but we caution there is a need to identify those for whom it is not. Typically, the patient who writes better than he or she copies is the one with bilateral brain damage or peripheral or central visual deficits. In these patients, one may shun visual stimuli for any treatment task. Frequently, these patients will reject writing treatment. For most patients, we lean on visual stimuli—forms, letters, words, sentences, pictures, and anagrams. The latter can be manipulated and arranged to form words that can be copied. Consideration of copying also reminds us of the relationship between writing and reading. The illiterate can copy; they do not write. Thus, writing progress with printed stimuli beyond copying relies on the patient's residual and premorbid reading ability. Fortunately, most aphasic patients read better than they write. The exception to this is the presence of alexia without agraphia (Dejerine, 1892), impaired ability to read with retained ability to write spontaneously and to dictation (Geschwind, 1974).

We realize that most writing is not copying or writing the names of pictures. But, most writing is monitored visually by the writer. Because we want our patients to become their own editors eventually, we like to keep them in the visual mode—looking at, checking, and correcting what they have put on paper.

Finally, visual stimuli may be more preferable for those patients who show Hatfield's (1985) lexical preservation and phonological deficit. These patients' word specific knowledge and their impaired ability to convert strings of phonemes into graphemes would argue against auditory treatment stimuli and in favor of visual treatment stimuli.

AUDITORY. Some of what we hear, we write. This includes phone messages, lecture notes, oral directions. Thus, the ability to write from auditory stimuli has its uses. However, in treating aphasic writing, one must ask whether filling the air with sound helps or hinders. For many clinicians, the next step beyond copying is writing to dictation. Again, Porch's (1967) group data support this assumption. Aphasic patients tend to write better to dictation than they do volitionally. And, again, if auditory stimulation helps, we use it. But, we keep things quiet for the patient who indicates our producing noise results in too much noise and erodes his or her writing.

Patients who benefit from auditory stimulation are those who do better on PICA Subtest C, writing words from dictation, and Subtest D, writing words from spelled dictation, than they do on Subtest B, writing the names of objects. Similarly, those with better phonological than lexical ability (Hatfield, 1985) may profit more from auditory stimuli than visual stimuli. An indication of this is better writing of pseudowords (trab, frub, moig) than irregularly spelled words (friend, sword, ocean). Finally, the patient who cannot arrange anagrams to form a word but improves when each letter is dictated to him or her may be indicating auditory stimuli should, at least, be combined with visual stimuli.

TACTILE-KINESTHETIC. We spend little time having patients trace letters or words with a finger or having them "get the feel" of a letter cut from sandpaper. Also, we seldom write a letter on a patient's palm as a tactile clue. But, some (Agranowitz & McKeown, 1964) do. We have used this approach with a patient who suffered alexia without agraphia (Wertz et al., 1979), but the tactile-kinesthetic stimuli were employed to improve reading, not writing. For most, visual and auditory stimuli are more efficient and sufficient than tactile-kinesthetic stimuli. But, again, if touching and feeling will obtain what does not come from looking or listening, we would not hesitate to move or lay on the patient's hands.

STIMULUS CONTENT

One, among many, of aphasia treatment's insufficiently tested tenants is that stimulus content—length, complexity, meaningfulness—will influence a patient's response. Hierarchies are constructed from short to long and from simple to complex. Single letters and nonsense words are eschewed in favor of "useful" words and phrases. Why? Well, it makes sense to us, but too seldom do we ask whether it makes sense to our patient. Of course, these parameters interact and, sometimes, cannot be manipulated independently. If one must write his or her address, is prognosis better for the patient who lives on 3rd St. and poor for the one who resides on Heggenberger Boulevard? We hope not. And, we know of no empirical evidence that indicates writing's future is preordained by geographical location. Nevertheless, we do attempt to exercise some control over stimulus content initially. But, we constantly monitor patient performance and let it tell us how *we* are doing.

LENGTH. Should aphasic writing be starved down to make it run or fattened up to make it communicate? The meager empirical evidence and abundant clinical preference suggest the former—shorten the length, at least in the initial stages of treatment. Bicker, Schuell, and Jenkins (1964) demonstrated aphasic people make fewer spelling errors in writing short words than in writing longer words. And, suggestions for treating writing (Brubaker, 1982; Collins, 1986; Darley, 1982) begin with letters and progress through words to sentences.

However, as indicated earlier, stimulus length cannot always be manipulated independently. For example, Bicker and colleagues (1964) also observed a word's frequency of occurrence also influences the probability of its being spelled correctly by aphasic people. Thus, some infrequently occurring short words are more often misspelled than longer frequently occurring words. Further, patient preference and premorbid practice can play havoc with our attempts to keep writing stimuli short. Aphasic patient Franklin Olszewski was more successful writing his name than in writing "pen," "fork," and "key" on PICA Subtest B. Lawrence Pendergrass and Arnold Worshawski were too.

Nevertheless, we do attempt to select writing treatment stimuli whose length are appropriate for a patient's residual language abilities. Thus, we begin with single, short words, for example, "eat" not "breakfast," "walk" not "ambulate," and "pain" not "a major irritation in the right upper extremity." Patient performance is monitored to determine when and whether to increase stimulus length. Similarly, length is shortened, when possible,

in our manipulation of stimulus complexity and meaningfulness. We start with "Concord" to derive a patient's address rather than "2255 Lincolnshire Way, Concord, California 94553." And, we urge shorter, error-free responses in spontaneous writing if longer attempts are loaded with mistakes. For example, the patient who elects to write "There mern and wolfun herpening a picnic" is encouraged to settle for "picnic" until time and training increase the probability of a correct longer response.

COMPLEXITY. Begin simple and gradually increase complexity is another cherished shibboleth in search of empirical support. Nevertheless, we use it until or unless patient performance proves us wrong. Often, we proceed as though easier is a synonym for complexity. It is not, but we forget. Thus, writing treatment hierachies frequently progress from copying to dictation to writing; or from copying words to finding two words embedded in one, for example, "gingerbread," to writing the name of a picture to writing a sentence that describes a picture. For most aphasic patients, the first step in each of the two hierarchies is easier than the succeeding steps. Is the first step less complex? Perhaps. But, in the first hierarchy length is controlled. The patient copies a set of words, then the same words are dictated, and, finally, the words are presented as pictures, and the patient writes the names of the pictures. However, in the second hierarchy, length changes among the steps. For example, writing a sentence describing a picture requires a longer response than writing the name of a picture. We do not know whether patient improvement or the lack of it results from manipulating complexity or length.

Other attempts to manipulate complexity include control of grammatic or semantic category, lexical composition, syntax, and redundancy. For example, stimuli may be restricted to one grammatic class (e.g., nouns) or one semantic category (e.g., animals) initially and gradually changed to include additional classes (e.g., nouns, verbs, adjectives, or animals, fruit, clothing). Or, initial stimuli may vary only the vowel (e.g., pet, pot, pat) and gradually change by varying the vowel and the final consonant (e.g., pen, pod, pal). Or, initial stimuli may include only objects (e.g., glass, box, book) and gradually change to prepositional phrases (e.g., in the glass, on the box, by the book) to sentences (e.g., Lift the glass, Open the box, Read the book), and so on. Or, redundancy can be gradually reduced by using paired pictures and spoken and printed cues. For example, initially the patient sees two pictures, one is an open door and the other is a closed door. Printed below the open door is "The door is open." The clinician points to the first picture and the sentence and says "The door is open. Now, write a sentence about the other picture." The minimal contrast, open-closed, and the spoken and printed cues, "The door is open," are designed to assist the patient in writing "The door is closed." Next, the pictures are retained, but the printed cue is removed. The clinician points to the first picture and says, "The door is open. Now, write a sentence about the other picture." Thus, difficulty, perhaps complexity, is gradually increased as the patient masters each previous step.

MEANINGFULNESS. We receive a lot of meaningless mail, but none of it consists of a series of perfectly formed ovals, the alphabet, days of the week, or the names of common objects. Writing treatment stimuli should be meaningful and permit a patient to write what people write—his or her name, address, telephone number, and other biographic information; notes to themselves and others: cards and letters; lists for shopping or things to do today. If it is necessary to drill at the letter or word or serial response level, the clinician should have a reason for it, and the reason should be explained and make sense to the patient. Further, this kind of drill should have an influence on meaningful writing tasks that utilize meaningful stimuli.

Thus, we select stimuli that patients can and want to use. These include the patients' biographic data—name, address, telephone number, occupation, names of spouse and children and friends. We include a list of words that represent daily needs or wants—pills, shave, bath, toilet, pain, smoke, drink, eat, etc. These may support, suggest, or substitute what cannot be said. Additional stimuli come from patients' occupations, hobbies, or interests. And, some stimuli are specific to how patients fill their day. For example, for an aphasic husband who took over the cooking for his working wife, we drilled eggs, bacon, milk, salt, fruit, etc. These found their way into shopping lists for his wife.

Not only should stimuli be meaningful, they should also be drilled in meaningful tasks as soon as possible. Copying of names, addresses, and telephone numbers is related to taking telephone messages, finding information in the yellow pages and copying it, and completing the address and return address on an envelope. For inpatients, completing menus for the dietician and copying or constructing a daily schedule has application. Signatures are encouraged on checks, forms, cards, and letters, and are not confined to 500 repetitions on a lined pad. Television shows and their days and times are listed from the newspaper TV schedule. Patients deserve demonstration that what and why clinicians drill in writing treatment transcends homework.

Frequently, severity or a lack of progress force us to set aside meaningfulness and drill until a hurdle can be cleared. For example, if our patient's graphic production is reduced to insoluble squiggles, we may practice copying geometric shapes or single letters to turn the unintelligible into something intelligible. We reason that what can be understood is more meaningful than something that cannot. Similarly, if our patient cannot make the leap from copying his or her address to writing it when we say it, we may insert a step that requires selecting and filling in missing letters or numbers to complete the address, for example, 2_5 L_mb_rd C_rcl_. But, we always attempt to explain why we deviate from meaningful activity to drill. Most of all, we never treat stimuli with reverence fit for a chasuble. If reasonable effort does not conquer a stimulus, we set it aside and try again later.

Differences in patients' history and

severity prevent prescribing a specific set of stimuli for treating writing. Nevertheless, one can establish criteria for stimulus selection. That is what we have done here. Attention to the stimulus modalities, stimulus length, and stimulus meaningfulness establish the criteria. A patient's history, interests, and severity dictate the specific stimuli selected under each criterion. This approach increases the probability that every word treated will earn its keep.

MECHANICS OF WRITING

Most aphasic writing can be explained as defects in syntax, semantics, and spelling. However, Benson (1979a) reminded us the aphasic patient's mechanics of writing, orthography, can be disrupted. This may result, in some patients, from using the non-preferred left hand, because dense hemiplegia renders the premorbidly preferred right hand useless. Or, poor aphasic orthography may be a residual of poor premorbid orthography. How much of the time spent in writing treatment must be devoted to a patient's writing mechanics? Is it necessary to teach left-handed writing to patients with right hemiplegia? Should patients be encouraged to print, or is cursive writing preferable? If patients have a choice, should they be encouraged to use one hand or the other? And, if they do not have a choice, will a writing prosthesis provide one? Answers to some of these questions are yes or no. Answers to others are it depends or we do not know.

We try to remind ourselves that a hole in the head does not explain all errors. Hansen and McNeil (1986) and Hansen and colleagues (1987) have provided some data to support this belief. In an exhaustive analysis of writing with the preferred hand and nonpreferred hand in normal geriatric persons, they found normal writing was not error-free in either hand, and significant differences in errors between hands were few. Thus, some of an aphasic patient's orthographic errors may have been present before he or she became aphasic, and if right hemiplegia forces use of the non-preferred left hand, writing will not be grossly

different than it would be if the patient could use his or her right hand. Golper, Fisher, Gordon, and Marshall (1984) supported Hansen and McNeil's observations in nonaphasic writers with a small sample of aphasic patients. Golper and colleagues found no significant differences in writing between patients using their premorbidly preferred hand and those with hemiplegia who were forced to use their nonpreferred hand. Thus, the hand a patient uses to write does not seem to influence greatly the patient's writing. However, recent results with a writing prosthesis that will be discussed later indicate this issue may need additional consideration.

Do we teach left-handed writing to the premorbidly right-handed patients who are currently right hemiplegic? The means are available. Every clinician who has seen an aphasic patient has probably seen a copy of Gardner's (1958) *Left Handed Writing Instructional Manual*. But, we suspect few clinicians employ it systematically. We do not. Fifty-one exercises distributed over nine lessons would teach a nonaphasic right-handed writer to write with his or her left hand. However, giving Gardner's manual to an aphasic patient would have no more influence on writing than giving him or her a book on phonics to improve reading. We do review Gardner's manual from time to time to remind us that paper and body are positioned differently for the left-handed writer than for the right-handed writer, that there are drills available to improve sliding movements and slant, and that formation of different letters can be derived by different drills. Usually, our patients do not need these lessons or drills. For those who do, we enlist the aid of an occupational therapist, or we construct brief bouts of homework to be completed under the watchful eye of a trained family member or friend.

One of us writes, one of us prints and writes, and one of us does not do either very legibly. We observe that aphasic patients display the same variety. Boone and Friedman (1976) did too. They found no significant group differences in correctness between aphasic patients' cursive and printed writing. However, they did see individual differences among patients. Their advice is sage—writing style should be determined by each patient's preference and best performance—and we accept it.

Brown, Leader, and Blum (1983) have provided evidence that the hand aphasic patients use in writing may influence performance. Using the skateboard prosthesis shown in Figure 11-11, Brown and colleagues observed three severely aphasic patients with right hemiplegia wrote better to dictation with the right hand in the prosthesis than they did with the nonhemiplegic left hand. Few differences between hands emerged on copying tasks, but right-handed writing with the prosthesis was superior in content and similar in orthography compared with nonhemiplegic left-handed writing. Brown and colleagues suggested that the prosthesis may permit access to submerged levels in language representation through use of an older axial and proximal motor system. The marked differences they observed between hands within patients contrasts with the lack of differences between hands reported by Golper and colleagues (1984) among patients. The theoretical implications of Brown and

coleagues' results are interesting. The potential application in treatment is exciting.

The existing evidence indicates aphasic patients' orthography has less influence on disrupted writing than their language deficits. For example, Selinger, Prescott, and Katz (1987) found no differences between aphasic patients, handwritten and computer typed responses on PICA graphic subtests. Poor orthography did not mask their patients' written language abilities. Moreover, patients took almost twice as much time to type responses on the computer as they did to write. So, we devote little treatment time to mending orthography. Most of our efforts are invested in improving written language. We do, however, anticipate additional information on the efficacy of Brown and colleagues' skateboard prosthesis.

METHODS

Methods for treating aphasic writing abound. Some are better than others, and some are better for some patients than others. The best are those that have been tried and

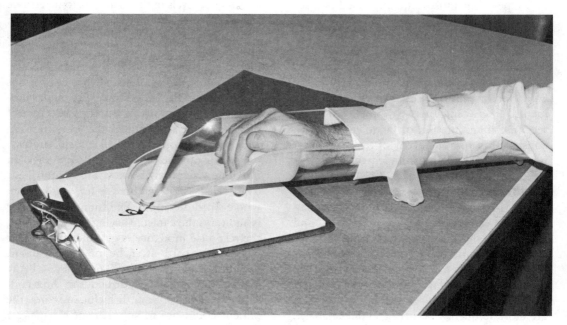

Figure 11-11. A skateboard prosthesis developed by Brown and colleagues (1983) that permits writing with the hemiplegic hand.

have succeeded. The very best are those that have been tried with a variety of patients and we know with whom they will succeed and with whom they will fail. The worst are those that imply they will help all patients. Because we continue to find out what works best with whom, we try different methods, and watch patient performance. Then we mix what we have tried and what we have seen and pursue connections that have sprouted from the mulch. We do this quickly and keep our wondering and wandering brief.

Here, we will discuss a variety of methods, not *the* method. We are yet to find it, and our patients convince us *it* does not exist. So, what follows are some things that have improved writing in some patients. For convenience, we divide what we discuss into traditional writing treatment, writing programs, and computer applications. Astute readers will notice quickly that the boundaries among these divisions are porous and easily disputed. Convenient organization is often controversial.

TRADITIONAL WRITING TREATMENT

One of the most frequently used phrases in aphasia therapy is "traditional treatment." It is also the least seldom defined. Most clinicians say traditional treatment means doing what Hildred Schuell did. If pressed to elaborate, most clinicians could provide the components that constitute traditional treatment. These include: a direct stimulus-response manipulation of language abilities, construction of a hierarchy of tasks within a performance modality from least to most difficult, intervention in the hierarchy at the level where a patient begins to experience difficulty, stimulus-response drill at that level until a criterion for correctness is reached, and moving up the hierarchy to a more difficult level each time criterion performance is attained. To this may be added what is done to improve the patient's probability of a correct response, for example, employing stimuli that are short, frequently occurring in the language, and minimally varied or using the patient's strongest stimulus modality—auditory, visual,

or both. And, one could elaborate by explaining what is done when a patient makes an error; for example, the stimulus is repeated, a cue is provided, or the patient is given the correct response. Certainly, none of this is new. Perhaps that is why it is called traditional. It fills a lot of the time clinicians devote to treating writing, and, for many patients, it works.

LaPointe (1978a) has elaborated the clear, straightforward, traditional treatment for aphasic writing shown in Table 11-3. It follows his Base-10 Programmed Response format (LaPointe, 1977a) in which the task, stimulus modality, and response modality are specified. Ten stimuli that conform to the task specification are selected, baselined, and drilled in treatment, and patient performance is plotted over several sessions. A criterion performance, for example, 90 percent correct or PICA scores of 13 and above in three consecutive sessions, is selected. The tasks are arranged in a presumed order of difficulty from easiest to most difficult. The clinician uses the patient's performance on appraisal measures to select the hierarchical level where treatment begins. Or, the clinician could probe with items from a variety of levels in the hierarchy to determine the level for intervention. Within task assistance, for example, combining stimulus modalities, repeats, cues, can be employed to increase the probability of a correct response and to mend errors. This is what constitutes the treatment. Patient performance guides progression, for example, if a patient succeeds at one level and cannot master the next, intervening tasks are constructed that yield success.

An example Base-10 for one task in LaPointe's hierarchy is shown in Figure 11-12. The task is writing three-letter words from whole-word dictation. The stimulus modality is auditory; the clinician saying the word. And, the response modality is graphic; the patient writes the word after he or she hears it. Criterion performance is 90 percent at a PICA 13, correct but delayed, or better in three consecutive sessions. Stimuli included words the patient could use to supplement his meager speech—"yes," "bad," "hot"—and names of family members—his son, "Bob," his wife,

TABLE 11-3.

LaPointe Base-10 Programmed Stimulation Treatment for Aphasic Writing.

Task	Input	Output	Example Stimuli
Copying geometric forms and letters	Visual	Graphic	X, △, T, □, V
Copying words	Visual	Graphic	tie, car, bed, comb, pills
Writing single letters to dictation	Auditory	Graphic	i, m, w, h, d
Writing three-letter words from dictated spelling	Auditory	Graphic	yes, sit, hot, bad, top
Writing three-letter words from whole word dictation	Auditory	Graphic	yes, sit, hot, bad, top
Writing five-letter words from whole word dictation	Auditory	Graphic	tired, happy, please, again, start
Writing two-word phrases from dictation	Auditory	Graphic	I can, She did, I'm tired, Don't yell
Writing two-word responses to questions	Auditory	Graphic	Q: Who can? R: I can. Q: Who did? R: She did. Q: How do you feel? R: I'm tired.

Adapted from LaPointe (1978a).

"Nan," his daughter, called "Sis," and the name of the family pet, "Dog." Performance was baselined in three sessions and was stable at 50 percent. Part of each day's treatment included about 20 minutes devoted to this task. Thirty treatment trials were run each day. Correct responses were applauded. Incorrect responses were followed with a repeat. If the response remained incorrect, the patient was shown the correct printed form of the error word simultaneously with the clinician saying the word, and he tried again. If the error persisted, the printed form of the word was presented, and the patient copied it. At the end of each session, a daily criterion run was completed. The only assistance provided was a repeat if the patient requested one. The data in Figure 11-12 show baseline performance and performance in daily criterion runs after each of five treatment sessions. Criterion performance was reached after the fifth session. Treatment moved up to the next step in the hierarchy, writing five-letter words from whole-word dictation. We continued to test

three-letter words from whole-word dictation in an untreated condition in three subsequent sessions. Performance held at 90 to 100 percent correct.

Haskins (1976) has presented a similar hierarchy for treating writing in severely aphasic patients. It includes additional steps in the lowest levels—tracing alphabet letters as they are named by the clinician, connecting dots to form letters, and writing the alphabet in serial order from dictation. Haskins also included some reading tasks—pointing to printed words when named—and some combined response modalities—tracing and spelling a word aloud after the clinician said the word. And, she extended the upper levels by adding writing words in specified categories spontaneously and formulating and writing short sentences containing previously practiced words. Haskins reported results for one patient who improved from the 36th to 88th PICA Graphic Percentile during five months of her traditional writing treatment.

Traditional writing treatment is sometimes

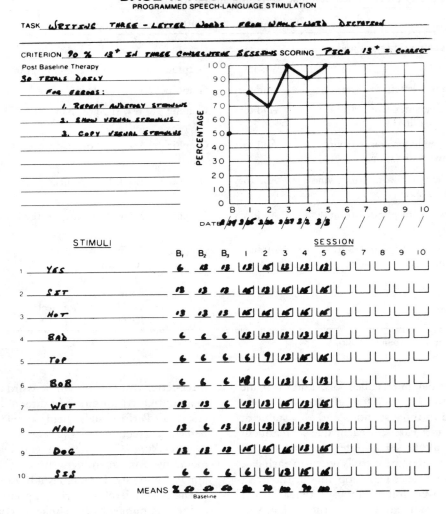

Figure 11-12. Base-10 performance at one level in a traditional treatment writing hierarchy. Reprinted with permission from PRO-ED.

based on a model of language processing, for example, one similar to that posited by Wepman, Jones, Bock, and Van Pelt (1960). These models typically plot language processing and performance along a transmission, sensory input, to integration, symbolic formulation, to transmission, motor output path. Within each stage are assumed various levels of function, for example, perceptual, association, and conceptual. These levels form a hier-

archy, and one can establish a hierarchical series of treatment tasks within each level. The result might resemble what is shown in Table 11-4.

A task hierarchy is provided for each of three levels—perceptual, association, and conceptual. At the perceptual level, meaning is not necessary to complete the tasks. The patient only needs adequate visual ability to see the stimuli and sufficient motor ability to copy. The hierarchy begins with nonlanguage

TABLE 11-4.
Writing Treatment Based on a Model of Language Processing and Performance.

Level	Task Hierarchy
Perceptual	1. Copying geometric forms
	2. Copying letters
	3. Copying words
	4. Copying phrases
Association	1. Transposing upper case letters into lower case letters, e.g., "T" to "t"
	2. Transposing printed stimuli into cursive stimuli, e.g., "L" to "$\mathcal{L}$"
	3. Transposing the printed name of a number into the arabic numeral, e.g., "Two" to "2"
Conceptual	Writing words to dictation
	1. Auditory, spoken word, and visual, printed word, stimulus with an auditory and visual repeat during performance
	2. Auditory, spoken word, and visual, printed word, stimulus with an auditory only repeat during performance
	3. Auditory, spoken word, stimulus only with an auditory repeat during performance
	4. Auditory, spoken word, stimulus with no repeat during performance

stimuli, geometric forms, and progresses through language stimuli that gradually increase in length—letters, words, and phrases.

The next level, association, requires the patient to develop some relationships between stimuli. The stimulus is presented in one form, for example, a capital "T," and the patient responds by producing a related form, for example, a lower case "t." Similar requirements are used to turn printed stimuli into cursive and relate the name of a number to its arabic counterpart.

At the conceptual level, a task is selected, for example, writing words to dictation. A series of steps utilize previous training at the perceptual and association levels, and, eventually, end with reproducing a spoken word in writing. The first step uses perception, copying the printed stimulus that is present throughout performance, and association, the pairing of the spoken word with the printed stimulus. Next, the perceptual cue, printed word, is present only during the initial stimulus, and the association cue, spoken word, is present during the initial stimulus and repeated during performance. Then,

the perceptual cue, printed word, is removed, and the patient must rely on only the association cue, spoken word, during the initial stimulus and its repeat during performance. Finally, criterion performance requires the patient to do what the hierarchy was designed to accomplish, write words to dictation. The clinician says the word, and the patient writes it.

These methods certainly do not exhaust what might be called traditional writing treatment. Our intent was to provide the rationale and some recipes. The former is more important than the latter. Competent clinicians become that way by spending a lot of time mixing and mastering. They decide where they want to go, and they plan how to get there. The best know, immediately, when they are lost. They know when to reorder a hierarchy, when to invent some intervening steps, and what help a patient needs to get him or her over the hill on which he or she has stalled. They develop an amazing command of the zigs and zags of disrupted writing behavior and how to mend it. They work as if they are sneaking up on something. And, they are.

WRITING PROGRAMS

When convictions become rubbed smooth by familiarity, we may need to rough them up. Traditional writing treatment gets roughed up by the creation of a writing program. The line between traditional writing treatment and a writing program is as slim as that between twilight and dusk. Usually, they differ in writing programs being more systematic, more based in a specific point of view, more focused on a specific stimulus or response, or more appropriate for a specific patient or group of patients. If you cannot always see the difference between traditional treatment and a program, we caution you not to worry. Frequently, we can't either.

One of the ingredients in traditional treatment is to select a group of stimuli, drill these at one level on a hierarchy until criterion performance is reached, and then move up to the next level in the hierarchy and drill the same stimuli at this new level. An alternative approach would be to select a single stimulus and move it up the hierarchy until it has been mastered and can be used functionally and then return and make the trip with another stimulus. The latter approach was developed by Basso (1978), and she called it *laddering*. Although laddering is most popular as a treatment for oral-expressive language deficits, we have modified it and present it here as a treatment for aphasic writing.

The principle behind laddering is to take a response that a patient can produce automatically and make it volitional. This is done through a series of steps, up the ladder, from automatic to voluntary. Along the way, the patient achieves what Basso called automatic-voluntary dissociation. Initially, the response can only be produced automatically with strong stimulation, but eventually it can be produced voluntarily with no or minimal stimulation. Table 11-5 shows the application of laddering in a writing program.

First, a stimulus is selected, for example, "key." In Step I, the clinician uses auditory cues—says the name, spells the name, and associates the object with its function—and visual cues—presents the printed word "key" and a picture of a key—to evoke an automatic response. In Step II, the auditory functional cue is dropped, and the spoken and spelled word cues are retained. Similarly, the visual printed word cue is dropped, and the picture is retained. In Step III, only the auditory name is retained and is paired with the picture. And finally, in Step IV the patient is required to write the name of the picture. Thus, performance has been led from automatic writing to dictation and perhaps copying, through writing to spelled dictation, to writing to whole-word dictation, to voluntarily writing the name of a picture. Then, the clinician selects another stimulus and repeats the process.

Basso's laddering procedure, unlike traditional hierarchical treatment, may leave the

TABLE 11-5.
The Use of Laddering in Treating Aphasic Writing.

Step	Stimulus	Response
I	Clinician says, "You lock a door with a key. Write key. K-E-Y" and shows the printed stimulus "KEY" and a picture of a key.	Patient writes or copies "KEY"
II	Clinician says, "This is a key. Write key. K-E-Y" and shows a picture of a key.	Patient writes "key" to spelled dictation
III	Clinician says, "This is a key. Write Key" and shows a picture of a key.	Patient writes "key" to whole-word dictation
IV	Clinician says, "What is this? Write its name" and shows a picture of a key.	Patient writes "key"

patient at the end of a treatment session with the ability to write 5 to 10 words volitionally. Of course, the patient's use and ability to write the words brought up the ladder in one session must be checked in subsequent sessions. And, treatment may need to be dynamic, ascending and descending the ladder with a stimulus depending on success at the next step.

A second treatment program to improve writing is the modificaton of LaPointe's (1984) verbal sequential treatment of split lists. Originally developed to improve confrontation naming in a patient who suffered aphasia and apraxia of speech, we apply it here as a treatment for written confrontation naming.

The stimuli consist of 20 pictures of objects. The ability to write the names of the pictures is baselined in three sessions. If performance is stable, the stimuli are divided into two equally difficult sets of 10 each. One set is treated for 10 sessions, and the other set is not treated. However, performance on both sets is measured at the end of each treatment session. After 10 sessions, the untreated set of pictures is treated, and the previously treated set is untreated. Again, performance on both sets is measured after each treatment session.

Treatment follows the steps listed in Table 11-6. Each stimulus in the treated set is presented, and the patient is asked to write the name. If the response is correct, the next stimulus is presented. For incorrect responses in Step I, the sequence in Step II is followed. Initially, the clinician shows the patient his or her error or errors, and Step I is repeated. If the response is correct, the next stimulus is presented. However, if the response remains incorrect, the clinician says the word, and the patient writes from whole-word dictation. If the response is now correct, Step I is presented for that stimulus. But, if the patient continues to fail, the clinician has the patient copy the word from a printed stimulus. If success follows, writing to dictation, B, is repeated, and if performance continues to be successful, Step I, writing the name of the picture, is repeated for that stimulus. However, if the patient cannot copy the name correctly, we set that stimulus aside and go on to the next. We seldom need C, copying, in this treatment program. If we do, and if the patient cannot copy correctly, we have probably selected too difficult a task for that patient, and we look for something more appropriate. If at first one does not succeed, trying again is appropriate. But, if one continues to fail, it is time for his or her clinician to try something else.

Figure 11-13 shows a patient's performance during sequential writing treatment. of split lists. Each data point represents the percent correct in Step I performance, writing the names of pictures. The patient's baseline was stable, 20 percent correct on 20 stimuli. These were divided into two lists of equal

TABLE 11-6.
Steps Used in Sequential Writing Treatment of Split Lists.

Steps	Procedure
I	Patient is requested to write the name of a picture. If the response is correct, the next picture is presented.
II	If the response is incorrect, the clinician employs the following sequence:
	A. Clinician shows the patient the error or errors and repeats the stimulus. If response is correct, clinician returns to Step I and presents the next stimulus.
	B. If response remains incorrect, clinician says the word, and the patient writes it to dictation. If the response is correct, clinician repeats Step I for that stimulus.
	C. If response remains incorrect, clinician has the patient copy the word from a printed stimulus. If the response is correct, clinician repeats B above and then Step I for that stimulus.
	D. If the response remains incorrect, clinician goes on to the next stimulus in Step I.

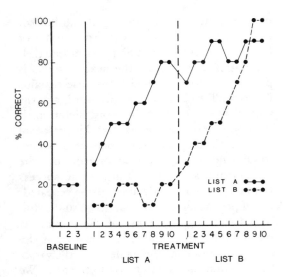

Figure 11-13. Patient performance in sequential writing treatment of split lists. List A treated during first 10 sessions and List B treated during the second 10 sessions.

difficulty, List A and List B, based on baseline performance. List A was treated for 10 sessions using the program in Table 11-6, and List B was untreated. Both lists were tested at the end of each session. During treatment, performance on List A rose to 80 percent correct. During the period of nontreatment, performance on List B fluctuated from 10 to 20 percent correct. After the tenth treatment session, List B was treated for 10 sessions, and List A was untreated. During this period, performance on List B rose to 100 percent correct, and performance on List A remained at 80 to 90 percent correct.

For this patient, our adaptation of LaPointe's (1984) sequential treatment of split lists approach into a sequential writing treatment for split lists was effective. When treated, performance on a list improved. When not treated, performance remained essentially unchanged.

We will discuss one additional writing program to show writing treatment need not be limited to the severely or moderately impaired patients, or to writing single words. More importantly, this program indicates

treatment of writing, like all treatment, is limited only by the creativity of the clinician.

One of our treatment principles is to make the aphasic writer his or her own editor. Rau (1973) did that by providing an immediate knowledge of results. Her patient was aphasic subsequent to a left hemisphere cerebral vascular accident and made substantial improvement during the first seven months postonset. However, continued improvement waned, and her performance had remained stable for almost 18 months. At about two years postonset, Rau designed a program to accomplish what her patient wanted to do: improve her writing. Overall PICA performance at the beginning of this treatment was at the 85th percentile, and writing performance on Subtest A was at the 89th percentile.

Rau designed a task to improve writing sentences. Thirty common objects were randomized into 12 10-item lists for presentation in three baseline, six treatment, and three posttreatment sessions. In each session, the patient was required to write a sentence that indicated the function of each of 10 objects. No feedback was provided during baseline and posttreatment sessions. During the treatment sessions, each sentence was given a numerical rating on a 15-point adequacy scale similar to the PICA multidimensional scoring system immediately after the patient produced each sentence. The patient's task was to use the rating to improve performance on subsequent sentences. For example, a "6" indicated an error or errors had been made, a "10" indicated an error had been made and self-corrected, and a "13" indicated performance was complete and correct but delayed. This immediate knowledge of results was used by the patient to plan, edit, and improve her performance on subsequent sentences.

Figure 11-14 shows the results of pretreatment, treatment, and posttreatment performance. Baseline performance stabilized at the 91st percentile. During treatment, performance rose to the 98th percentile, and when treatment was withdrawn, performance dropped to the 87th percentile. These results indicated the treatment was effective—performance

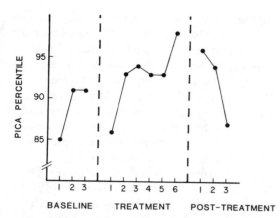

Figure 11-14. Patient performance in a sentence writing treatment that provided immediate knowledge of results (after Rau, 1973).

improved during treatment and declined during withdrawal. They also indicated a need for more treatment. Additional information to document the treatment effect was fewer errors in each sentence during the treatment condition than in baseline and posttreatment, more complete and accurate sentences written during the treatment condition, and longer sentences produced during the treatment condition. Independent confirmation was seen in PICA Subtest A performance—89th percentile pretreatment, 98th percentile performance immediately posttreatment, and 98th percentile performance in a six-month follow-up after treatment. Thus, Rau demonstrated a writing program that provided an immediate knowledge of results improved sentence production in her mildly aphasic patient.

The writing programs described here certainly do not exhaust what is available. Further, they only suggest two (Basso, 1978; LaPointe, 1984) of many possibilities for converting a treatment designed for another modality to the treatment of writing. Most of all, they are offered as an outline for the development of appropriate programs for appropriate patients. Clinicians have an apprehension of limits. They also have a sense that the attempt must, nevertheless, be made. Our examples document some attempts that were successful.

COMPUTERIZED TREATMENT

Some have been steering the treatment of aphasic writing from the calm waters of tradition into the more controversial seas of change. Finding themselves at sea in a sieve, they say, "Look here, a team of user-friendly porpoises with trailer hitches attached may haul aphasic writing to a shore where it communicates." These folks advocate utilizing microcomputers to accomplish what may not be possible with pencil and paper. And, some (Steele, Weinrich, Kleczewska, Wertz, & Carlson, 1987) have suggested computers may permit communication by severely aphasic people who are globally impaired in all traditional modalities.

Katz (1986) has presented the most complete discussion thus far on the use of microcomputers in aphasia treatment. Their application, at present, appears more appropriate for improving reading and writing than for treating auditory comprehension and oral expressive language. Computerized treatment for writing requires the patient to type on the computer keypad and view the results on the computer monitor. The writing treatment is contained in the computer program. Like all writing treatment, except for copying, computer writing treatment relies on the patients' ability to read. Several attempts have been made to improve aphasic writing (typing) using microcomputers. These are discussed here.

Seron, Deloche, Moulard, and Rousselle (1980) employed a microcomputer in a single word writing to dictation task. The clinician said the word and the patient typed it using the computer keypad. If the correct letter was selected, it was displayed on the computer monitor. If an incorrect letter was selected, a buzzer sounded. However, if the incorrect letter was contained in the word, it was displayed on the computer monitor in dashed lines in its correct position in the word. If the incorrect letter was not contained in the word, nothing appeared on the computer monitor. Thus, the patient typed the word spoken by the clinician, letter by letter, and used the computer feedback to make choices after producing an error.

Five aphasic patients were treated in seven to 30 sessions with Seron and colleagues' treatment. Pretreatment and posttreatment tests in which the patients wrote single words to dictation were used to determine the treatment's efficacy. A significant reduction in the number of words misspelled and the number of total errors made on a posttest at the end of treatment indicated the computerized treatment had improved spelling ability and that this improvement had transferred to handwritten responses. A second posttest, six weeks after treatment had ended, showed five of the six patients continued to perform above pretest performance.

Katz and Nagy (1984) developed "Speller" as a computerized treatment task for written confrontation naming. Drawings of objects are displayed on the computer monitor, and the patient's task is to type the name of the object on the computer keypad. If the response is correct, auditory and visual feedback are given and a new picture is displayed. If the response is incorrect, auditory and visual feedback indicate an error has been made, and treatment begins with a hierarchy of six cues. These range from simple repetition of the stimulus, presentation of anagrams with and without feedback, selection of the target word from a multiple-choice array, to copying the target word. The computer program selects which cue to present based on the patient's previous attempts to type the target word. Thus, the patient's response influences the kind of help he or she receives.

Eight aphasic patients were treated with Speller in 4 to 15 sessions. Handwritten confrontation naming was measured in pre- and posttreatment tests. Seven of the eight patients showed marked improvement in their computer typed responses during the treatment trial, and the group displayed significant improvement on the handwritten posttest compared with performance on the pretest. Thus, the aphasic patient's written confrontation naming improved, and computer treatment resulted in improved writing.

The positive results obtained by Seron and colleagues (1980) and Katz and Nagy (1984) suggest microcomputers may be appropriate tools for mending aphasic writing. Loverso and colleagues (1985) and Loverso (1987), however, suggest caution in the growing tendency to embrace technology.

Success with a clinician presented program (Loverso, Selinger, & Prescott, 1979) that used the "verb as core" to improve verbal and written performance led Loverso and colleagues (1985) to compare the same program administered in two different modes, one by a clinician and one by a microcomputer. The treatment utilizes verbs as "pivots" and WH-questions (who, what, when, where, and why) as cues to elicit actor-agent-object spoken and written sentences. Using a random assignment of treatments design, Loverso and colleagues compared an aphasic patient's progress through the six steps in the program. Their results indicated both modes were effective. The patient improved his ability to say and write sentences, however, criterion performance was reached in 36 treatment sessions with the clinician compared with 67 treatment sessions with the computer.

Katz's (1986, 1987) and Loverso's (1987) cautions are sage. Presently, the microcomputer is one of the clinician's tools. It is not a clinician. Its potential lies in its economy, providing more treatment at a reduced cost, and its quality, providing efficacious treatment. But, use of the microcomputer to treat aphasic writing to date has produced promise, not proof.

Additional potential applications of microcomputers exist at both ends of the aphasic severity continuum. One is to lessen the mildly aphasic patient's burden in editing what he or she has written, and the other is to provide the severely aphasic person with an alternative mode of communication. We offer an example of each application.

Some aphasic people improve writing performance markedly. They transcend writing to dictation tasks, confrontation written naming drills, and even written sentence formulation treatment. For these, we apply our principle of making the patient his or her own editor. Reading performance and general language abilities have risen to a level where the patient is ready to detect and correct writing errors.

Doing this with pencil and paper is laborious, time consuming, and erodes the patient's patience. Enter the word processor! The production of printed hard copy for editing and the ease of revision permitted by word processing reduces the time and effort in writing and rewriting, avoids deciphering illegible orthography, and for most patients, is fun. Enjoyment in treatment, we find, is a great alternative to psychosis.

W. B. was ready to write cards and letters and—his choice— maintain a diary. Doing this with pen and ink was unacceptable. Although his aphasic errors had waned and he was good at detecting them, a sufficient number persisted to require him to write and rewrite and rewrite some more. In addition, his orthography made us suspect he had been a physician and not the engineer he claimed to have been. For W. B., the microcomputer and its word processing capabilities was "love at first byte." He wanted to write letters to friends and family, so these became the treatment stimuli. He mastered the computer's word processing mechanics in five sessions and needed only an occasional reminder of procedural requirements in subsequent sessions. We encouraged him to compose and type his letters on the computer. After each effort, we calculated the percent of errors he made in every 100 words. A printed copy of his performance after each session permitted us to do this. It also permitted us to determine W. B.'s ability to detect and correct errors. Thus, we were able to derive the data shown in Figure 11-15.

Baseline performance in his ability to recognize his errors was around 50 percent. This rose to 84 percent during 10 treatment sessions, and it remained at that level after treatment ended. W. B.'s total errors in 100 words typed on the computer keypad were approximately 40 percent. This dropped to 14 percent at the end of 10 treatment sessions, and it stayed there after treatment stopped. He could correct about 20 percent of the errors he made during baseline. After 10 treatment sessions, he was correcting 50 percent of the errors he made, and he maintained this performance after treatment had ended. Thus,

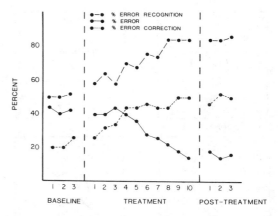

Figure 11-15. W. B.'s performance in word processing treatment, showing the percent of errors, percent of error recognition, and percent of error correction.

W. B. could produce letters to friends and family on the word processor that were 86 percent correct. Eighty-four percent of the errors he made, he recognized. And, 50 percent of these he corrected. What he posted, therefore, contained approximately seven percent errors; slightly better than the correspondence exchanged among the coauthors of this book.

Finally, the computer may come to the aid of those who cannot communicate in any modality. We had our doubts about this, and although we remain skeptical, we are becoming convinced. Initially, we reasoned that computer-aided communication worked for those who could do everything but talk. The problem in aphasia is language, not speech. Therefore, if computers required aphasic patients to use language, the results would be no better than the patient's performance in oral-expressive or written language. One needs something to say before one can say it orally, graphically, or with a computer. Thus, the computer may be a treatment tool, but an alternative means of communication? Not likely. Then we became acquainted with the work of Steele and his colleagues (Steele et al., 1986, 1987).

Several years ago Gardner and colleagues (1976) demonstrated severely aphasic patients who possessed little or no ability to communicate in natural language could learn and

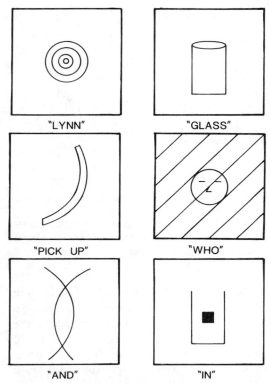

Figure 11-16. VIC symbols developed by Gardner and colleagues (1976) for communication by severely aphasic patients.

use a visual communication system (VIC) that employed pictures and symbols similar to those shown in Figure 11-16. The patients learned to understand and respond to VIC symbols on index cards and to use them to create commands, ask questions, form simple declaratives, and express photic or emotional utterances. After 2 to 11 weeks of training, comprehension of VIC symbols exceeded comprehension of spoken English by 17 to 77 percent among five of the patients studied. And, responsive naming with VIC symbols exceeded responsive naming in spoken English by 53 to 89 percent. Thus, the severely aphasic patients improved their communicative abilities with VIC, but the system was seldom used outside of the treatment sessions. Family members reported that the stacks of index cards were too cumbersome for use in most situations and difficult for patients with hemiplegia to manage.

Steele and his colleagues (1986, 1987) have adapted the VIC concept to the microcomputer to reduce the motoric, cognitive, and organizational demands on aphasic patients. This adaptation, Computer-based Visual Communication System (C-VIC), utilizes the Apple Macintosh and its "mouse" device. Icons are organized in "stacks" and can be accessed, selected, and arranged in syntactic strings by the patient. Figure 11-17 shows the basic "stacks" that are grouped into proper nouns, common nouns, verbs, prepositions, modifiers, and interjections. In addition, punctuation, numbers, and time symbols are available. The patient or clinician begins a string with a punctuation mark to indicate the type (command, question, etc.) of string to be constructed. Then, the mouse cursor is placed on a stack and clicked to display the alternatives in the stack. For example, the common noun stack contains symbols for cup, pencil, apple, etc. One of these is selected and placed in one of the response windows after the punctuation mark. Then, the user goes to another stack to select the next symbol in the utterance being created. Eventually, a string is created as shown in Figure 11-18. The patient or clinician can respond to the string by carrying out an action or constructing a C-VIC string in the lower response windows. Printed English equivalents are displayed below the string to ease translation for those not familiar with the C-VIC vocabulary and syntax.

The results with C-VIC thus far are amazing. Globally aphasic patients learn and use C-VIC to communicate. However, they remain severely impaired in natural language. Thus, C-VIC appears to be a potential alternative mode of communication and not a treatment to improve natural language. J. S. is a representative example. A left hemisphere thromboembolic infarct left him severely aphasic, overall PICA performance at the 9th percentile and a WAB AQ of 7.3. Eight months of traditional treatment resulted in some improvement, PICA Overall at the 28th percentile and WAB AQ of 10.4, but he remained a nonfunctional communicator. Five weeks of C-VIC training obtained the results shown in Figure 11-19. Auditory comprehen-

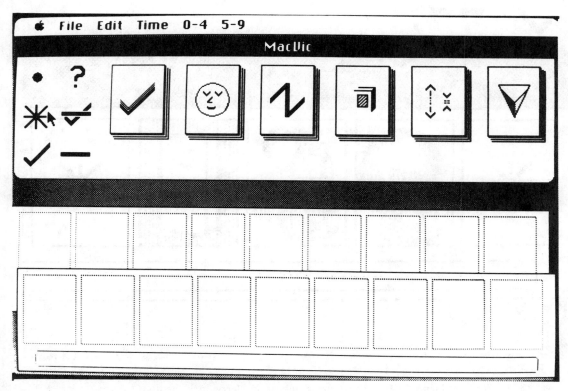

Figure 11-17. C-VIC "stacks" that can be explored by the patient for construction of syntactic strings.

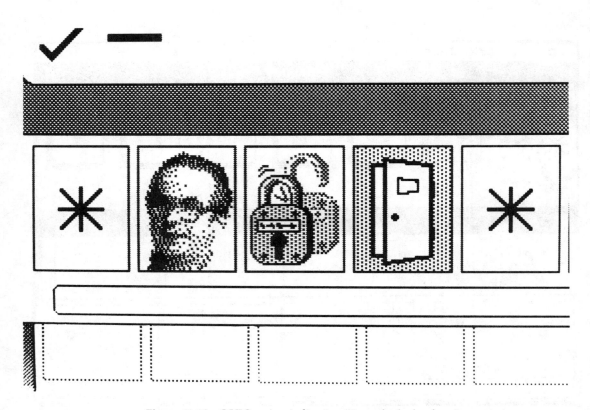

Figure 11-18. C-VIC string indicating "Jerry, lock the door."

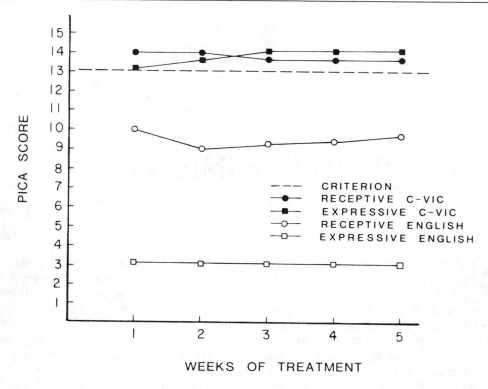

Figure 11-19. J. S.'s performance in C-VIC and in natural language.

sion and confrontation naming in C-VIC became functional, but both remained severely impaired in natural language. J. S. continues to have difficulty understanding the spoken phrase "Put the pencil in the glass" and his verbal production remains limited to a recurring unintelligible utterance, "Tee ne." But, he can leave the room while 1 of 20 objects is removed from the array; return and scan the objects; construct in C-VIC, "Who has the pencil?"; read the clinician's C-VIC response, "Dick has the pencil"; and go to Dick and collect the missing object. That, to us, is amazing.

SUMMARY

Writing can be improved by treatment in most, not all, aphasic patients. For some, the gains are small but noticeable. For others, the gains are marked and useful. Although treatment will not return writing to its premorbid proficiency, clinicians and patients seek what can be salvaged. To do this, a patient must want to write. If he or she does, the clinician appraises to find where strengths and deficits reside. Once these are identified, a prognosis for improvement is stated and sought. Treatment utilizes appropriate stimuli and follows tradition, uses a specific writing program, or employs a microcomputer. Constantly, throughout treatment, the efficacy of the effort is evaluated. All gains are identified clearly for the patient, encouraged into use, and applauded. When everything is out of reach, something can be a lot, and it can satisfy.

12

IN RECOGNITION

Deciding to write is the easiest decision authors make about a book. Deciding when to stop is the hardest. In describing the aphasic person, we stopped short of describing the nonlanguage strengths and weaknesses of aphasic men and women. We avoided excruciating detail of aphasic signs and symptoms. We did not describe all the tests, all the methods, or all discharge and follow-up options. We did not describe group treatment, counseling, bibliotherapy, or vocational planning. We stopped short of describing all these, despite their importance, because the description of a clinical approach to aphasia, if it were to be complete, would require several volumes. Indeed, several volumes have been written and doubtless, the easy decision has been made about others.

Although we did not consciously create criteria for deciding what to include and what not to include, we must have done so unconsciously. Now that we have seen the product, it appears that our main criterion was tradition. We included the traditional topics. A second criterion was experience. We included what we have experience with. We know that aphasia is more than a language disorder and that aphasia treatment is more than, and often different from, what happens between two people sitting across a clinic table. What we hope for with this book is that it helps some aphasiologists or potential aphasiologists get started. Where they stop will be guided by their unique experiences, education, and reading.

REFERENCES

Ackerman, R. H. (1980). Editorial—A new image for the neuroradiologist. *American Journal of Neuroradiology, 1,* 271–273.

Adamovich, B., & Henderson, J. (1984). Can we learn more from word fluency measures with aphasic, right brain injured, and closed head trauma patients? In R. H. Brookshire (Ed.), *Proceedings of the Conference on Clinical Aphasiology* (pp. 124–131). Minneapolis: BRK Publishers.

Adams, R. D., & Victor, M. (1981). *Principles of neurology.* New York: McGraw-Hill.

Agranowitz, A., & McKeown, M. R. (1964). *Aphasia handbook for adults and children.* Springfield, IL: Charles C Thomas.

Alajouanine, T. (1956). Verbal realization in aphasia. *Brain, 79,* 1–28.

Alajouanine, T., Castaigne, P., Lhermitte, F., Escourolle, R., & Ribancourt, B. D. (1957). Etude de 43 cas d'aphasie post traumatique. *Encephale, 46,* 1–45.

Albert, M. L., & Bear, D. (1974). Time to understand: A case study of word deafness with reference to the role of time in auditory comprehension. *Brain, 97,* 373–384.

Albert, M. L., Goodglass, H., Helm, N. A., Rubens, A. B., & Alexander, M. P. (1981). *Clinical aspects of dysphasia.* New York: Springer-Verlag.

Alexander, M. P., & LoVerme, S. R. (1980). Aphasia following left hemisphere intracerebral hemorrhage. *Neurology, 30,* 1193–1202.

Alexander, M. P., & Schmidt, M. A. (1980). The aphasia syndromes of stroke in the left anterior cerebral artery territory. *Archives of Neurology, 37,* 97–100.

Anderson, E. T., & Ulatowska, H. K. (1977). Letters from an aphasic individual: A linguistic investigation. In R. H. Brookshire (Ed.), *Proceedings of the Conference on Clinical Aphasiology* (pp. 226–233). Minneapolis: BRK Publishers.

Anderson, P. P., Bourestom, N., & Greenberg, F. R. (1970). *Rehabilitation predictors in completed stroke: Final report.* Minneapolis: American Rehabilitation Foundation.

Apel, K., Newhoff, M., & Browning-Hall, J. (1982). *Contingent queries in Broca's aphasia.* Paper presented at the Annual Convention of the American Speech-Language-Hearing Association, Toronto, Canada.

Appell, J., Kertesz, A., & Fisman, M. (1982). A study of language functioning in Alzheimer patients. *Brain and Language, 17,* 73–81.

Archibald, Y. M., & Wepman, J. M. (1968). Language disturbance and nonverbal cognitive performance in eight patients following injury to the right hemisphere. *Brain, 91,* 117–127.

Armstrong, E. (1987). Cohesive harmony in aphasic discourse and its significance to listener perception of coherence. In R. H. Brookshire (Ed.), *Proceedings of the Conference on Clinical Aphasiology* (pp. 210–215). Minneapolis: BRK Publishers.

Arvedson, J., McNeil, M., & West, T. (1985). Prediction of revised Token Test overall, subtest, and linguistic unit scores by two shortened versions. In R. H. Brookshire (Ed.), *Proceedings of the Conference on Clinical Aphasiology* (pp. 57–63). Minneapolis: BRK Publishers.

ASHA Committee on Language, Subcommittee on Cognition and Language. (1987). The role of speech-language pathologists in the habilitation and rehabilitation of cognitively-impaired individuals. *Asha, 29,* 53–55.

Assal, G., Buttet, J., & Jolivet, R. (1981). Dissociations in aphasia: A case report. *Brain and Language, 13,* 223–240.

Aten, J. (1972). *Auditory memory and auditory sequencing.* Paper presented to the Symposium on Auditory Processing, Las Vegas, NV.

Aten, J., & Lyon, J. (1978). Measures of PICA

subtest variance: A preliminary assessment of their value as predictors of language recovery in aphasic patients. In R. H. Brookshire (Ed.), *Proceedings of the Conference on Clinical Aphasiology* (pp. 106–116). Minneapolis: BRK Publishers.

Baer, W. P. (1976). *The aphasic patient: A program for auditory comprehension and language training.* Springfield, IL: Charles C Thomas.

Baker, H. L., Berquist, T., Kispert, D., Reese, D., Houser, W., Earnest, F., Forbes, G., & May, G. (1985). Magnetic resonance imaging in a routine clinical setting. *Mayo Clinic Proceedings, 60,* 75–90.

Barlow, D. H., & Hayes, S. C. (1979). Alternating treatments design: One strategy for comparing the effects of two treatments in a single subject. *Journal of Applied Behavior Analysis, 12,* 199–210.

Barlow, D. H., Hayes, S. C., & Nelson, R. O. (1984). *The scientist practitioner.* New York: Pergamon Press.

Barton, M., Maruszewski, M., & Urrea, D. (1969). Variation of stimulus context and its effect on word-finding ability in aphasics. *Cortex, 5,* 351–365.

Basso, A. (1978). Aphasia rehabilitation. In Y. Lebrun & R. Hoops (Eds.), *The management of aphasia* (pp. 9–21). Amsterdam: Swets & Zeitlinger B.V.

Basso, A., Capitani, E., & Moraschini, S. (1982). Sex differences in recovery from aphasia. *Cortex, 18,* 469–475.

Basso, A., Capitani, E., & Vignolo, L. (1979). Influence of rehabilitation of language skills in aphasic patients: A controlled study. *Archives of Neurology, 36,* 190–196.

Basso, A., Capitani, E., & Zanobio, E. (1982). Pattern of recovery of oral and written expression and comprehension in aphasic patients. *Behavioral Brain Research, 6,* 115–128.

Bayles, K. A. (1984). Language and dementia. In A. L. Holland (Ed.), *Language disorders in adults: Recent advances* (pp. 209–244). Austin, TX: PRO-ED.

Bayles, K. A., & Kaszniak, A. W. (1987). *Communication and cognition in normal aging and dementia.* Austin, TX: PRO-ED.

Bayles, K. A., Tomoeda, C. K., & Caffrey, J. T. (1982). Language and dementia producing diseases. *Communicative Disorders: A Journal for Continuing Education, 7,* 131–146.

Benedikt, M. (1865). Uber aphasie, agraphie and verwandte pathologische Zustande. *Wiener Mediznesche Presse, 6,* 897–1265.

Bennett, C., & Alter, K. (1985). *Referential semantic analysis.* San Diego: College-Hill Press.

Benson, D. F. (1967). Fluency in aphasia: Correlation with radioactive scan localization. *Cortex, 3,* 373–394.

Benson, D. F. (1973). Psychiatric aspects of aphasia. *British Journal of Psychiatry, 123,* 555–556.

Benson, D. F. (1975). Disorders of verbal expression. In D. F. Benson & D. Blumer (Eds.), *Psychiatric aspects of neurologic disease* (pp. 121–137). New York: Grune & Stratton.

Benson, D. F. (1977). The third alexia. *Archives of Neurology, 34,* 327–331.

Benson, D. F. (1979a). *Aphasia, alexia, and agraphia.* New York: Churchill Livingstone.

Benson, D. F. (1979b). Aphasia rehabilitation. *Archives of Neurology, 36,* 187–189.

Benson, D. F. (1979c). Neurological correlates of anomia. In H. Whitaker & H. Whitaker (Eds.), *Studies in neurolinguistics* (Vol. 4, pp. 93–328). New York: Academic Press.

Benson, D. F., & Geschwind, N. (1969). The alexias. In P. J. Vinken & G. W. Bruyn (Eds.), *Handbook of clinical neurology* (Vol. 4, pp. 112–140). Amsterdam: North Holland Publishing Company.

Benson, D. F., & Geschwind, N. (1976). Aphasia and related disturbances. In A. B. Baker (Ed.), *Clinical neurology* (Vol. 1, pp. 1–28). New York: Harper & Row.

Benton, A. L. (1967). Problems of test construction in the field of aphasia. *Cortex, 3,* 32–53.

Benton, A. L. (1973). *The measurement of aphasic disorders.* Aspectos patologicos del lenguaje. Actas de las Primeras Jornadas Internacionales del lenguaje, Lima, Peru.

Benton, A., Smith, K., & Lang, M. (1972). Stimulus characteristics and object naming in aphasic patients. *Journal of Communication Disorders, 5,* 19–24.

Berko-Gleason, J. B., Goodglass, H., Obler, L., Green, E., Hyde, M., & Weintraub, S. (1980). Narrative strategies of aphasic and normal speaking subjects. *Journal of Speech and Hearing Research, 23,* 370–382.

Berman, M., & Peele, L. M. (1967). Self-generated cues: A method for aiding aphasic and apractic patients. *Journal of Speech and Hearing Disorders, 32,* 372–376.

Berndt, R. S., & Caramazza, A. (1980). A redefinition of the syndrome of Broca's aphasia: Implications for a neuropsychological model of language. *Applied Psycholinguistics, 1,* 225–278.

Berndt, R. S., Caramazza, A., & Zurif, E. (1983).

Language functions: Syntax and semantics. In S. J. Segalowitz (Ed.), *Language function and brain organization* (pp. 5–28). New York: Academic Press.

Bernstein-Ellis, E. G., Wertz, R. T., Dronkers, N. F., & Milton, S. B. (1985). PICA performance by traumatically brain injured and left hemisphere CVA patients. In R. H. Brookshire (Ed.), *Proceedings of the Conference on Clinical Aphasiology* (pp. 97–106). Minneapolis: BRK Publishers.

Beyn, E. S., & Shokhor-Trotskaya, M. L. (1966). The preventive method of speech rehabilitation in aphasia. *Cortex, 2,* 96–108.

Bicker, A. L., Schuell, H., & Jenkins, J. J. (1964). Effect of word frequency and word length on aphasic spelling errors. *Journal of Speech and Hearing Research, 7,* 183–192.

Binder, G. (1984). *Aphasia: A societal and clinical appraisal of pragmatic and linguistic behaviors.* Unpublished master's thesis, University of California, Santa Barbara.

Bisiach, E. (1966). Perceptual factors in the pathogenesis of anomia. *Cortex, 2,* 690–695.

Bisiach, E. (1976). Characteristics of visual stimuli and naming performance in aphasic adults: Comments on the paper by Corlew and Nation. *Cortex, 12,* 74–75.

Blau, A. F. (1983). Vocabulary selection in augmentative communication: Where do we begin? In H. Winitz (Ed.), *Treating language disorders: For clinicians by clinicians* (pp. 205–233). Austin, TX: PRO-ED.

Blumstein, S. E., Milberg, W., & Shrier, R. (1982). Semantic processing in aphasia: Evidence from an auditory lexical decision task. *Brain and Language, 17,* 301–315.

Boehme, G. (1984). Aphasia: Causes, age distribution and hearing function. *Laryngology, Rhinology, Otology, 63,* 79–81.

Bogdanoff, M. G., & Katz, R. C. (1983). Modification of the CLOZE procedure for measuring reading levels in aphasic adults. In R. H. Brookshire (Ed.), *Proceedings of the Conference on Clinical Aphasiology* (pp. 28–34). Minneapolis: BRK Publishers.

Boller, F. (1973). Destruction of Wernicke's area without language disturbance: A fresh look at crossed aphasia. *Neuropsychologia, 11,* 243–246.

Boller, F. (1979). Introduction: Testing for comprehension: A short history of comprehension tests up to the Token Test. In F. Boller & M. Dennis (Eds.), *Auditory comprehension: Clinical and experimental studies with the Token Test* (pp. 3–13). New York: Academic Press.

Boller, F., & Dennis, M. (Eds.). (1979). *Auditory comprehension: Clinical and experimental studies with the Token Test.* New York: Academic Press.

Boller, F., Kim, Y., & Mack, J. L. (1977). Auditory comprehension in aphasia. In H. Whitaker & H. A. Whitaker (Eds.), *Studies in neurolinguistics* (Vol. 3, pp. 1–63). New York: Academic Press.

Boller, F., & Vignolo, L. (1966). Latent sensory aphasia in hemisphere-damaged patients: An experimental study with the Token Test. *Brain, 89,* 815–830.

Bond, S., & Ulatowska, H. (1985). Methodology for assessing auditory comprehension of discourse in aphasia. In R. H. Brookshire (Ed.), *Proceedings of the Conference on Clinical Aphasiology* (pp. 272–279). Minneapolis: BRK Publishers.

Boone, D. R., & Friedman, H. M. (1976). Writing in aphasia rehabilitation: Cursive vs manuscript. *Journal of Speech and Hearing Disorders, 41,* 523–529.

Borkowski, J. G., Benton, A. L., & Spreen, D. (1967). Word fluency and brain damage. *Neuropsychologia, 5,* 135–140.

Bowman, C., Hodson, B., & Simpson, R. (1980). Oral apraxia and aphasic misarticulation. In R. H. Brookshire (Ed.), *Proceedings of the Conference on Clinical Aphasiology* (pp. 89–95). Minneapolis: BRK Publishers.

Brain, R. (1961). *Speech disorders: Aphasia, apraxia, and agnosia.* Washington, DC: Butterworth.

Bramwell, B. (1899, June 3). On crossed aphasia. *Lancet,* 803–805.

Branch, C., Milner, B., & Rasmussen, T. (1964). Intercarotid sodium amytal for the lateralization of cerebral dominance. *Journal of Neurosurgery, 21,* 399–405.

Broca, P. (1861). Remarques sur le siege de la faculte du langage articule suivies d'une observation d'aphemie (perte de la parole). *Bull, Soc. D'Anat., (2nd series),* 330–337.

Broca, P. (1865). Sur le siege de la faculte du langage articule. *Bulletin de la Societe de'Anthropoligie, 6,* 337–393.

Brookshire, R. H. (1971). Effects of trial time and inter-trial interval on naming by aphasic subjects. *Journal of Communication Disorders, 3,* 289–301.

Brookshire, R. H. (1972). *Differences in auditory processing deficits among aphasic patients.*

Paper presented at the Annual Convention of American Speech-Language-Hearing Association, San Francisco, CA.

Brookshire, R. H. (1978a). *An introduction to aphasia* (2nd ed.). Minneapolis: BRK Publishers.

Brookshire, R. H. (1978b). Auditory comprehension and aphasia. In D. F. Johns (Ed.), *Clinical management of neurogenic communicative disorders* (pp. 103–128). Boston: Little, Brown.

Brookshire, R. H. (1985). Clinical research in aphasiology. In R. H. Brookshire (Ed.), *Proceedings of the Conference on Clinical Aphasiology* (pp. 9–14). Minneapolis: BRK Publishers.

Brookshire, R. H., & Nicholas, L. E. (1982). Comprehension of directly and indirectly pictured verbs by aphasic and non-aphasic listeners. In R. H. Brookshire (Ed.), *Proceedings of the Conference on Clinical Aphasiology* (pp. 200–206). Minneapolis: BRK Publishers.

Brown, D. A. (1982). *Reading diagnosis and remediation.* Englewood Cliffs, NJ: Prentice Hall.

Brown, J. W. (1972). *Aphasia, apraxia, and agnosia: Clinical and theoretical aspects.* Springfield, IL: Charles C Thomas.

Brown, J. W. (1977). *Mind, brain and consciousness: The neuropsychology of cognition.* New York: Academic Press.

Brown, J. W., Leader, B. J., & Blum, C. S. (1983). Hemiplegic writing in severe aphasia. *Brain and Language, 19,* 204–215.

Brown, J. W., & Perecman, E. (1985). Neurological basis of language processing. In J. K. Darby (Ed.), *Speech and language evaluation in neurology: Adult disorders* (pp. 45–82). Orlando: Grune & Stratton.

Brown, L., Sherbenou, R., & Johnsen S., (1984). *Test of nonverbal intelligence–TONI.* Austin, TX: PRO-ED.

Brownell, G. L., Budinger, T. F., Lauterbur, P. C., & McGeer, P. L. (1982). Positron tomography and nuclear magnetic resonance imaging. *Science, 215,* 619–626.

Brubaker, S. (1982). *Sourcebook for aphasia.* Detroit: Wayne State University Press.

Buck, M. (1968). *Dysphasia: Professional guidance for family and patient.* Englewood Cliffs, NJ: Prentice Hall.

Buckingham, H. W. (1979). Linguistic aspects of lexical retrieval disturbances in the posterior fluent aphasias. In H. Whitaker & H. A. Whitaker (Eds.), *Studies in neurolinguistics* (Vol. 4, pp. 269–291). New York: Academic Press.

Burger, L. H., & Wertz, R. T. (1984). The effect of a token training program on auditory comprehension in a case of Wernicke's aphasia. In R. H. Brookshire (Ed.), *Proceedings of the Conference on Clinical Aphasiology* (pp. 173–180). Minneapolis: BRK Publishers.

Burger, L. H., Wertz, R. T., & Woods, D. (1983). A response to treatment in a case of cortical deafness. In R. H. Brookshire (Ed.), *Proceedings of the Conference on Clinical Aphasiology* (pp. 127–136). Minneapolis: BRK Publishers.

Butfield, E., & Zangwill, O. (1946). Re-education in aphasia: A review of 70 cases. *Journal of Neurology, Neurosurgery, and Psychiatry, 9,* 75–79.

Butterworth, B., Howard, D., & McLoughlin, P. (1984). The semantic deficit in aphasia: The relationship between semantic errors in auditory comprehension and picture naming. *Neuropsychologia, 22,* 409–426.

Candelise, L., Landi, G., Orazio, E. N., & Boccardi, E. (1985). Prognostic significance of hyperglycemia in acute stroke. *Archives of Neurology, 42,* 661–663.

Canter, G. (1973). Some thoughts on the problem of word-finding. *Hearing and Speech News, 41,* 6–7.

Caramazza, A., & Berndt, R. S. (1978). Semantic and syntactic processes in aphasia. A review of the literature. *Psychological Bulletin, 85,* 898–918.

Carmon, A., Gordon, H. W., Bental, E., & Harness, B. Z. (1977). Retraining in literal alexia: Substitution of a right hemisphere perceptual strategy for impaired left hemispheric processing. *Bulletin of the Los Angeles Neurological Society, 42,* 41–50.

Carpenter, M. B. (1978). *Core text of neuroanatomy* (2nd ed.). Baltimore: Williams & Wilkins.

Chapey, R. (1981). The assessment of language disorders in adults. In R. Chapey (Ed.), *Language intervention strategies in adult aphasia* (pp. 31–84). Baltimore: Williams & Wilkins.

Chapman, J. (1966). The early symptoms of schizophrenia. *British Journal of Psychiatry, 112,* 225–251.

Chedru, F., & Geschwind, N. (1972). Disorders of higher cortical functioning in acute confusional states. *Cortex, 8,* 395–411.

Chesher, E. C. (1937). Aphasia: I. Technique of clinical examination. *Bulletin of the Neurological Institute of New York, 6,* 134–144.

Chusid, J. G. (1979). *Correlative neuroanatomy and functional neurology* (17th ed.). Los Altos, CA: Lange Medical Publishing.

Cicone, M., Wapner, W., Foldi, N., Zurif, E., & Gardner, H. (1979). The relation between gesture and language in aphasic communication. *Brain and Language, 8,* 324–349.

Clark, C., Crockett, D. J., & Klonoff, H. (1979). Empirically derived groups in the assessment of recovery from aphasia. *Brain and Language, 7,* 240–251.

Clark, H. H., & Clark, E. V. (1977). *Psychology and language: An introduction to psycholinguistics.* New York: Harcourt Brace Jovanovich.

Coelho, C. A., & Duffy, R. J. (1985). Communicative use of signs in aphasia: Is acquisition enough? In R. H. Brookshire (Ed.), *Proceedings of the Conference on Clinical Aphasiology* (pp. 222–228). Minneapolis: BRK Publishers.

Cohen, J. (1969). *Statistical power analysis for the behavioral sciences.* New York: Academic Press.

Colby, K. M., Christinaz, D., Parkison, R. C., Graham, S., & Karpf, C. (1981). A word-finding computer program with a dynamic lexical-semantic memory for patients with anomia using an intelligent speech prosthesis. *Brain and Language, 14,* 272–281.

Collins, M. (1983). Treatment of global aphasia. In W. H. Perkins (Ed.), *Current therapy of communication disorders: Language handicaps in adults* (pp. 25–33). New York: Thieme-Stratton.

Collins, M. (1986). *Diagnosis and treatment of global aphasia.* San Diego: College-Hill Press.

Collins, M., McNeil, M., Lentz, S., Shubitowski, Y., & Rosenbek, J. (1984). Word fluency and aphasia: Some linguistic and not-so-linguistic considerations. In R. H. Brookshire (Ed.), *Proceedings of the Conference on Clinical Aphasiology* (pp. 78–84). Minneapolis: BRK Publishers.

Coltheart, M. (1980). A right-hemisphere hypothesis. In M. Coltheart, K. Patterson, & J. Marshall (Eds.), *Deep dyslexia* (pp. 326–380). London: Routledge & Kegan Paul.

Coltheart, M. (1983). Aphasia therapy research: A single case study approach. In C. Code & D. J. Muller (Eds.), *Aphasia therapy* (pp. 193–202). London: Edward Arnold.

Connell, P. J., & Thompson, C. K. (1986). Flexibility of single-subject experimental designs. Part III: Using flexibility to design or modify experiments. *Journal of Speech and Hearing Disorders, 51,* 214–225.

Corlew, M., & Nation, J. (1975). Characteristics of visual stimuli and naming performance in aphasic adults. *Cortex, 11,* 186–191.

Cotman, C. W., & McGaugh, J. L. (1980). *Behavioral neuroscience.* New York: Academic Press.

Cousins, N. (1982). The physician as communicator. *Journal of the American Medical Association, 248,* 587–589.

Cronbach, L. J. (1970). *Essentials of psychological testing* (3rd ed.). New York: Harper & Row.

Crystal, D. (1982). *Profiling linguistic disability.* New York: Elsevier.

Crystal, D., Fletcher, P., & Garman, M. (1976). *The grammatical analysis of language disability.* London: Edward Arnold.

Culton, G. L. (1969). Spontaneous recovery from aphasia. *Journal of Speech and Hearing Research, 12,* 825–832.

Czvik, P. S. (1976). The application of an auditory approach using nonvariable materials in the treatment of aphasia: Two case studies. In R. H. Brookshire (Ed.), *Proceedings of the Conference on Clinical Aphasiology* (pp. 291–302). Minneapolis: BRK Publishers.

Dabul, B. (1979). *Apraxia battery for adults.* Austin, TX: PRO-ED.

Damasio, A. (1981). The nature of aphasia: Signs and syndromes. In M. T. Sarno (Ed.), *Acquired aphasia* (pp. 51–65). New York: Academic Press.

Damasio, A., Damasio, H., Rizzo, M., Varney, N., & Gersh, F. (1982). Aphasia with nonhemorrhagic lesions in the basal ganglia and internal capsule. *Archives of Neurology, 39,* 15–20.

Damasio, H. (1981). Cerebral localization of the aphasias. In M. T. Sarno (Ed.), *Acquired aphasia* (pp. 27–50). New York: Academic Press.

Darby, J. K. (Ed.). (1985). *Speech and language evaluation in Neurology: Adult disorders.* Orlando: Grune & Stratton.

Darley, F. L. (1969). *Aphasia: Input and output disturbances in speech and language processing.* Paper presented to the American Speech and Hearing Association, Chicago, IL.

Darley, F. L. (1972). The efficacy of language rehabilitation in aphasia. *Journal of Speech and Hearing Disorders, 37,* 3–21.

Darley, F. L. (1975). Treatment of acquired aphasia. In W. J. Friedlander (Ed.), *Advances in neurology: Vol. 7. Current reviews of higher nervous sytem dysfunction* (pp. 111–145). New York: Raven Press.

Darley, F. L. (1979). Treat or neglect? *Asha, 21,* 628–631.

Darley, F. L. (1982). *Aphasia.* Philadelphia: W. B. Saunders.

Darley, F. L., Aronson, A. E., & Brown, J. R. (1975). *Motor speech disorders.* Philadelphia: W. B. Saunders.

David, R. M. (1983). Researching into the efficacy of aphasia therapy. In C. Code & D. J. Muller (Eds.), *Aphasia therapy* (pp. 15–24). London: Edward Arnold.

David, R. M., Enderby, P., & Bainton, D. (1982). Treatment of acquired aphasia: Speech therapists and volunteers compared. *Journal of Neurology, Neurosurgery, and Psychiatry, 45,* 957–961.

Davis, G. A. (1978). The clinical application of withdrawal, single-case research designs. In R. H. Brookshire (Ed.), *Proceedings of the Conference on Clinical Aphasiology* (pp. 11–19). Minneapolis: BRK Publishers.

Davis, G. A. (1983). *A survey of adult aphasia.* Englewood Cliffs, NJ: Prentice Hall.

Davis, G. A., & Wilcox, J. (1981). Incorporating parameters of natural conversation in aphasia. In R. Chapey (Ed.), *Language intervention strategies in adult aphasia* (pp. 169–194). Baltimore: Williams & Wilkins.

Davis, G. A., & Wilcox, M. J. (1985). *Adult aphasia rehabilitation: Applied pragmatics.* Austin, TX: PRO-ED.

Deal, J. L., & Deal, L. A. (1978). Efficacy of aphasia rehabilitation: Preliminary results. In R. H. Brookshire (Ed.), *Proceedings of the Conference on Clinical Aphasiology* (pp. 66–77). Minneapolis: BRK Publishers.

Deal, J. L., Deal, L. A., Wertz, R. T., Kitselman, K., & Dwyer, C. (1979). Right hemisphere PICA percentiles: Some speculations about aphasia. In R. H. Brookshire (Ed.), *Proceedings of the Conference on Clinical Aphasiology* (pp. 30–37). Minneapolis: BRK Publishers.

Deal, J. L., Wertz, R. T., & Spring, C. (1981). Differentiating aphasia and the language of generalized intellectual impairment. In R. H. Brookshire (Ed.), *Proceedings of the Conference on Clinical Aphasiology* (pp. 166–173). Minneapolis: BRK Publishers.

Dejerine, J. (1891). Contribution a l'etude des troubles de l'ecriture chez les aphasiques. (A propos d'une observation d'aphasie motrice avec paragraphie pour l'ecriture spontanee et sous dictec.). *Comptes Rendus des seances de la Societe de Biologie et de ses Filales, 9,* 97–113.

Dejerine, J. (1892). Des differentes varietes de cecite verbale. *Memories de la Societe Biologique, 4,* 1–30.

Deloche, G., & Seron, X. (1981). Sentence understanding and knowledge of the world: Evidence from a sentence-picture matching task performed by aphasic patients. *Brain and Language, 14,* 57–69.

DeRenzi, E., & Faglioni, P. (1978). Normative data and screening power of a shortened version of the Token Test. *Cortex, 14,* 41–49.

DeRenzi, E., & Ferrari, C. (1978). The Reporter's Test: A sensitive test to detect expressive disturbances in aphasics. *Cortex, 14,* 279–293.

DeRenzi, E., Motti, F., & Nichelli, P. (1980). Imitating gestures. *Archives of Neurology, 37,* 6–10.

DeRenzi, E., & Vignolo, L. A. (1962). The Token Test: A sensitive test to detect receptive disturbances in aphasics. *Brain, 85,* 665–678.

DeWitt, L. D., Grek, A. J., Buonanno, F. S., Levine, D. N., & Kistler, J. P. (1985). MRI and the study of aphasia. *Neurology, 35,* 861–865.

DiSimoni, F. G., Darley, F. L., & Aronson, A. E. (1977). Patterns of dysfunction in schizophrenic patients on an aphasia test battery. *Journal of Speech and Hearing Disorders, 42,* 498–513.

DiSimoni, F. G., Keith, R. L., & Darley, F. L. (1980). Prediction of PICA overall score by short versions of the test. *Journal of Speech and Hearing Research, 23,* 511–516.

DiSimoni, F. G., Keith, R. L., Holt, D. L., & Darley, F. L. (1975). Practicality of shortening the Porch Index of Communicative Ability. *Journal of Speech and Hearing Research, 18,* 491–497.

Doyle, P., & Holland, A. (1982). Clinical management of a patient with pure word deafness. In R. H. Brookshire (Ed.), *Proceedings of the Conference on Clinical Aphasiology* (pp. 138–146). Minneapolis: BRK Publishers.

Dronkers, N. F. (1987). Crossed aphasia. In R. H. Brookshire (Ed.), *Proceedings of the*

Conference on Clinical Aphasiology (pp. 339–348). Minneapolis: BRK Publishers.

Duffy, J. R. (1979). Boston diagnostic aphasia examination (BDAE). In F. L. Darley (Ed.), *Evaluation of appraisal techniques in speech and language pathology* (pp. 198–202). Reading, MA: Addison-Wesley.

Duffy, J. R. (1981). Schuell's stimulation approach to rehabilitation. In R. Chapey (Ed.), *Language intervention strategies in adult aphasia*. Baltimore: Williams & Wilkins.

Duffy, J. R. (1984). Nuclear magnetic resonance (NMR): Background and potential impact on the practice of speech and language pathology. In R. H. Brookshire (Ed.), *Proceedings of the Conference on Clinical Aphasiology* (pp. 7–13). Minneapolis: BRK Publishers.

Duffy, J. R. (1987). Slowly progressive aphasia. In R. H. Brookshire (Ed.), *Proceedings of the Conference on Clinical Aphasiology* (pp. 349–356). Minneapolis: BRK Publishers.

Duffy, J. R., & Keith, R. (1980). Performance of non brain-injured adults on the PICA: Descriptive data and comparison to patients with aphasia. *Aphasia Apraxia Agnosia, 2,* 1–30.

Duffy, R. J., & Duffy, J. R. (1981). Three studies of deficits in pantomimic expression and pantomime recognition in aphasia. *Journal of Speech and Hearing Research, 46,* 70–84.

Duffy, R., & Duffy, J. (1984). *The New England pantomime tests.* Austin, TX: PRO-ED.

Dunn-Rankin, P. (1977). The visual characteristics of words. *Scientific-American, 238,* 122–130.

Editorial. (1977). Progress in aphasia. *Lancet, 2,* 24.

Edwards, S., Ellams, J., & Thompson, J. (1976). Language and intelligence in dysphasia: Are they related? *British Journal of Disorders of Communication, 11,* 83–94.

Eggert, G. (1977). *Wernicke's works on aphasia.* The Hague: Mouton Publishers.

Eisenson, J. (1946). *Examining for aphasia.* New York: The Psychological Corporation.

Eisenson, J. (1949). Prognostic factors relating to language rehabilitation in aphasic patients. *Journal of Speech and Hearing Disorders, 14,* 262–264.

Eisenson, J. (1954). *Examining for aphasia, revised.* New York: The Psychological Corporation.

Eisenson, J. (1964). Aphasia: A point of view as to the nature of the disorder and factors that determine prognosis for recovery. *International Journal of Neurology, 4,* 287–295.

Eisenson, J. (1984). *Adult aphasia,* (2nd ed.). Englewood Cliffs, NJ: Prentice-Hall.

Ekman, P. & Friesen, W. V. (1972). Hand movements. *Journal of Communication, 22,* 353–374.

Emerick, L. (1971). *Appraisal of language disturbance.* Marquette, MI: Northern Michigan University Press.

Enderby, P. (1983). *Frenchay dysarthria assessment.* San Diego: College-Hill Press.

Exner, S. (1881). *Lokalisation des Funktion der Grosshirnrinde des Menschen.* Wien: Braunmuller.

Faber, M. M., & Aten, J. L. (1979). Verbal performance in aphasic patients in response to intact and altered pictorial stimuli. In R. H. Brookshire (Ed.), *Proceedings of the Conference on Clinical Aphasiology* (pp. 177–186). Minneapolis: BRK Publishers.

Farber, R., & Reichstein, M. B. (1981). Language dysfunction in schizophrenia. *British Journal of Psychiatry, 139,* 519–522.

Fedio, P., & Van Buren, J. M. (1975). Memory deficits during electrical stimulation in the left and right thalamus and parietal subcortex. *Brain and Language, 2,* 78–100.

Fisher, C. M. (1959). The pathological and clinical aspects of thalamic hemorrhage. *Transactions of the American Neurological Association, 84,* 56–59.

Fitch-West, J., & Sands, E. S. (1987). *The bedside evaluation screening test (BEST).* Austin, TX: PRO-ED.

Fleiss, J. L. (1981). *Statistical methods for rates and proportions.* New York: John Wiley & Sons.

Florance, C. L., & Deal, J. L. (1977). A treatment protocol for nonverbal stroke patients. In R. H. Brookshire (Ed.), *Proceedings of the Conference on Clinical Aphasiology* (pp. 59–67). Minneapolis: BRK Publishers.

Flowers, C. R., & Danforth, L. C. (1979). A stepwise auditory comprehension improvement program administered to aphasic patients by family members. In R. H. Brookshire (Ed.), *Proceedings of the Conference on Clinical Aphasiology* (pp. 196–202). Minneapolis: BRK Publishers.

Fodor, J. A. (1983). *The modularity of mind.* Cambridge, MA: The MIT Press.

Frazier, C. H., & Ingham, S. D. (1920). A review of the effects of gunshot wounds of the head: Based on the observation of two hundred cases at U. S. General Hospital No. 11, Cape May, N. J. *Archives of Neurology, 3,* 17–40.

Fromm, D., Holland, A. L., Swindell, C. S., & Reinmuth, O. M. (1985). Various consequences of subcortical stroke. Prospective study of 16 consecutive cases. *Archives of Neurology, 42*, 943–950.

Gainotti, G. (1976). The relationship between semantic impairment in comprehension and naming in aphasic patients. *British Journal Disorders of Communication, 11*, 57–61.

Gainotti, G., Caltagirone, C., & Ibba, A. (1975). Semantic and phonemic aspects of auditory comprehension in aphasia. *Linguistics, 154*, 15–29.

Gainotti, G., Caltagirone, C., & Miceli, G. (1979). Semantic disorders of auditory language comprehension in right brain-damaged patients. *Journal of Psycholinguistic Research, 8*, 13–20.

Gallaher, A. J., & Canter, G. J. (1982). Reading and listening comprehension in Broca's aphasia: Lexical versus syntactical errors. *Brain and Language, 17*, 183–192.

Gardiner, G., & Brookshire, R. H. (1972). Effects of unisensory and multisensory presentation of stimuli upon naming by aphasic subjects. *Language and Speech, 15*, 342–357.

Gardner, H. (1973). The contribution of operativity to naming capacity in aphasic patients. *Neuropsychologia, 11*, 213–220.

Gardner, H. (1974). The naming of objects and symbols by children and aphasic patients. *Journal of Psycholinguistic Research, 3*, 133–149.

Gardner, H. (1985). *The mind's new science: A history of the cognitive revolution.* New York: Basic Books, Inc.

Gardner, H., Albert, M. L., & Weintraub, S. (1975). Comprehending a word: The influence of speed and redundancy on auditory comprehension in aphasia. *Cortex, 11*, 155–162.

Gardner, H., & Winner, E. (1978). A study of repetition in aphasic patients. *Brain and Language, 6*, 168–178.

Gardner, H., & Winner, E. (1981). Artistry and aphasia. In M. T. Sarno (Ed.), *Acquired aphasia* (pp. 361–384). New York: Academic Press.

Gardner, H., Zurif, E., Berry, T., & Baker, E. (1976). Visual communication in aphasia. *Neuropsychology, 14*, 275–292.

Gardner, W. H. (1958). *Left handed writing instructional manual.* Danville, IL: Interstate.

Gates-MacGinitie Reading Tests. (1965). New York: Teachers College Press.

Gazzaniga, M. S., & LeDoux, J. E. (1978). *The integrated mind.* New York: Plenum Press.

Geschwind, N. (1965). Disconnection syndromes in animals and man. *Brain, 88*, 237–294, 585–644.

Geschwind, N. (1967). The varieties of naming errors. *Cortex, 3*, 97–112.

Geschwind, N. (1970). The organization of language and the brain. *Science, 170*, 940–944.

Geschwind, N. (1973). *Writing and its disorders.* Paper presented at the Second Pan-American Congress of Audition and Language, Lima, Peru.

Geschwind, N. (1974). The development of the brain and the evolution of language. In N. Geschwind (Ed.), *Selected papers on language and the brain.* Dordrecht, Holland: D. Reidel.

Geschwind, N., Quadfasel, F., & Segarra, J. (1968). Isolation of the speech area. *Neuropsychologia, 6*, 327–340.

Gheorghita, N. (1981). Vertical reading: A new method for reading disturbances in aphasics. *Journal of Clinical Neuropsychology, 3*, 161–164.

Glass, A. V., Gazzaniga, M., & Premack, D. (1973). Artificial language training in aphasia. *Neuropsychologia, 11*, 95–103.

Gleason, J. B., Goodglass, H., Green, E., Ackerman, N., & Hyde, M. R. (1975). The retrieval of syntax in Broca's aphasia. *Brain and Language, 2*, 451–471.

Gloning, K., Trappl, R., Heiss, W., & Quatember, R. (1976). Prognosis and speech therapy in aphasia. In Y. Lebrun & R. Hoops (Eds.), *Neurolinguistics 4: Recovery in aphasics* (pp. 57–64). Amsterdam: Swets & Zeitlinger B.V.

Glosser, G., Kaplan, E., & LoVerme, S. (1982). Longitudinal neuropsychological report of aphasia following left-subcortical hemorrhage. *Brain and Language, 15*, 95–116.

Godfrey, C. M., & Douglass, E. (1959). The recovery process in aphasia. *Canadian Medical Association Journal, 80*, 618–624.

Goldberg, S. (1979). *Clinical neuroanatomy made ridiculously simple.* Miami: MedMaster, Inc.

Goldstein, K. (1948). *Language and language disturbances.* New York: Grune & Stratton.

Golper, L. A., Fisher, B., Gordon, M. E., & Marshall, R. C. (1984). *Mortoric and linguistic features in aphasic writing.* Paper presented at the Annual Convention of the

American Speech-Language-Hearing Association, San Francisco, CA.

Goodglass, H. (1973). Studies on the grammar of aphasics. In H. Goodglass & S. Blumstein (Eds.), *Psycholinguistics and aphasia* (pp. 183–215). Baltimore: Johns Hopkins University Press.

Goodglass, H. (1981). The syndromes of aphasia: Similarities and differences in neurolinguistic features. *Topics in Language Disorders, 1,* 1–14.

Goodglass, H., & Baker, E. (1976). Semantic field naming and auditory comprehension in aphasia. *Brain and Language, 3,* 359–374.

Goodglass, H., & Blumstein, S. (1973). *Psycholinguistics and aphasia.* Baltimore: The Johns Hopkins University Press.

Goodglass, H., & Geschwind, N. (1976). Language disorders (aphasia). In E. C. Carterette & M. P. Friedman (Ed.), *Handbook of perception: Vol. 7. Speech and Language* (pp. 389–428). New York: Academic Press.

Goodglass, H., Gleason, J. B., Bernholtz, N. D., & Hyde, M. R. (1972). Some linguistic structures in the speech of a Broca's aphasic. *Cortex, 8,* 191–212.

Goodglass, H., Gleason, J. B., & Hyde, M. R. (1970). Some dimensions of auditory language comprehension in aphasia. *Journal of Speech and Hearing Research, 13,* 595–606.

Goodglass, H., & Hunter, M. (1970). A linguistic comparison of speech and writing in two types of aphasia. *Journal of Communication Disorders, 3,* 28–35.

Goodglass, H., Hyde, M. R., & Blumstein, S. (1969). Frequency, picturability, and availability of nouns in aphasia. *Cortex, 5,* 104–119.

Goodglass, H., & Kaplan, E. (1972). *The assessment of aphasia and related disorders.* Philadelphia: Lea & Febiger.

Goodglass, H., & Kaplan, E. (1983a). *Boston diagnostic examination for aphasia.* Philadelphia: Lea & Febiger.

Goodglass, H., & Kaplan, E. (1983b). *The assessment of aphasia and related disorders* (2nd ed.). Philadelphia: Lea & Febiger.

Goodglass, H., Kaplan, E., Weintraub, S., & Ackerman, N. (1976). The "tip-of-the-tongue" phenomenon in aphasia. *Cortex, 12,* 145–153.

Goodglass, H., Klein, B., Carey, P., & Jones, K. (1966). Specific semantic word categories in aphasia. *Cortex, 2,* 74–89.

Goodglass, H., Quadfasel, F. A., & Timberlake, W. H. (1964). Phrase length and the type and severity of aphasia. *Cortex, 1,* 133–153.

Goodglass, H., & Stuss, D. T. (1979). Naming to picture versus description in three aphasic subgroups. *Cortex, 15,* 199–211.

Graham, L. F., Holtzapple, P., & LaPointe, L. L. (1987). Does contextually related action facilitate auditory comprehension? Performance across three conditions by high and low comprehenders. In R. H. Brookshire (Ed.), *Proceedings of the Conference on Clinical Aphasiology* (pp. 180–187). Minneapolis: BRK Publishers.

Grant, D. A. (1954). *Test manual for the Wisconsin card-sorting task.* Madison, WI: University of Wisconsin, Department of Psychology.

Gravel, J., & LaPointe, L. L. (1982). Rate of speech of health care providers during interactions with aphasic and nonaphasic individuals. In R. H. Brookshire (Ed.), *Proceedings of the Conference on Clinical Aphasiology* (pp. 208–211). Minneapolis: BRK Publishers.

Gravel, J., & LaPointe, L. L. (1983). Length and redundancy in health care providers' speech during interactions with aphasic and nonaphasic individuals. In R. H. Brookshire (Ed.), *Proceedings of the Conference on Clinical Aphasiology* (pp. 211–217). Minneapolis: BRK Publishers.

Gravel, J., & LaPointe, L. L. (1984). *Rate, length, and redundancy of physicians' speech during in-hospital interactions with aphasic patients.* Paper presented at the Annual Convention of the American Speech-Language-Hearing Association, San Francisco, CA.

Green, E. (1970). On the contribution of studies in aphasia to psycholinguistics. *Cortex, 6,* 216–235.

Green, E., & Boller, F. (1974). Features of auditory comprehension in severely impaired aphasics. *Cortex, 10,* 133–145.

Grossman, M. (1981). A bird is a bird is a bird: Making reference within and without superordinate categories. *Brain and Language, 12,* 313–331.

Gunderson, C. H. (1982). *Quick reference to clinical neurology.* Philadelphia: J. B. Lippincott Company.

Gurland, G., Chwat, S., & Wollner, S. (1982). Establishing a communication profile in adult-aphasia. In R. H. Brookshire (Ed.), *Proceedings of the Conference on Clinical Aphasiology* (pp. 18–27). Minneapolis: BRK Publishers.

Hageman, C. F., McNeil, M. R., Rucci-Zimmer, S., & Cariski, D. M. (1982). The reliability of patterns of auditory processing deficits: Evidence from the Revised Token Test. In R. H. Brookshire (Ed.), *Proceedings of the Conference on Clinical Aphasiology* (pp. 230–234). Minneapolis: BRK Publishers.

Hagen, C. (1973). Communication abilities in hemiplegia: Effect of speech therapy. *Archives of Physical Medicine and Rehabilitation, 54,* 454–463.

Halstead, W. C., & Wepman, J. M. (1949). The Halstead-Wepman aphasia screening test. *Journal of Speech and Hearing Disorders, 14,* 9–15.

Hansen, A. M., & McNeil, M. R. (1986). Differences between writing with the dominant and nondominant hand by normal geriatric subjects on a spontaneous writing task: Twenty perceptual and computerized measures. In R. H. Brookshire (Ed.), *Proceedings of the Conference on Clinical Aphasiology* (pp. 116–122). Minneapolis: BRK Publishers.

Hansen, A. M., McNeil, M. R., & Vetter, D. K. (1987). More differences between writing with the dominant and nondominant hand by normal geriatric subjects: Eight perceptual and eight computerized measures. In R. H. Brookshire (Ed.), *Proceedings of the Conference on Clinical Aphasiology* (Vol. 17, pp. 152–157). Minneapolis: BRK Publishers.

Hanson, W., Metter, E. J., Riege, W. H., Kuhl, D. E., & Phelps, M. E. (1984). Positron emission tomography. In R. H. Brookshire (Ed.), *Proceedings of the Conference on Clinical Aphasiology* (pp. 14–23). Minneapolis: BRK Publishers.

Hart, S., Berndt, R. S., & Caramazza, A. (1985). Category-specific naming deficit following cerebral infarction. *Nature, 316,* 439–440.

Hartman, J. (1981). Measurement of early spontaneous recovery of aphasia with stroke. *Annals of Neurology, 9,* 89–91.

Hartman, J., & Landau, W. M. (1987). Comparison of formal language therapy with supportive counseling for aphasia due to acute vascular accident. *Archives of Neurology, 24,* 646–649.

Hartmann, D. P., & Hall, R. V. (1976). The changing criterion design. *Journal of Applied Behavior Analysis, 9,* 527–532.

Haskins, S. (1976). A treatment procedure for writing disorders. In R. H. Brookshire (Ed.), *Proceedings of the Conference on Clinical Aphasiology* (pp. 192–199). Minneapolis: BRK Publishers.

Hatfield, F. M. (1983). Aspects of acquired dysgraphia and implications for re-education. In C. Code & D. J. Muller (eds.), *Aphasia therapy* (pp. 157–169). London: Edward Arnold.

Hatfield, F. M. (1985). Visual and phonological factors in acquired dysgraphia. *Neuropsychologia, 23,* 13–29.

Hatfield, G. M., & Zangwill, O. L. (1974). Ideation in aphasia: The picture-story method. *Neuropsychologia, 12,* 389–393.

Hayward, R., Naeser, M., & Zatz, L. J. (1977). Cranial computed tomography in aphasia. *Radiology, 123,* 653–660.

Head, H. (1926). *Aphasia and kindred disorders of speech.* Cambridge, MA: Cambridge University Press.

Hecaen, H. (1972). *Introduction á la Neuropsychologie.* Paris: Larousse.

Hecaen, H., & Albert, M. L. (1978). *Human neuropsychology.* New York: John Wiley & Sons.

Hecaen, H., Angelergues, R., & Douzens, J. (1963). Les agraphies. *Neuropsychologia, 1,* 179–208.

Hecaen, H., Mazurs, G., & Ramier, A. (1971). Aphasi croiseé chez un sujet droiter bilingue. *Revue Neurologique, 124,* 319–323.

Heinemann, A. W., Roth, E. J., Cichowski, K., & Betts, H. B. (1987). Multivariate analysis of improvement and outcome following stroke rehabilitation. *Archives of Neurology, 44,* 1167–1172.

Helm, N. (1979). Management of palilalia with a pacing board. *Journal of Speech and Hearing Disorders, 44,* 350–353.

Helm, N. (1981). *Helm elicited language program for syntax stimulation.* Austin, TX: Exceptional Resources, Inc.

Helm-Estabrooks, N. (1981). Show me the... whatever: Some variables affecting auditory comprehension scores of aphasic patients. In R. H. Brookshire (Ed.), *Proceedings of the Conference on Clinical Aphasiology* (pp. 105–107). Minneapolis: BRK Publishers.

Helm-Estabrooks, N., & Barresi, B. (1980). Voluntary control of involuntary utterances: A treatment approach for severe aphasia. In R. H. Brookshire (Ed.), *Proceedings of the Conference on Clinical Aphasiology* (pp. 208–330). Minneapolis: BRK Publishers.

Helm-Estabrooks, N., Fitzpatrick, P. M., &

Barresi, B. (1981). Responses of an agrammatic patient to a syntax stimulation program for aphasia. *Journal of Speech and Hearing Disorders, 46,* 422–427.

Helm-Estabrooks, N., Fitzpatrick, P. M., & Barresi, B. (1982). Visual action therapy for global aphasia. *Journal of Speech and Hearing Disorders, 47,* 385–389.

Helm-Estabrooks, N., & Ramsberger, G. (1986). Treatment of agrammatism in long-term Broca's aphasia. *British Journal of Disorders of Communication, 21,* 39–45.

Helmich, J., & Wipplinger, M. (1975). Effects of stimulus presentation on the naming behavior of an aphasic adult: A clinical report. *Journal of Communication Disorders, 8,* 23–29.

Henri, B. P., & Canter, G. J. (1975). *A longitudinal investigation of patterns of language recovery in eight recent aphasics.* Paper presented at the Annual Convention of the American Speech-Language-Hearing Association, Washington, DC.

Hersen, M., & Barlow, D. H. (1976). *Single case experimental designs: Strategies for studying behavior change.* New York: Pergamon Press.

Hier, D. B., & Mohr, J. P. (1977). Incongruous oral and written naming. Evidence for a subdivision of the syndrome of Wernicke's aphasia. *Brain and Language, 4,* 115–126.

Hodson, B. (1981). *Assessment of phonological processes.* Danville: Interstate.

Holland, A. L. (1977). Some practical considerations in aphasia rehabilitation. In M. Sullivan & M. Kommers (Eds.), *Rationale for adult aphasia therapy.* Omaha: University of Nebraska Medical Center.

Holland, A. L. (1980a). *Communicative abilities in daily living.* Austin, TX: PRO-ED.

Holland, A. L. (1980b). The usefulness of treatment for aphasia: A serendipitous study. In R. H. Brookshire (Ed.), *Proceedings of the Conference on Clinical Aphasiology* (pp. 240–247). Minneapolis: BRK Publishers.

Holland, A. L. (1982). When is aphasia aphasia: The problem of closed head injury. In R. H. Brookshire (Ed.), *Proceedings of the Conference on Clinical Aphasiology* (pp. 345–349). Minneapolis: BRK Publishers.

Holland, A. L. (1983). Remarks on observing aphasic people. In R. H. Brookshire (Ed.), *Proceedings of the Conference on Clinical Aphasiology* (pp. 1–3). Minneapolis: BRK Publishers.

Holland, A. L., Greenhouse, J. B., Fromm, D., &

Swindell, C. S. (in press). Predictors of language restitution following stroke: A multivariate analysis. *Journal of Speech and Hearing Research.*

Holland, A. L., & Sondermon, J. C. (1974). Effects of a program based on the Token Test for teaching comprehension skills to aphasics. *Journal of Speech and Hearing Research, 17,* 589–598.

Holland, A. L., Swindell, C. S., & Forbes, M. M. (1985). The evolution of initial global aphasia: Implications for prognosis. In R. H. Brookshire (Ed.), *Proceedings of the Conference on Clinical Aphasiology* (pp. 169–175). Minneapolis: BRK Publishers.

Holtzapple, P. (1972). The influence of illiteracy on predicting recovery from aphasia. In R. H. Brookshire (Ed.), *Proceedings of the Conference on Clinical Aphasiology* (pp. 48–54). Minneapolis: BRK Publishers.

Horner, J. (1983). Treatment of Broca's aphasia. In W. H. Perkins (Ed.), *Current therapy of communication disorders: Language handicaps in adults* (pp. 3–13). New York: Thieme-Stratton.

Horner, J., & Chacko, R. (1984). Cerebral blood flow. In R. H. Brookshire (Ed.), *Proceedings of the Conference on Clinical Aphasiology* (pp. 24–33). Minneapolis: BRK Publishers.

Horner, J., & Fedor, K. H. (1983). Minor hemisphere mediation in aphasia treatment. In H. Winitz (Ed.), *Treating language disorders: For clinicians by clinicians* (pp. 181–204). Austin, TX: PRO-ED.

Howard, D. (1986). Beyond randomised controlled trials: The case for effective case studies of the effects of treatment in aphasia. *British Journal of Disorders of Communication, 21,* 89–102.

Howard, D., Patterson, K. E., Franklin, S., Orchard-Lisle, V. M., & Morton, J. (1985). Treatment of word retrieval deficits in aphasia: A comparison of two therapy methods. *Brain, 108,* 817–829.

Howes, D., & Geschwind, N. (1969). Quantitative studies of aphasic language. In D. M. Risch & E. A. Weinstein (Eds.), *Disorders of communication* (Vol. 17, pp. 2219–2243). New York: Haffner Publishing Co.

Huizinga, J. (1982). *Looking at American signs.* Skokie, IL: Voluntad Publishing Co.

Hynd, G. W., & Cohen, M. (1983). *Dyslexia: Neuropsychological theory, research, and clinical differentiation.* New York: Grune & Stratton.

Ingram, D. (1976). *Phonological disability in children.* New York: Elsevier.

Isgur, J. (1975). Establishing letter-sound associations by an object-imaging-projection method. *Journal of Learning Disorders, 8,* 349–353.

Jackson, J. H. (1866). On a case of loss of power of expression: Inability to talk, to write, and to read correctly after convulsive attacks. *British Medical Journal, 192,* 326–330.

Jaffe, J. (1981). The psychiatrists's approach to managing the aphasic patient. In R. T. Wertz (Ed.), *Aphasia: Interdisciplinary approach. Seminars in speech, language, and hearing* (pp. 249–258). New York: Thieme-Stratton.

Johns, D. F., & Darley, F. L. (1970). Phonemic variability in apraxia of speech. *Journal of Speech and Hearing Research, 13,* 556–583.

Kandel, E. R., & Schwartz, J. H. (Eds.). (1981). *Principles of neural science.* New York: Elsevier/North-Holland.

Kaplan, E., Goodglass, H., & Weintraub, S. (1983). *Boston naming test.* Philadelphia: Lea & Febiger.

Katz, R. C. (1983a). *Understanding questions.* Tucson: Communication Skill Builders.

Katz, R. C. (1983b). *Understanding stories.* Tucson: Communication Skill Builders.

Katz, R. C. (1986). *Aphasia treatment and microcomputers.* San Diego: College-Hill Press.

Katz, R. C. (1987). Efficacy of aphasia treatment using microcomputers. *Aphasiology, 1,* 141–149.

Katz, R. C., & LaPointe, L. L. (1983). *Understanding sentences: Absurdities.* Tucson: Communication Skill Builders.

Katz, R. C., & Nagy, V. T. (1984). An intelligent computer-based spelling task for chronic aphasic patients. In R. H. Brookshire (Ed.), *Proceedings of the Conference on Clinical aphasiology* (pp. 65–72). Minneapolis: BRK Publishers.

Katz, R. C., & Porch, B. E. (1983). *PICA pad.* Palo Alto, CA: Consulting Psychologists Press.

Katz, R. C., & Tong Nagy, V. (1982). A computerized treatment system for chronic aphasic patients. In R. H. Brookshire (Ed.), *Proceedings of the Conference on Clinical Aphasiology* (pp. 153–160). Minneapolis: BRK Publishers.

Katz, R., & Tong Nagy, V. (1983). Computerized approach for improving word recognition in chronic aphasic adults. In R. H. Brookshire (Ed.), *Proceedings of the Conference on*
Clinical Aphasiology (pp. 65–72). Minneapolis: BRK Publishers.

Katz, R. C., & Tong Nagy, V. (1985). A self-modifying computerized reading program for severely-impaired aphasic patients. In R. H. Brookshire (Ed.), *Proceedings of the Conference on Clinical Aphasiology* (pp. 184–188). Minneapolis: BRK Publishers.

Kean, M. L. (1977). The linguistic interpretation of aphasic syndromes. Agrammatism in Broca's aphasia, an example. *Cognition, 5,* 9–46.

Kean, M. L. (1985). *Agrammatism.* New York: Academic Press.

Kearns, K. P. (1980). The application of phonological process analysis to adult neuropathologies. In R. H. Brookshire (Ed.), *Proceedings of the Conference on Clinical Aphasiology* (pp. 187–195). Minneapolis: BRK Publishers.

Kearns, K. P. (1986). Flexibility of single-subject experimental designs. Part II: Design selection and arrangement of experimental phases. *Journal of Speech and Hearing Disorders, 51,* 204–213.

Kearns, K. P., & Hubbard, D. (1977). A comparison of auditory comprehension tasks in aphasia. In R. H. Brookshire (Ed.), *Proceedings of the Conference on Clinical Aphasiology* (pp. 32–45). Minneapolis: BRK Publishers.

Kearns, K. P., & Simmons, N. (1983). A practical procedure for the grammatical analysis of aphasic language impairments: The LARSP. In R. H. Brookshire (Ed.), *Proceedings of the Conference on Clinical Aphasiology* (pp. 4–14). Minneapolis: BRK Publishers.

Kearns, K. P., Simmons, N. N., & Sisterhen, C. (1982). Gestural sign (Amer-Ind) as a facilitator of verbalization in patients with aphasia. In R. H. Brookshire (Ed.), *Proceedings of the Conference on Clinical Aphasiology* (pp. 183–191). Minneapolis: BRK Publishers.

Keenan, J. S. (1966). A method for eliciting naming behavior from aphasic patients. *Journal of Speech and Hearing Disorders, 31,* 261–266.

Keenan, J. S. (1971). The detection of minimal dysphasia. *Archives of Physical Medicine and Rehabilitation, 52,* 227–232.

Keenan, J. S., & Brassell, E. G. (1974). A study of factors related to prognosis for individual aphasic patients. *Journal of Speech and Hearing Disorders, 39,* 257–269.

Keenan, J. S., & Brassell, E. G. (1975). *Aphasia*

language performance scales. Murfreesboro, TN: Pinnacle Press.

Keith, R. L. (1980). *Graduated language training for patients with aphasia.* Danville, IL: Interstate Printers & Publishers.

Kenin, J., & Swisher, L. P. (1972). A study of patterns of recovery in aphasia. *Cortex, 8,* 56–68.

Kent, R. D. (1984). Brain mechanisms of speech and language with special reference to emotional interaction. In R. Vandemore (Ed.), *Language science: Recent advances.* San Diego: College-Hill Press.

Kent, R. D. (1985). Science and the clinician: The practice of science and the science of practice. In R. D. Kent (Ed.), *Application of research to assessment and therapy. Seminars in speech and language, 6* (pp. 1–12). New York: Thieme-Stratton.

Kent, R. D., & Fair, J. (1985). Clinical research: Who, when, and how. In R. D. Kent (Ed.), *Application of research to assessment and therapy. Seminars in speech and language, 6* (pp. 23–24). New York: Thieme-Stratton.

Kent, R. D., & Rosenbek, J. C. (1982). Prosodic disturbance and neurologic lesion. *Brain and Language, 15,* 259.

Kent, R. D., & Rosenbek, J. C. (1983). Acoustic patterns of apraxia of speech. *Journal of Speech and Hearing Research, 26,* 231–248.

Kertesz, A. (1979). *Aphasia and associated disorders: Taxonomy, localization, and recovery.* New York: Grune & Stratton.

Kertesz, A. (1982). *Western aphasia battery.* New York: Grune & Stratton.

Kertesz, A. (1983). *Localization in neuropsychology.* New York: Academic Press.

Kertesz, A., & Black, S. E. (1985). Cerebrovascular disease and aphasia. In J. K. Darby (Ed.), *Speech and language evaluation in neurology: adult disorders* (pp. 83–122). Orlando: Grune & Stratton.

Kertesz, A., Black, S. E., Nicholson, L., & Carr, T. (1987). The sensitivity and specificity of MRI in stroke. *Neurology, 37,* 1580–1585.

Kertesz, A., Harlock, W., & Coates, R. (1979). Computer tomographic localization, lesion size, and prognosis in aphasia and nonverbal impairment. *Brain and Language, 8,* 34–50.

Kertesz, A., & McCabe, P. (1977). Recovery patterns and prognosis in aphasia. *Brain, 100,* 1–18.

Kertesz, A., & Phipps, J. (1980). The numerical taxonomy of acute and chronic aphasia syndromes. *Psychological Research, 41,* 179–198.

Kertesz, A., & Sheppard, A. (1981). The epidemiology of cognitive and aphasic impairment in stroke. *Brain, 104,* 117–128.

Kirk, R. E. (1982). *Experimental design.* Monterey, CA: Brooks/Cole Publishing Company.

Kirschner, H., & Webb, W. (1981). Selective involvement of the auditory verbal modality in an acquired communication disorder: Benefit from sign language therapy. *Brain and Language, 5,* 161–170.

Kitselman, K. P., Deal, J. L., & Wertz, R. T. (1981). The application of statistical analysis to single-case designs (A discussion session). In R. H. Brookshire (Ed.), *Proceedings of the Conference on Clinical Aphasiology* (pp. 339–341). Minneapolis: BRK Publishers.

Klor, B. M., & Ratusnik, D. L. (1980). Semantic relations in aphasic adults. In R. H. Brookshire (Ed.), *Proceedings of the Conference on Clinical Aphasiology* (pp. 47–52). Minneapolis: BRK Publishers.

Kneebone, C. S., & Burns, R. J. (1981). A case of cortical deafness. *Clinical Experimental Neurology, 18,* 91–97.

Knopman, D. S., Selnes, O. A., Niccum, N., & Rubens, A. B. (1983). A longitudinal study of speech fluency in aphasia: CT scan correlates of recovery and persistent nonfluency. *Neurology, 33,* 1170–1178.

Knopman, D. S., Selnes, O. A., Niccum, N., & Rubens, A. B. (1984). Recovery of naming in aphasia: Relationship to fluency, comprehension, and CT findings. *Neurology, 34,* 1461–1470.

Kohn, S. E., & Goodglass, H. (1985). Picture-naming in aphasia. *Brain and Language, 24,* 266–283.

Kreindler, A., & Fradis, A. (1968). *Performances in aphasia. A neurodynamical, diagnostic and psychological study.* Paris: Gauthier-Villars.

Kurtzke, J. F. (1982). On the role of clinicians in the use of drug trial data. *Neuroepidemiology, 1,* 124–136.

Kurtzke, J. F., & Kurland, L. T. (1973). The epidemiology of neurologic disease. In A. B. Baker (Ed.), *Clinical neurology* (Vol. 3, pp. 1–80). New York: Harper & Row.

Lambrecht, K. J., & Marshall, R. (1983). Comprehension in severe aphasia: A second look. In R. H. Brookshire (Ed.), *Proceedings of the Conference on Clinical Aphasiology* (pp. 186–192). Minneapolis: BRK Publishers.

LaPointe, L. L. (1977a). Base-10 programmed stimulation: Task specification, scoring and plotting performance in aphasia therapy. *Journal of Speech and Hearing Disorders, 42*, 90–105.

LaPointe, L. L. (1977b). *Diagnosis and treatment of reading disturbances associated with aphasia.* Paper presented at the third annual course in behavioral neurology and neuropsychology, Florida Neurology Society, Orlando, FL.

LaPointe, L. L. (1978a). Aphasia therapy: Some principles and strategies for treatment. In D. F. Johns (Ed.), *Clinical management of neurogenic communicative disorders* (pp. 129–190). Boston: Little, Brown & Company.

LaPointe, L. L. (1978b). Multiple baseline designs. In R. H. Brookshire (Ed.), *Proceedings of the Conference on Clinical Aphasiology* (pp. 20–29). Minneapolis: BRK Publishers.

LaPointe, L. L. (1982). *Movement toward volitional control in aphasia treatment: Laddering and self-cueing strategies.* Paper presented at Assessment and Diagnosis-based Treatments for Aphasia, University of Wisconsin, Madison, WI.

LaPointe, L. L. (1983). Aphasia intervention with adults: Historical, present, and future approaches. In J. Miller, D. E. Yoder, & R. Schiefelbusch (Eds.), *Contemporary issues in language intervention.* Rockville, MD: ASHA Reports, 12.

LaPointe, L. L. (1984). Sequential treatment of split lists: A case report. In J. C. Rosenbek, M. R. McNeil, & A. E. Aronson (Eds.), *Apraxia of speech: Physiology, acoustics, linguistics, management* (pp. 277–286). San Diego: College-Hill Press.

LaPointe, L. L. (1985). Aphasia therapy: Some principles and strategies for treatment. In D. F. Johns (Ed.), *Clinical management of neurogenic communicative disorders* (2nd ed.). Boston: Little, Brown.

LaPointe, L. L., & Culton, G. L. (1969). Visual-spatial neglect subsequent to brain injury. *Journal of Speech and Hearing Disorders, 34*, 82–86.

LaPointe, L. L., Holtzapple, P., & Graham, L. (1985). The relationships among two measures of auditory comprehension and daily living communicative skills. In R. H. Brookshire (Ed.), *Proceedings of the Conference on Clinical Aphasiology* (pp. 38–46). Minneapolis: BRK Publishers.

LaPointe, L. L., Holtzapple, P., & Graham, L. (1986). Comprehension of three-part commands by aphasic subjects: Analysis of error location. In R. H. Brookshire (Ed.), *Proceedings of the Conference on Clinical Aphasiology* (pp. 65–72). Minneapolis: BRK Publishers.

LaPointe, L. L., & Horner, J. (1978, Spring) The functional auditory comprehension task (FACT): Protocol and test format. *FLASHA Journal*, 27–33.

LaPointe, L. L., & Horner, J. (1979). *Reading comprehension battery for aphasia.* Austin, TX: PRO-ED.

LaPointe, L. L., Horner, J., & Lieberman, R. J. (1978). Effects of ear presentation and delayed response on the processing of Token Test commands by aphasic adults. In R. H. Brookshire (Ed.), *Proceedings of the Conference on Clinical Aphasiology* (pp. 112–123). Minneapolis: BRK Publishers.

LaPointe, L. L., Horner, J., Lieberman, R. J., & Riske, J. E. (1974). *Assessing patterns of auditory perception and comprehension impairment in aphasia.* Paper presented at the annual meeting of the Academy of Aphasia, Warrenton, VA.

LaPointe, L. L., & Kraemer, I. T. (1983). Treatment of alexia without agraphia. In W. Perkins (Ed.), *Current therapy of communication disorders: Language handicaps in adults* (pp. 77–85). New York: Thieme-Stratton.

Lasky, E. Z., Weidner, W. E., & Johnson, J. P. (1976). Influence of linguistic complexity, rate of presentation, and interphrase pause time on auditory-verbal comprehension of adult aphasic patients. *Brain and Language, 3*, 386–395.

Lebrun, Y. (1976). Neurolinguistic models of language and speech. In H. Whitaker & H. A. Whitaker (Eds.), *Studies in neurolinguistics* (Vol. 1, pp. 1–30). New York: Academic Press.

Lebrun, Y., & Hoops, R. (Eds.). (1974). *Intelligence and aphasia. Neurolinguistics 2.* Amsterdam: Swets & Zeitlinger B.V.

Lecours. A. (1966). Serial order in writing: A study of misspelled words in "Developmental Dysgraphia." *Neuropsychologia, 4*, 221–241.

Lee, L. (1969). *Northwestern syntax screening test.* Evanston, IL: Northwestern University Press.

Lemme, M. L., Hedberg, N. L., & Bottenberg, D. E. (1984). Cohesion in narratives of aphasic adults. In R. H. Brookshire (Ed.), *Proceedings of the Conference on Clinical Aphasiology* (pp. 215–222). Minneapolis: BRK Publishers.

Lendrem, W., & Lincoln, N. B. (1985). Spontaneous recovery of language in patients with aphasia between 4 and 34 weeks after stroke. *Journal of Neurology, Neurosurgery, and Psychiatry, 48*, 743–748.

Lentz, S., Shubitowski, Y., Rosenbek, J. C., & McNeil, M. R. (1983). *Treating spontaneous speech production in transcortical motor aphasia.* Paper presented at the Annual Convention of the American Speech-Language-Hearing Association, Cincinnati, OH.

Lesser, R. (1978). *Linguistic investigations of aphasia.* London: Arnold.

Lezak, M. (1983). *Neuropsychological assessment* (2nd ed.). New York: Oxford University Press.

Li, E. C., & Canter, G. (1983). Phonemic cueing: An investigation of subject variables. In R. H. Brookshire (Ed.), *Proceedings of the Conference on Clinical Aphasiology* (pp. 96–103). Minneapolis: BRK Publishers.

Lincoln, N. B., McGuirk, E., Mulley, G. P., Lendrem, W., Jones, A. C., & Mitchell, J. R. A. (1984). Effectiveness of speech therapy for aphasic stroke patients: A randomised controlled trial. *Lancet, 1*, 1197–1200.

Linebaugh, C. W., & Lehner, L. H. (1977). Cueing hierarchies and word retrieval: A therapy program. In R. H. Brookshire (Ed.), *Proceedings of the Conference on Clinical Aphasiology* (pp. 19–31). Minneapolis: BRK Publishers.

Logue, R. D., & Dixon, M. M. (1979). Word association and the anomic response: Analysis and treatment. In R. H. Brookshire (Ed.), *Proceedings of the Conference on Clinical Aphasiology* (pp. 248–260). Minneapolis: BRK Publishers.

Lomas, J., & Kertesz, A. (1978). Patterns of spontaneous recovery in aphasic groups: A study of adult stroke patients. *Brain and Language, 5*, 388–401.

Longstreth, W. T., Jr., Koepsell, T. D., & van Belle, G. (1987). Clinical neuroepidemiology: II. Outcomes. *Archives of Neurology, 44*, 1196–1202.

Love, R. J., & Webb, W. G. (1977). The efficiency of cueing techniques in Broca's aphasia. *Journal of Speech and Hearing Disorders, 42*, 170–178.

Love, R. J., & Webb, W. G. (1986). *Neurology for the speech-language pathologist.* London: Butterworth.

Loverso, F. L. (1987). Unfounded expectations: Computers in rehabilitation. *Aphasiology, 1*, 157–159.

Loverso, F. L., & Prescott, T. E. (1981). The effect of alerting signals on left brain-damaged (aphasic) and normal subjects' accuracy and response time to visual stimuli. In R. H. Brookshire (Ed.), *Proceedings of the Conference of Clinical Aphasiology* (pp. 55–67). Minneapolis: BRK Publishers.

Loverso, F. L., Prescott, T. E., Selinger, M., Wheeler, K. M., & Smith, R. (1985). The application of microcomputers for the treatment of aphasic adults. In R. H. Brookshire (Ed.), *Proceedings of the Conference on Clinical Aphasiology* (pp. 189–195). Minneapolis: BRK Publishers.

Loverso, F. L., Selinger, M., & Prescott, T. E. (1979). Application of verbing strategies to aphasia treatment. In R. H. Brookshire (Ed.), *Proceedings of the Conference on Clinical Aphasiology* (pp. 229–238). Minneapolis: BRK Publishers.

Lubinski, R. (1981). Speech language and audiology programs in home health care agencies and nursing homes. In D. S. Beasley & G. A. Davis (Eds.), *Aging: Communication processes and disorders* (pp. 339–356). New York: Grune & Stratton.

Ludlow, C. L. (1977). Recovery from aphasia: A foundation for treatment. In M. Sullivan & M. S. Kommers (Eds.), *Rationale for adult aphasia therapy* (pp. 97–134). Omaha: University of Nebraska Medical Center.

Ludlow, C. L., Rosenberg, J., Fair, C., Buck, D., Schesselman, S., & Salazar, A. (1986). Brain lesions associated with nonfluent aphasia fifteen years following penetrating head injury. *Brain, 109*, 55–80.

Luria, A. R. (1963). *Restoration of function after brain injury.* New York: Macmillan.

Luria, A. R. (1964). Factors and forms of aphasia. In A. V. S. d. Reuck & M. O'Connor (Eds.), *Disorders of communication* (pp. 143–161). Boston: Little, Brown & Company.

Luria, A. R. (1970) *Traumatic aphasia: Its syndromes, psychology, and treatment.* The Hague: Mouton.

Luria, A. R. (1977). On quasi-aphasic speech disturbances in lesions of the deep structures of the brain. *Brain and Language, 4*, 432–459.

Luria, A. R. (1981). *Language and cognition.* New York: John Wiley & Sons.

Lyon, J. G. (1984). *An augmentative means of communication for the functionally nonverbal aphasic adult.* Paper presented at the Third Annual Southeastern Aphasiology Conference, Ft. Walton Beach, FL.

Lyon, J. G. (1986). Standardized test batteries: Advances in aphasia testing. In L. L. LaPointe (Ed.), *Aphasia: Nature and assessment. Seminars in speech and language, 7* (pp. 159–180). New York: Thieme-Stratton.

Major, B. J., & Wilson, K. J. (1985). *Computerized reading for aphasics.* San Diego: College-Hill Press.

Marcé, P. (1856). Mémoire sur quelques observations de physiologie tendant à demontrer l'existence d'un principe coordinateur de l'écriture et ses rapports avec le principe coordinateur de la parole. *Comptes Rendus des Séances de la Société de Biologie et de ses Filiales, 3,* 93–115.

Marie, P. (1883). De l'aphasie, cécite verbale, surdite verbale, aphasie motire, agraphie. *Revue Medicale, 3,* 693–702.

Marks, M., Taylor, M., & Rusk, H. A. (1957). Rehabilitation of the aphasic patient: A summary of three years' experience in a rehabilitation setting. *Archives of Physical Medicine and Rehabilitation, 38,* 219–226.

Marquardsen, J. (1969). The natural history of cerebrovascular disease. A retrospective study of 769 patients. *Acta Neurologica Scandinavia, 45,* 1–192.

Marshall, J. C., & Newcombe, F. (1966). Syntactic and semantic errors in paralexia. *Neuropsychologia, 4,* 169–176.

Marshall, J. C., & Newcombe, F. (1973). Stages in recovery from dyslexia following a left cerebral abscess. *Cortex, 3,* 329–332.

Marshall, J. C., & Newcombe, F. (1980). The conceptual status of deep dyslexia: An historical perspective. In M. Coltheart, K. Patterson, & J. C. Marshall (Eds.), *Deep dyslexia* (pp. 1–21). London: Routledge & Kegan Paul.

Marshall, N., & Holtzapple, P. A. (1976). Melodic intonation therapy: Variations on a theme. In R. H. Brookshire (Ed.), *Proceedings of the Conference on Clinical Aphasiology* (pp. 115–141). Minneapolis: BRK Publishers.

Marshall, R. C. (1975). Word retrieval strategies of aphasic adults in conventional speech. In R. H. Brookshire (Ed.), *Proceedings of the Conference on Clinical Aphasiology* (pp. 165–174). Minneapolis: BRK Publishers.

Marshall, R. C. (1976). Word retrieval behavior of aphasic adults. *Journal of Speech and Hearing Disorders, 41,* 444–451.

Marshall, R. C. (1978). *Clinician controlled auditory stimulation for aphasic adults.* Tigard, OR: C. C. Publications.

Marshall, R. C. (1981). Heightening auditory comprehension for aphasic patients. In R. Chapey (Ed.), *Language intervention strategies in adult aphasia* (pp. 297–328). Baltimore: Williams & Wilkins.

Marshall, R. C., & Neuburger, S. (1984). Extended comprehension training reconsidered. In R. H. Brookshire (Ed.), *Proceedings of the Conference on Clinical Aphasiology* (pp. 181–187). Minneapolis: BRK Publishers.

Marshall, R. C., & Phillips, D. S. (1983). Prognosis for improved verbal communication in aphasic stroke patients. *Archives of Physical Medicine and Rehabilitation, 64,* 597–600.

Marshall, R. C., Tompkins, C. A., & Phillips, D. S. (1982). Improvement in treated aphasia: Examination of selected prognostic factors. *Folia Phoniatrica, 34,* 305–315.

Marshall, R. C., Tompkins, C. A., Rau, M. T., Phillips, D. S., Golper, L. A., & Lambrecht, K. J. (1980). Verbal self-correction behavior of aphasic subjects for single word tasks. In R. H. Brookshire (Ed.), *Proceedings of the Conference on Clinical Aphasiology* (pp. 39–46). Minneapolis: BRK Publishers.

Martin, A. D. (1974). Some objections to the term apraxia of speech. *Journal of Speech and Hearing Disorders, 39,* 53–64.

Martin, A. D. (1981a). An examination of Wepman's thought centered therapy. In R. Chapey (Ed.), *Language intervention strategies in adult aphasia* (pp. 141–154). Baltimore: Williams & Wilkins.

Martin, A. D. (1981b). The role of theory in therapy: A rationale. *Topics in Language Disorders, 1,* 63–72.

Martin, A. D. (1981c). Therapy with the jargonaphasic. In J. W. Brown (Ed.), *Jargonaphasia* (pp. 305–326). New York: Academic Press.

Martinoff, J. T., Martinoff, R., & Stokke, V. (1980). *Language rehabilitation: Auditory comprehension.* Austin, TX: PRO-ED.

Martinoff, J. T., Martinoff, R. & Stokke, V. (1983). *Language rehabilitation: Reading.* Austin, TX: PRO-ED.

Mazzocchi, R., & Vignolo, L. (1979). Localization of lesions in aphasia: Clinical CT scan correlations in stroke patients. *Cortex, 15,* 627–654.

McGlone, J. (1977). Sex differences in the cerebral organization of verbal functions in patients with unilateral brain lesions. *Brain, 100,* 775–793.

McHenry, L. C. (1969). *Garrison's history of neurology.* Springfield, IL: Charles C Thomas.

McKeever, M., Holmes, G. L., & Russman, B. S. (1983). Speech abnormalities in seizures: A comparison of absence and partial complex seizures. *Brain and Language, 19,* 25–32.

McNeil, M. R. (1977). *Effects of diotic and selective binaural intensity variation on auditory processing in aphasia.* Unpublished doctoral dissertation, University of Denver.

McNeil, M. R. (1979). Porch Index of Communicative Ability. In F. L. Darley (Ed.), *Evaluation of appraisal techniques in speech and language pathology* (pp. 223–235). Reading, MA: Addison-Wesley.

McNeil, M. R. (1982). The nature of aphasia in adults. In N. J. Lass, L. V. McReynolds, J. L. Northern, & D. E. Yoder (Eds.), *Speech, language, and hearing: Volume III. Pathologies of speech and language* (pp. 692–740). Philadelphia: W. B. Saunders Company.

McNeil, M. R., & Hageman, C. F. (1979). Auditory processing deficits in aphasia evidenced on the Revised Token Test: Incidence and prediction of across subtest and across item within subtest patterns. In R. H. Brookshire (Ed.), *Proceedings of the Conference on Clinical Aphasiology* (pp. 47–69). Minneapolis: BRK Publishers.

McNeil, M. R., & Kimelman, M. D. Z. (1986). Toward an integrative information processing structure of auditory comprehension and processing in adult aphasia. In L. LaPointe (Ed.), *Aphasia: Nature and assessment. Seminars in Speech and Language, 7* (pp. 123–146). New York: Thieme Stratton.

McNeil, M. R., & Prescott, T. E. (1978). *Revised Token Test.* Baltimore: University Park Press.

McReynolds, L. V., & Kearns, K. P. (1983). *Single-subject experimental designs in communicative disorders.* Austin, TX: PRO-ED.

McReynolds, L. V., & Thompson, C. K. (1986). Flexibility of single-subject experimental designs. Part I: Review of the basics of single-subject designs. *Journal of Speech and Hearing Disorders, 51,* 194–203.

Meikle, M., Wechsler, E., Tupper, A., Benenson, M., Butler, J., Mulhall, D., & Stern, G. (1979). Comparative trial of volunteer and professional treatments of dysphasia after stroke. *British Medical Journal, 2,* 87–89.

Messerli, P., Tissot, A., & Rodriguez, J. (1976). Recovery from aphasia: Some factors of prognosis. In Y. Lebrun & R. Hoops (Eds.), *Neurolinguistics 4: Recovery in aphasics* (pp. 124–135). Amsterdam: Swets & Zeitlinger B.V.

Mesulam, M. M. (1982). Slowly progressive aphasia without generalized dementia. *Annals of Neurology, 11,* 592–598.

Metter, E. J., & Hanson, W. R. (1985). Brain imaging as related to speech and language. In J. K. Darby (Ed.), *Speech and language evaluation in neurology: Adult disorders* (pp. 123–160). Orlando: Grune & Stratton.

Metter, E. J., Riege, W. H., Hanson, W. R., Camras, L. R., Phelps, M. E., & Kuhl, D. E. (1984). Correlations of glucose metabolism and structural damage to language function in aphasia. *Brain and Language, 21,* 187–207.

Michel, F., & Andreewohy, E. (1983). Deep dysphasia: An analog of deep dyslexia in the auditory modality. *Brain and Language, 18,* 212–223.

Milberg, W., & Blumstein, S. E. (1981). Lexical decision and aphasia: Evidence for semantic processing. *Brain and Language, 14,* 371–385.

Mills, R. H. (1977). The effects of environmental sound on the naming performance of aphasic subjects. In R. H. Brookshire (Ed.), *Proceedings of the Conference on Clinical Aphasiology* (pp. 68–79). Minneapolis: BRK Publishers.

Mills, R. H. (1982). Microcomputerized auditory comprehension training. In R. H. Brookshire (Ed.), *Proceedings of the Conference on Clinical Aphasiology* (pp. 147–152). Minneapolis: BRK Publishers.

Milner, B. (1964). Some effects of frontal lobectomy in man. In J. M. Warren & K. Akert (Eds.), *The frontal granular cortex and behavior* (pp. 313–334). New York: McGraw-Hill.

Minckler, J. (1972). *Introduction to neuroscience.* St. Louis: C. V. Mosby Co.

Mohr, J. P. (1973). Rapid amelioration of motor aphasia. *Archives of Neurology, 28,* 77–82.

Mohr, J. P. (1980). Revision of Broca aphasia and the syndrome of Broca's area infarction and its implications in aphasia therapy. In R. H. Brookshire (Ed.), *Proceedings of the Conference on Clinical Aphasiology* (pp. 1–16). Minneapolis: BRK Publishers.

Mohr, J. P., Pessin, M. S., Finkelstein, S., Funkenstein, H. H., Duncan, G. W., & Davis, K. R. (1978). Broca aphasia: Pathological and clinical aspects. *Neurology, 28,* 311–324.

Moss, C. S. (1972). *Recovery with aphasia: The aftermath of my stroke.* Urbana, IL: University of Illinois Press.

Moyer, S. B. (1979). Rehabilitation of alexia: A case study. *Cortex, 15,* 139–144.

Mulley, G. P. (1986). *Current issues in adult aphasia*. Paper presented to the St. Mary's Medical Center, San Francisco, CA.

Myers, P. S. (1979). Profiles of communication deficits in patients with right cerebral hemisphere damage. In R. H. Brookshire (Ed.), *Proceedings of the Conference on Clinical Aphasiology* (pp. 38–46). Minneapolis: BRK Publishers.

Myers, P. S. (1980). Visual imagery in aphasia treatment. A new look. In R. H. Brookshire (Ed.), *Proceedings of the Conference on Clinical Aphasiology* (pp. 68–77). Minneapolis: BRK Publishers.

Myers, P. S. (1984). Right hemisphere impairment. In A. L. Holland (Ed.), *Language disorders in adults: Recent advances* (pp. 177–208). Austin, TX: PRO-ED.

Myers, P. S., & Linebaugh, C. W. (1984). The use of context-dependent pictures in aphasia rehabilitation. In R. H. Brookshire (Ed.), *Proceedings of the Conference on Clinical Aphasiology* (pp. 145–158). Minneapolis: BRK Publishers.

Naeser, M. A., Alexander, M. P., Helm-Estabrooks, N., Levin, H. L., Laughlin, S. A., & Geschwind, N. (1982). Aphasia with predominantly subcortical lesion sites: Description of three capsular/putamenal syndromes. *Archives of Neurology, 39*, 1–14.

Naeser, M. A., & Hayward, R. W. (1978). Lesion localization in aphasia with cranial computed tomography and the Boston Aphasia Exam. *Neurology, 28*, 545–551.

Naeser, M., Hayward, R., Laughlin, S., Becker, J., Jernigan, T., & Zatz, L. (1981). Quantitative CT scan studies in aphasia: II. Comparison of the right and left hemispheres. *Brain and Language, 12*, 165–189.

Neisser, U. (1966). *Cognitive psychology*. New York: Appleton-Century-Crofts.

Nelson reading test. (1962). Boston: Houghton-Mifflin Co.

Nicholas, L. E., & Brookshire, R. H. (1983). Syntactic simplification and context: Effects on sentence comprehension by aphasic adults. In R. H. Brookshire (Ed.), *Proceedings of the Conference on Clinical Aphasiology* (pp. 166–172). Minneapolis: BRK Publishers.

Nicholas, L. E., & Brookshire, R. H. (1985). Consistency of the effects of rate of speech on brain-damaged subjects' comprehension of four types of information in narrative discourse. In R. H. Brookshire (Ed.),

Proceedings of the Conference on Clinical Aphasiology (pp. 262–271). Minneapolis: BRK Publishers.

Nielsen, J. M. (1946). *Agnosia, apraxia, aphasia*. New York: Hoeber.

Obler, L. K., & Albert, M. L. (1981). Language and aging: A neurobehavioral analysis. In D. S. Beasley & G. A. Davis (Eds.), *Aging: Communication processes and disorders* (pp. 107–122). New York: Grune & Stratton.

Obler, L. K., Albert, M. L., Caplass, L. R., Mohr, J. P., & Geer, D. E. (1980). *Stroke type, sex differences and aging*. Paper presented at the 18th Academy of Aphasia Annual Meeting, Bass River, MA.

Ojemann, G. A. (1975). Language and the thalamus: Object naming and recall during and after thalamic stimulation. *Brain and Language, 2*, 101–120.

Oldendorf, W. H. (1978). The quest for an image of brain: A brief historical and technical review of brain imaging techniques. *Neurology*, 517–533.

Olsen, T. S., Bruhn, P., & Oberg, R. G. E. (1986). Cortical hypoperfusion as a possible cause of subcortical aphasia. *Brain, 109*, 393–410.

Orgass, B., & Poeck, K. (1966). Clinical validation of a new test for aphasia: An experimental study of the Token Test. *Cortex, 2*, 222–243.

Paradis, M. (1987). *The assessment of bilingual aphasia*. Hillsdale, NJ: Lawrence Erlbaum Associates.

Pasternack, K., & LaPointe, L. L. (1982). *Test-retest and intertester reliability of the Reading Comprehension Battery for Aphasia*. Paper presented at the annual convention of the American Speech-Language-Hearing Association, Toronto, Canada.

Patterson, K. (1980). Derivational errors in deep dyslexia. In M. Coltheart, K. Patterson, & J. Marshall (Eds.), *Deep dyslexia* (pp. 286–306). London: Routledge & Kegan Paul.

Pease, D., & Goodglass, H. (1978). The effects of cueing on picture naming in aphasia. *Cortex, 14*, 178–189.

Peele, T. L. (1977). *The neuroanatomic basis for clinical neurology* (3rd ed.). New York: McGraw-Hill Book Co.

Penfield, W., & Roberts, L. (1959). *Speech and brain mechanisms*. Princeton: Princeton University Press.

Penn, M. A. C. (1983). *Syntactic and pragmatic aspects of aphasic language*. Unpublished doctoral dissertation, University of the Witwatersrand, Johannesburg, South Africa.

Perkins, W. H., & Kent, R. (1986). *Functional anatomy of speech, language and hearing: A primer.* San Diego: College-Hill Press.

Piehler, M., & Holland, A. (1984). Cohesion in aphasic language. In R. H. Brookshire (Ed.), *Proceedings of the Conference on Clinical Aphasiology* (pp. 208–214). Minneapolis: BRK Publishers.

Pierce, R. S. (1983a). *Aphasia treatment manual: A research-directed guide.* Kent, OH: Blaca Enterprises.

Pierce, R. S. (1983b). Decoding syntax during reading in aphasia. *Journal of Communication Disorders, 16,* 181–188.

Pierce, R. S., & Beekman, L. A. (1985). Effects of linguistic and extralinguistic context on semantic and syntactic processing in aphasia. *Journal of Speech and Hearing Research, 28,* 250–254.

Pirozzolo, F. J. (1979). *The neuropsychology of developmental reading disorders.* New York: Praeger Press.

Plumridge, T. S., LaPointe, L. L., & Lombardino, L. (1985). *Perceptions and definitions of aphasia by spouses of aphasic individuals.* Paper presented at the annual convention of the American Speech-Language-Hearing Association, Washington, DC.

Podraza, B. L., & Darley, F. L. (1977). Effects of auditory prestimulation on naming in aphasia. *Journal of Speech and Hearing Research, 20,* 669–683.

Poeck, K. (1983). What do we mean by "aphasic syndromes?" A neurologist's view. *Brain and Language, 20,* 79–89.

Poeck, K., DeBlesser, R., & Graf von Keyserlingk, D. (1984). Neurolinguistic status and localization of lesion in aphasic patients with exclusively consonant-vowel recurring utterances. *Brain, 107,* 199–217.

Poeck, K., Huber, W., & Willmes, K. (1986). *Outcome of intensive speech therapy in aphasia.* Paper presented to the 24th Annual Meeting of the Academy of Aphasia, Nashville, TN.

Poeck, K., Kerschensteiner, M., & Hartje, W. (1972). A quantitative study on language understanding in fluent and nonfluent aphasia. *Cortex, 8,* 229–304.

Pogacar, S., & Williams, R. S. (1984). Alzheimer's disease presenting as slowly progressive aphasia. *Rhode Island Medical Journal, 67,* 181–185.

Porch, B. E. (1967). *Porch index of communicative ability.* Palo Alto, CA: Consulting Psychologists Press.

Porch, B. E. (1969). *An introduction to clinical aphasiology.* Paper presented to the First Conference on Clinical Aphasiology, Albuquerque, NM.

Porch, B. E. (1981). *Porch index of communicative ability* (3rd ed.). Palo Alto, CA: Consulting Psychologists Press.

Porch, B. E., & Callaghan, S. (1981). Making predictions about recovery: Is there HOAP? In R. H. Brookshire (Ed.), *Proceedings of the Conference on Clinical Aphasiology* (pp. 187–200). Minneapolis: BRK Publishers.

Porch, B. E., Collins, M., Wertz, R. T., & Friden, T. P. (1980). Statistical prediction of change in aphasia. *Journal of Speech and Hearing Research, 23,* 312–321.

Porrazzo, S. A. (1975). Evaluation and treatment of reading deficits in aphasic patients. In R. H. Brookshire (Ed.), *Proceedings of the Conference on Clinical Aphasiology* (pp. 89–95). Minneapolis: BRK Publishing.

Powell, G. E., Clark, E., & Bailey, S. (1979). Categories of aphasia: A cluster-analysis of Schuell test profiles. *British Journal of Disorders of Communication, 14,* 111–122.

Prins, R. S., Snow, C. E., & Wagenaar, E. (1978). Recovery from aphasia: Spontaneous speech versus language comprehension. *Brain and Language, 6,* 192–211.

Prinz, P. (1980). A note on requesting strategies in adult aphasics. *Journal of Communication Disorders, 12,* 65–73.

Prutting, C., & Kirchner, D. (1983). Applied pragmatics. In T. Gallagher & C. Prutting (Eds.), *Pragmatic assessment and intervention issues in language* (pp. 29–64). San Diego: College-Hill Press.

Prutting, C., & Kirchner, D. (1983). Applied pragmatics. In T. Gallagher & C. Prutting (Eds.), *Pragmatic assessment and intervention issues in language* (pp. 29–64). Austin, TX: PRO-ED.

& Pickering, M. (1984). The costs of using trained and supervised volunteers as part of a speech therapy service for dysphasic patients. *British Journal of Disorders of Communication, 19,* 205–212.

Rau, J. (1973). *The effects of immediate feedback on the graphic performance of an aphasic adult.* Paper presented at the Clinical Aphasiology Conference, Albuquerque, NM.

Raven, J. C. (1962). *Coloured progressive matrices.* London: H. K. Lewis.

Raymer, A. M., & LaPointe, L. L. (1983). *Comprehension of live voice versus telephone transmission in aphasia.* Paper presented at the Annual Conference of the American Speech-Language-Hearing Association, Cincinnati, OH.

Raymer, A. M., & LaPointe, L. L. (1986). The nature and assessment of the mildly-impaired aphasic person. In L. L. LaPointe (Ed.), *Aphasia: Nature and assessment. Seminars in speech and language, 7* (pp. 207–221). New York: Thieme-Stratton.

Revusky, S. H. (1967). Some statistical treatments compatible with individual organism methodology. *Journal of the Experimental Analysis of Behavior, 10,* 319–330.

Riedel, K. (1981). Auditory comprehension in aphasia. In M. T. Sarno (Ed.), *Acquired aphasia* (pp. 215–270). New York: Academic Press.

Rinnert, C., & Whitaker, H. A. (1973). Semantic confusions by aphasic patients. *Cortex, 9,* 56–81.

Risser, A. H., & Spreen, O. (1985). Test review: The Western Aphasia Battery. *Journal of Clinical and Experimental Neuropsychology, 7,* 463–470.

Roberts, J. A., Wertz, R. T., Bernstein-Ellis, E., & Shubitowski, Y. (1987). Pragmatic and syntactic improvement in fluent and nonfluent aphasia. In R. H. Brookshire (Ed.), *Proceedings of the Conference on Clinical Aphasiology* (pp. 29–34). Minneapolis: BRK Publishers.

Rochford, G., & Williams, M. (1962). Studies in the development and breakdown of the use of names. *Journal of Neurology, Neurosurgery, and Psychiatry, 25,* 222–233.

Rochford, G., & Williams, M. (1965). Studies in the development and breakdown of the use and names: IV. The effects of word frequency. *Journal of Neurology, Neurosurgery, and Psychiatry, 28,* 407–413.

Rosenbek, J. C. (1979). Wrinkled feet. In R. H. Brookshire (Ed.), *Proceedings of the Conference on Clinical Aphasiology* (pp. 163–176). Minneapolis: BRK Publishers.

Rosenbek, J. C. (1982). When is aphasia aphasia? In R. H. Brookshire (Ed.), *Proceedings of the Conference on Clinical Aphasiology* (pp. 360–366). Minneapolis: BRK Publishers.

Rosenbek, J. C. (1983). Some challenges for clinical aphasiologists. In J. Miller, D. Yoder, & R. Schiefelbusch (Eds.), *Contemporary Issues in Language Intervention, ASHA Reports 12* (pp. 317–325). Rockville, MD: The American Speech-Language-Hearing Association.

Rosenbek, J. C. (1985). Treating apraxia of speech. In D. F. Johns (Ed.), *Clinical management of neurogenic communicative disorders* (2nd ed., pp. 267–312). Boston: Little, Brown & Company.

Rosenbek, J. C. (1987). *A changing criterion design in the treatment of aphasia.* Paper presented to the conference on the Adult Aphasic: A Management Approach, Long Beach, CA.

Rosenbek, J. C., Green, E. F., Flynn, M., Wertz, R. T., & Collins, M. J. (1977). Anomia: A clinical experiment. In R. H. Brookshire (Ed.), *Proceedings of the Conference on Clinical Aphasiology* (pp. 103–111). Minneapolis: BRK Publishers.

Rosenbek, J. C., & LaPointe, L. L. (1981). Motor speech disorders and the aging process. In D. S. Beasley & G. A. Davis (Eds.), *Aging: Communication processes and disorders* (pp. 159–174). New York: Grune & Stratton.

Rosenbek, J. C., & LaPointe, L. L. (1985). The dysarthrias: Description, diagnosis, and treatment. In D. F. Johns (Ed.), *Clinical management of neurogenic communication disorders* (2nd ed., pp. 97–152). Boston: Little, Brown & Company.

Rosenbek, J. C., Lemme, M. L., Ahern, M. B., Harris, E. H., Wertz, R. T. (1973). A treatment for apraxia of speech in adults. *Journal of Speech and Hearing Disorders, 38,* 462–472.

Rosenbek, J. C., Robbins, J., & Levine, R. (1985). *Neurologic, speech-language, and swallowing findings in angular-gyrus plus syndrome.* Paper presented to the American Speech-Language-Hearing Association, Washington, DC.

Rosenbek, J. C., & Shimon, D. (1984). Computerized axial tomography in aphasiology. In R. H. Brookshire (Ed.), *Proceedings of the Conference on Clinical Aphasiology* (pp. 1–6). Minneapolis: BRK Publishers.

Ross, D., & Spencer, S. (1981). *Reading and writing task hierarchy.* Springfield, IL: Charles C Thomas.

Rubeck, P. F. (1977). Decoding procedures: Pupil self-analysis and observed behaviors. *Reading Improvement, 14,* 187–192.

Rubens, A. B. (1976). Transcortical motor aphasia. In H. Whitaker & H. A. Whitaker (Eds.), *Studies in neurolinguistics* (Vol. 1, pp. 293–303). New York: Academic Press.

Rubens, A. B. (1979). Agnosia. In K. Heilman & E. Valenstein (Eds.), *Clinical neuropsychology* (pp. 233–267). New York: Oxford University Press.

Rubow, R. T., Rosenbek, J. C., Collins, M. J., & Longstreth, D. (1982). Vibrotactile stimulation for intersystemic reorganization in the treatment of apraxia of speech. *Archives of Physical Medicine and Rehabilitation, 63,* 150–153.

Rushakoff, G. E. (1984). Clinical applications in communication disorders. In A. H. Schwartz (Ed.), *Handbook of micro-computer applications in communication disorders* (pp. 147–171). San Diego: College-Hill Press.

Ryan, W. J. (1982). *The nurse and the communicatively impaired adult.* New York: Springer Publishing Company.

Saffron, E. M., Bogyo, L. C., Schwartz, M. F., & Marin, O. S. M. (1980). Does deep dyslexia reflect right-hemisphere reading? In M. Coltheart, K. Patterson, & J. C. Marshall (Eds.), *Deep dyslexia* (pp. 381–406). London: Routledge & Kegan Paul.

Sahs, A. L., Hartman, E. C., & Aronson, S. M. (1979). *Stroke: Cause, prevention, treatment, and rehabilitation.* London: Castle House Publishers, Ltd.

Salvatore, A. P. (1974). *An investigation of the effects of pause duration on sentence comprehension by aphasic subjects.* Unpublished doctoral dissertation, University of Minnesota.

Salvatore, A. P. (1982). Artificial language training in brain damaged adults using a matrix training procedure. In R. H. Brookshire (Ed.), *Proceedings of the Conference on Clinical Aphasiology* (pp. 298–307). Minneapolis: BRK Publishers.

Salvatore, A. P., Trunzo, M. J., Holtzapple, P., & Graham, L. (1983). Investigation of the sentence hierarchy of the Helm Elicited Language Program for Syntax Stimulation. In R. H. Brookshire (Ed.), *Proceedings of the Conference on Clinical Aphasiology* (pp. 73–84). Minneapolis: BRK Publishers.

Sands, E., Sarno, M. T., & Shankweiler, D. (1969). Long-term assessment of language function in aphasia due to stroke. *Archives of Physical Medicine and Rehabilitation, 50,* 202–206.

Sarno, M. T. (1969). *The Functional Communication Profile: Manual of directions* (Rehabilitation Monograph 42). New York: New York University Medical Center, Institute of Rehabilitation Medicine.

Sarno, M. T. (1980). The nature of verbal impairment after closed head injury. *Journal of Nervous and Mental Disease, 168,* 685–692.

Sarno, M. T. (1983). *Understanding aphasia: A guide for family and friends.* New York: The Institute of Rehabilitation Medicine, New York University Medical Center.

Sarno, M. (1984). Verbal impairment after closed head injury: Report of a replication study. *Journal of Nervous and Mental Disease, 172,* 475–479.

Sarno, M. T., & Levita, E. (1971). Natural course of recovery in severe aphasia. *Archives of Physical Medicine and Rehabilitation, 52,* 175–178.

Sarno, M. T., & Levita, E. (1979). Recovery in aphasia during the first year post stroke. *Stroke, 10,* 663–370.

Sarno, M. T., & Levita, E. (1981). Some observations on the nature of recovery in global aphasia after stroke. *Brain and Language, 13,* 1–12.

Sarno, M. T., Silverman, M., & Sands, E. (1970). Speech therapy and language recovery in severe aphasia. *Journal of Speech and Hearing Research, 13,* 607–623.

Sasanuma, S. (1980). Acquired dyslexia in Japanese: Clinical features and underlying mechanisms. In M. Coltheart, K. Patterson, & J. Marshall (Eds.), *Deep dyslexia* (pp. 48–90). London: Routledge & Kegan Paul.

Schuell, H. (1957). A short examination for aphasia. *Neurology (Minneapolis), 7,* 625–634.

Schuell, H. (1965a). *The Minnesota test for differential diagnosis of aphasia.* Minneapolis: University of Minnesota Press.

Schuell, H. (1965b). *Differential diagnosis of aphasia with the Minnesota test.* Minneapolis: University of Minnesota Press.

Schuell, H. (1966). A re-evaluation of the short examination for aphasia. *Journal of Speech and Hearing Disorders, 31,* 137–147.

Schuell, H., & Jenkins, J. J. (1959). The nature of language deficit in aphasia. *Psychological Review, 66,* 45–67.

Schuell, H., Jenkins, J. J., & Carroll, J. B. (1962). A factor analysis of the Minnesota Test for Differential Diagnosis of Aphasia. *Journal of Speech and Hearing Research, 5,* 349–369.

Schuell, H., Jenkins, J. J., & Jiménez-Pabón, E. (1964). *Aphasia in adults: Diagnosis, prognosis and treatment.* New York: Hoeber Medical Division, Harper & Row Publishers.

Schuell, H., & Sefer, H. (1973). *Differential diagnosis of aphasia: Revised*. Minneapolis: University of Minnesota.

Segalowitz, S. J. (Ed.). (1983). *Language function and brain organization*. New York: Academic Press.

Selinger, M. S. (1982). *Auditory event related potentials, cerebral specialization, and language comprehension in aphasia*. Unpublished doctoral dissertation, University of Denver.

Selinger, M. S. (1984). Using cortical evoked potentials in aphasiology. In R. H. Brookshire (Ed.), *Proceedings of the Conference on Clnical Aphasiology* (pp. 34–39). Minneapolis: BRK Publishers.

Selinger, M. S., Prescott, T., & Katz, R. (1987). Handwritten vs computer typed responses on Porch Index of Communicative Ability graphic subtests. In R. H. Brookshire (Ed.), *Proceedings of the Conference on Clinical Aphasiology* (pp. 136–142). Minneapolis: BRK Publishers.

Selnes, O. A., Knopman, D. S., Niccum, N., Rubens, A. B., & Larson, D. (1983). Computed tomographic scan correlates of auditory comprehension deficits in aphasia: A prospective recovery study. *Annals of Neurology, 13,* 558–566.

Selnes, O. A., Niccum, N., Knopman, D. S., & Rubens, A. B. (1984). Recovery of single word comprehension: CT-scan correlates. *Brain and Language, 21,* 72–84.

Selnes, O. A., Niccum, N., & Rubens, A. B. (1982). CT scan correlates of recovery in auditory comprehension. In R. H. Brookshire (Ed.), *Proceedings of the Conference on Clinical Aphasiology* (pp. 112–118). Minneapolis: BRK Publishers.

Seron, X., Deloche, G., Bastard, V., Chassin, G., & Hermand, N. (1979). Word-finding difficulties in learning transfer in aphasic patients. *Cortex, 15,* 149–155.

Seron, X., Deloche, G., Moulard, G., & Rousselle, M. (1980). A computer-based therapy for the treatment of aphasic subjects with writing disorders. *Cortex, 45,* 45–58.

Shewan, C. M., & Bandur, D. L. (1986). *Treatment of aphasia: A language-oriented approach*. Austin, TX: PRO-ED.

Shewan, C. M., & Bandur, D. L. (1986). *Treatment of aphasia: A language-oriented approach*. San Diego: College-Hill Press.

Shewan, C. M., & Canter, G. J. (1971). Effects of vocabulary, syntax, and sentence length on auditory comprehension in aphasic patients. *Cortex, 7,* 209–226.

Shewan, C. M., & Kertesz, A. (1980). Reliability and validity characteristics of the Western Aphasia Battery (WAB). *Journal of Speech and Hearing Disorders, 45,* 308–324.

Shewan, C. M., & Kertesz, A. (1984). Effects of speech and language treatment on recovery from aphasia. *Brain and Language, 23,* 272–299.

Shriberg, L. D., & Kwiatkowski, J. (1980). *Natural process analysis (NPA): A procedure for phonological analysis of continuous speech samples*. New York: John Wiley & Sons.

Shubitowski, Y., Lentz, S. E., Rosenbek, J. C., & McNeil, M. R. (1983). *Treating written naming in a severe, chronic Wernicke's aphasic person*. Paper presented at the Annual Convention of the American Speech-Language-Hearing Association, Cincinnati, OH.

Sidman, M. (1960). *Tactics of scientific research: Evaluating experimental data in psychology*. New York: Basic Books, Inc.

Siegel, G. M. (1987). The limits of science in communication disorders. *Journal of Speech and Hearing Disorders, 52,* 306–312.

Siegel, G. M., & Spradlin, J. E. (1985). Therapy and research. *Journal of Speech and Hearing Disorders, 50,* 226–230.

Sies, L. F. (1974). *Aphasia theory and therapy: Selected lectures and papers by Hildred Schuell*. Baltimore: University Park Press.

Silverman, F. H. (1977). *Research design in speech pathology and audiology*. Englewood Cliffs, NJ: Prentice Hall.

Simmons, N. N. (1980). Choice of stimulus modes in treating apraxia of speech: A case study. In R. H. Brookshire (Ed.), *Proceedings of the Conference on Clinical Aphasiology* (pp. 302–307). Minneapolis: BRK Publishers.

Simmons, N. N. (1983). Treatment of conduction aphasia. In W. H. Perkins (Ed.), *Current therapy of communication disorders: Language handicaps in adults* (pp. 45–55). New York: Thieme-Stratton.

Simmons, N. N. (1984). Experimental analysis of a treatment program for alexia without agraphia. In R. H. Brookshire (Ed.), *Proceedings of the Conference on Clinical Aphasiology* (pp. 166–172). Minneapolis: BRK Publishers.

Simmons, N. N. (1986). Beyond standardized measures: Special tests, language in context, and discourse analysis in aphasia. In

L. L. LaPointe (Ed.), *Aphasia: Nature and assessment. Seminars in speech and language,* 7 (pp. 181–206). New York: Thieme-Stratton.

Skelly, M. (1975). Aphasic patients talk back. *American Journal of Nursing, 75,* 1140–1142.

Skelly, M. (1979). *Amerind gestural code based on universal American Indian hand talk.* New York: Elsevier North-Holland.

Sklar, M. (1966). *Sklar aphasia scale.* Los Angeles: Western Psychological Services.

Smith, A. (1972). *Diagnosis, intelligence, and rehabilitation of chronic aphasics: Final report.* Ann Arbor: University of Michigan, Department of Physical Medicine & Rehabilitation.

Smith, A. (1973). *Symbol digit modalities test.* Los Angeles: Western Psychological Services.

Spreen, O., & Benton, A. L. (1969). *Neurosensory center comprehensive examination for aphasia* (rev. ed.). Victoria, BC: University of Victoria.

Spreen, O., & Benton, A. L. (1977). *Neurosensory center comprehensive examination for aphasia* (1977 rev.). Victoria, BC: University of Victoria.

Stanton, K., Yorkston, K. M., Talley-Kenyon, V., & Beukelman, D. (1981). Language utilization in teaching reading to left neglect patients. In R. H. Brookshire (Ed.), *Proceedings of the Conference on Clinical Aphasiology.* Minneapolis: BRK Publishers.

Steele, R. D., Weinrich, M., Kleczewska, M. K., Wertz, R. T., & Carlson, G. S. (1987). Evaluating performance of severely aphasic patients on a computer-aided visual communication system. In R. H. Brookshire (Ed.), *Proceedings of the Conference on Clinical Aphasiology* (pp. 46–54). Minneapolis: BRK Publishers.

Steele, R. D., Weinrich, M., Wertz, R. T., & Carlson, G. (1986). *A microcomputer based visual communication system for treating severe aphasia.* Paper presented at the 24th Annual Meeting of the Academy of Aphasia, Nashville, TN.

Tanridag, O., & Kirshner, H. S. (1985). Aphasia and agraphia in lesions of the posterior internal capsule and putamen. *Neurology, 35,* 1797–1801.

Thompson, C. K., Hall, H. R., & Sison, C. E. (1986). Effects of hypnosis and imagery training on naming behavior in aphasia. *Brain and Language, 28,* 141–153.

Thompson, C. K., & Kearns, K. D. (1981). An experimental analysis of acquisition, generalization, and maintenance of naming behavior in a patient with anomia. In R. H. Brookshire (Ed.), *Proceedings of the Conference on Clinical Aphasiology* (pp. 35–45). Minneapolis: BRK Publishers.

Thorndike, E., & Lorge, I. (1944). *Teacher's workbook of 30,000 words.* New York: Columbia University Press.

Tikofsky, R. S. (1984). Contemporary aphasia diagnostics. In N. J. Lass (Ed.), *Speech and language: Advances in basic research and practice* (Vol. 11, pp. 1–111). New York: Academic Press.

Tikofsky, R. S., & Reynolds, G. L. (1962). Preliminary study: Nonverbal learning and aphasia. *Journal of Speech and Hearing Research, 5,* 133–143.

Tikofsky, R. S., & Reynolds, G. L. (1963). Further studies of nonverbal learning and aphasia. *Journal of Speech and Hearing Research, 6,* 329–337.

Tissot, R., Lhermitte, F., & Ducarne, B. (1963). Etat intellectuel des aphasiques. Essai d'une nouvelle approche à travers des epreuves perceptives et operatoires. *L'Encephale, 52,* 285–320.

Tonkovich, J. (1979). Case relations in Broca's aphasia: Some considerations regarding treatment. In R. H. Brookshire (Ed.), *Proceedings of the Conference on Clinical Aphasiology* (pp. 239–247). Minneapolis: BRK Publishers.

Tonkovich, J., & Loverso, F. (1982). A training matrix approach for gestural acquisition by the agrammatic patient. In R. H. Brookshire (Ed.), *Proceedings of the Conference on Clinical Aphasiology* (pp. 283–288). Minneapolis: BRK Publishers.

Trousseau, M. (1864). De l'aphasie, maladie décrite recomment sous le nom impropre d'aphemie. *Gazette des Hopitaux Civils et Militaires, 1,* 13–14.

Tzeng, O. J. L., & Wang, W. S. Y. (1983). The first two r's. *American Scientist, 71,* 238–243.

Ulatowska, H. K., & Bond, S. (1983). Aphasia: Discourse considerations. *Topics in Language Disorders, 3,* 21–34.

Ulatowska, H. K., Doyel, A. W., Freedman-Stern, R. F., Macaluso-Hayes, S., & North, A. J. (1983). Production of procedural discourse in aphasia. *Brain and Language, 18,* 315–341.

Ulatowska, H. K., Freedman-Stern, R. F., Doyel, A. W., Macaluso-Haynes, S., & North, A. J. (1983). Production of narrative discourse in aphasia. *Brain and Language, 19,* 317–334.

Ulatowska, H. K., North, A. J., & Macaluso-Haynes, S. (1981). Production of discourse and communicative competence in aphasia. In R. H. Brookshire (Ed.), *Proceedings of the Conference on Clinical Aphasiology* (pp. 75–82). Minneapolis: BRK Publishers.

VanDemark, A. (1982). Predicting post-treatment scores on the Boston Diagnostic Aphasia Examination. In R. H. Brookshire (Ed.), *Proceedings of the Conference on Clinical Aphasiology* (pp. 103–110). Minneapolis: BRK Publishers.

VanDemark, A., Lemmer, E., & Drake, M. (1982). Measurement of reading comprehension in aphasia with the RCBA. *Journal of Speech and Hearing Disorders, 47,* 288–291.

Varney, N. R. (1984). Phonemic imperception in aphasia. *Brain and Language, 21,* 85–94.

Vellutino, F. R. (1979). *Dyslexia: Theory and research.* Boston: Alpine Press.

Vignolo, L. (1964). Evolution of phasia and language rehabilitation: A retrospective exploratory study. *Cortex,* 344–367.

Von Stockert, T. R. (1978). A standardized program for aphasia therapy. In V. Lebrun & R. Hoops (Eds.), *The management of aphasia* (pp. 97–107). Amsterdam: Swets & Zeitlinger B.V.

Waller, M., & Darley, F. L. (1978). The influence of context on the auditory comprehension of paragraphs by aphasic subjects. *Journal of Speech and Hearing Research, 21,* 732–745.

Waller, M., & Darley, F. L. (1979). Effect of prestimulation on sentence comprehension by aphasic subjects. *Journal of Communication Disorders, 12,* 461–479.

Wallesch, C. W., Kornhuber, H. H., Brunner, R. J., Kunz, T., Hollerbach, B., & Suger, G. (1983). Lesions of the basal ganglia, thalamus, and deep white matter: Differential effects on language functions. *Brain and Language, 20,* 286–304.

Wang, W. S. Y. (1982). *Human communication: Language and its psychobiological bases.* Salt Lake City: W. H. Freeman.

Warren, R. L., Gabriel, C., Johnston, A., & Gaddie, A. (1987). Efficacy during acute rehabilitation. In R. H. Brookshire (Ed.), *Proceedings of the Conference on Clinical Aphasiology* (pp. 1–11). Minneapolis: BRK Publishers.

Wechsler, A. F. (1977). Presenile dementia presenting as aphasia. *Journal of Neurology, Neurosurgery, and Psychiatry, 40,* 303–305.

Wechsler, D. (1955). *Manual for the Wechsler Adult Intelligence Scale.* New York: The Psychological Corporation.

Weidner, W. E., & Jinks, A. F. (1983). The effects of single versus combined cue presentations on picture naming by aphasic adults. *Journal of Communication Disorders, 16,* 111–121.

Weigl, E. (1968). On the problem of cortical syndromes: Experimental studies. In M. L. Simmel (Ed.), *The reach of mind* (pp. 143–159). New York: Springer Publishing Co.

Weigl, E. (1970). Neuropsychological studies of structure and dynamics of semantic fields with the deblocking method. In C. H. V. Schooneveld (Ed.), *Sign-language-culture* (pp. 287–290). The Hague: Mouton.

Weiner, F. (1983a). *Aphasia I: Noun association.* Baltimore: University Park Press.

Weiner, F. (1983b). *Aphasia II: Opposites and similarities.* Baltimore: University Park Press.

Weiner, F. (1984). *Phonological analysis by computer (PAG).* State College, PA: Parrot Software.

Weiner, H. L., & Levitt, L. P. (1978). *Neurology for the house officer,* (2nd ed.). Baltimore: Williams & Wilkins.

Weisenberg, T., & McBride, K. E. (1935). *Aphasia: A clinical and psychological study.* New York: Commonwealth Fund.

Wener, D., & Duffy, J. (1983). An investigation of the sensitivity of the Reporter's Test to expressive language disturbances. (Abstract). In R. H. Brookshire (Ed.), *Proceedings of the Conference on Clinical Aphasiology* (pp. 15–27). Minneapolis: BRK Publishers.

Wepman, J. M. (1951). *Recovery from aphasia.* New York: Ronald Press.

Wepman, J. M. (1972). Aphasia therapy: A new look. *Journal of Speech and Hearing Disorders, 37,* 203–214.

Wepman, J. M. (1976). Aphasia: Language without thought or thought without language. *Asha, 18,* 131–136.

Wepman, J. M., & Jones, L. V. (1961). *Studies in aphasia: An approach to testing.* Chicago: University of Chicago Education Industry Service.

Wepman, J. M., Jones, L. V., Bock, R. D., & Van Pelt, D. (1960). Studies in aphasia: Background and theoretical formulations. *Journal of Speech and Hearing Disorders, 25,* 323–332.

Wernicke, C. (1874). *Der Aphasische Symptomenkomplex.* Breslau, Poland: M. Cohn & Weigert.

Wertz, R. T. (1966). *The effects of interhemispheric and intrahemispheric lesions on nonverbal trial and error learning behavior in brain damaged adults.* Paper presented to the 42nd Annual American Speech and Hearing Association Convention, Washington, DC.

Wertz, R. T. (1967). *Behavior deficits associated with right hemispheric lesions.* Paper presented to the 43rd Annual American Speech and Hearing Association Convention, Chicago, IL.

Wertz, R. T. (1978). Neuropathologies of speech and language: An introduction to patient management. In D. F. Johns (Ed.), *Clinical management of neurogenic communicative disorders* (pp. 1–102). Boston: Little, Brown & Company.

Wertz, R. T. (1979). Word fluency measure (WF). In F. L. Darley (Ed.), *Evaluation of appraisal techniques in speech and language pathology* (pp. 243–246). Reading, MA: Addison-Wesley.

Wertz, R. T. (1982a). Response to treatment in a case of crossed aphasia. In R. H. Brookshire (Ed.), *Proceedings of the Conference on Clinical Aphasiology* (pp. 129–137). Minneapolis: BRK Publishers.

Wertz, R. T. (1982b). Language deficit in aphasia and dementia: The same as, different from, or both? In R. H. Brookshire (Ed.), *Proceedings of the Conference on Clinical Aphasiology* (pp. 350–359). Minneapolis: BRK Publishers.

Wertz, R. T. (1983). Language intervention context and setting for the aphasic adult: When? In J. Miller, D. E. Yoder, & R. Schiefelbusch (Eds.), *Contemporary issues in language intervention, ASHA Reports 12* (pp. 196–220). Rockville, MD: American Speech-Language-Hearing Association.

Wertz, R. T. (1985). Neuropathologies of speech and language: An introduction to patient management. In D. F. Johns (Ed.), *Clinical management of neurogenic communicative disorders* (2nd ed., pp. 1–96). Boston: Little, Brown & Company.

Wertz, R. T. (1986a). *Examining and explaining the efficacy of our efforts.* Paper presented to the Tenth Annual Speech-Language Pathology Symposium: Neurogenic Communication Disorders, Tempe, AZ.

Wertz, R. T. (1986b). Specialty recognition in neurogenic speech, language, and cognitive disorders: Clinical competence in aphasia and apraxia of speech. In R. H. Brookshire (Ed.), *Proceedings of the Conference on Clinical Aphasiology* (pp. 319–324). Minneapolis: BRK Publishers.

Wertz, R. T. (1987). Language treatment for aphasia is efficacious, but for whom? *Topics in Language Disorders, 8,* 1–10.

Wertz, R. T., Collins, M. J., Weiss, D., Kurtzke, J. F., Friden, T., Brookshire, R. H., Pierce, J., Holtzapple, P., Hubbard, D. J., Porch, B. E., West, J. A., Davis, L., Matovitch, V., Morley, G. K., & Resurreccion, E. (1981). Veterans Administration cooperative study on aphasia: A comparison of individual and group treatment. *Journal of Speech and Hearing Research, 24,* 580–594.

Wertz, R. T., Deal, J. L., & Robinson, A. J. (1984). Classifying the aphasias: A comparison of the Boston Diagnostic Aphasia Examination and the Western Aphasia Battery. In R. H. Brookshire (Ed.), *Proceedings of the Conference on Clinical Aphasiology* (pp. 40–47). Minneapolis: BRK Publishers.

Wertz, R. T., Deal, L., & Deal, J. (1980). Prognosis in aphasia: Investigation of the high-overall and the short-direct methods to predict change in PICA performance. In R. H. Brookshire (Ed.), *Proceedings of the Conference on Clinical Aphasiology* (pp. 164–173). Minneapolis: BRK Publishers.

Wertz, R. T., Flynn, M., Green, E., Rosenbek, J. C., & Collins, M. J. (1979). Alexia without agraphia: Some considerations for patient management. *Aphasia, Apraxia, Agnosia, 1,* 26–31.

Wertz, R. T., Kitselman, K. P., & Deal, L. A. (1981). *Classifying the aphasias: Contributions to patient management.* Paper presented to the Academy of Aphasia, London, Ontario.

Wertz, R. T., LaPointe, L. L., & Rosenbek, J. C. (1984). *Apraxia of speech in adults: The disorder and its management.* New York: Grune & Stratton.

Wertz, R. T., & Porch, B. E. (1970). Effects of masking noise on verbal performance of adult aphasics. *Cortex, 6,* 399–409.

Wertz, R. T., & Rosenbek, J. C. (1978). Group designs for the study of aphasia. In R. H. Brookshire (Ed.), *Proceedings of the Conference on Clinical Aphasiology* (pp. 1–10). Minneapolis: BRK Publishers.

Wertz, R. T., Shubitowski, Y., Dronkers, N. F., Lemme, M. L., & Deal, J. L. (1985). *Word fluency measure reliability in normal and brain damaged adults.* Paper presented to the American Speech-Language-Hearing Association, Washington, DC.

Wertz, R. T., Weiss, D. G., Aten, J. L., Brookshire, R. H., Garcia-Bunuel, L., Holland, A. L., Kurtzke, J. F., LaPointe, L. L., Milianti, F. J., Brannegan, R., Greenbaum, H., Marshall, R. C., Vogel, D., Carter, J., Barnes, N. S., & Goodman, R. (1986). Comparison of clinic, home, and deferred language treatment for aphasia: A Veterans Administration cooperative study. *Archives of Neurology, 43,* 653–658.

West, J. F. (1973). Auditory comprehension in aphasic adults: Improvement through training. *Archives of Physical Medicine and Rehabilitation, 54,* 78–86.

West, J. F. (1978). Heightening the action imagery of materials used in aphasia treatment. In R. H. Brookshire (Ed.), *Proceedings of the Conference on Clinical Aphasiology* (pp. 201–211). Minneapolis: BRK Publishers.

Whitaker, H., & Whitaker, H. A. (1976a). *Studies in neurolinguistics. Vol. 1.* New York: Academic Press.

Whitaker, H., & Whitaker, H. A. (1976b). *Studies in neurolinguistics. Vol. 2.* New York: Academic Press.

Whitaker, H., & Whitaker, H. A. (1977). *Studies in neurolinguistics. Vol. 3.* New York: Academic Press.

Whitaker, H., & Whitaker, H. A. (1979). *Studies in neurolinguistics. Vol. 4.* New York: Academic Press.

Whitehouse, P., Caramazza, A., & Zurif, E. (1978). Naming in aphasia: Interacting effects of form and function. *Brain and Language, 6,* 63–74.

Whurr, R. (1974). *Aphasia screening test.* (Obtainable from 2 Alwyne Road, London N1 2HH)

Wiederholt, W. C. (1982). *Neurology for non-neurologists.* San Diego: Academic Press.

Wiegel-Crump, C., & Koenigsknecht, R. A. (1973). Tapping the lexical store of the adult aphasic: Analysis of the improvement made in word retrieval skills. *Cortex, 9,* 410–418.

Wilcox, M. J. (1983). Aphasia: Pragmatic considerations. *Topics in Language Disorders, 3,* 34–48.

Wilcox, M. J., & Davis, G. A. (1977). Speech act analysis of aphasic communication in individual and group settings. In R. H. Brookshire (Ed.), *Proceedings of the Conference on Clinical Aphasiology* (pp. 166–174). Minneapolis: BRK Publishers.

Williams, S. E., & Canter, G. J. (1981). On the assessment of naming disturbances in adult aphasia. In R. H. Brookshire (Ed.), *Proceedings of the Conference on Clinical Aphasiology* (pp. 155-165). Minneapolis: BRK Publishers.

Wilson, M., & Fox, B. (1983). *Microcomputer language assessment and development system (MICRO-LADS).* Burlington, VT: Laureate Learning Systems, Inc.

Wilson, R. H., Fowler, C. G., & Shanks, J. E. (1981). Audiological assessment of the aphasic patient. In R. T. Wertz (Ed.), *Aphasia: Interdisciplinary approach. Seminars in Speech, Language, Hearing* (pp. 299–314). New York: Thieme-Stratton.

Wolf, P. A., Dawber, T. R., Thomas, H. E., Colton, T., & Kannel, W. B. (1977). Epidemiology of stroke. In R. A. Thompson & J. R. Green (Eds.), *Advances in neurology* (Vol. 16, pp. 5–18). New York: Raven Press.

Wolvin, A. D., & Coakley, C. G. (1985). *Listening.* Dubuque, IA: William C. Brown, Publishers.

Wood, M. L. (1986). *Private practice in communication disorders.* San Diego: College-Hill Press.

Wyke, M. (1962). An experimental study of verbal association in dysphasic subjects. *Brain, 85,* 679–686.

Yarnell, R., Monroe, P., & Sobel, L. (1976). Aphasia outcome in stroke: A clinical and neuroradiological correlation. *Stroke, 7,* 516–522.

Yorkston, K., & Beukelman, D. (1977). A system for quantifying verbal output of high-level aphasic patients. In R. H. Brookshire (Ed.), *Proceedings of the Conference on Clinical Aphasiology* (pp. 175–180). Minneapolis: BRK Publishers.

Yorkston, K. M., & Beukelman, D. R. (1980). An analysis of connected speech samples of aphasic and normal speakers. *Journal of Speech and Hearing Disorders, 45,* 27–36.

Yorkston, K. M., & Beukelman, D. R. (1981). *Assessment of intelligibility of dysarthric speech.* Austin, TX: PRO-ED.

Zangwill, O. L. (1967). Speech and the minor hemisphere. *Acta Neurologica et Psychiatrica Belgica, 67,* 1013–1020.

Zubrick, A., & Smith, A. (1979). Review of the Minnesota Test for Differential Diagnosis of Aphasia (MTDDA). In F. L. Darley (Ed.),

Evaluation of appraisal techniques in speech and language pathology (pp. 212–217). Reading, MA: Addison-Wesley.

Zurif, E. B., Caramazza, A., & Myerson, R. (1972). Grammatical judgments of agrammatic aphasics. *Neuropsychologia, 10*, 405–417.

Zurif, E., Caramazza, A., Myerson, R., & Galvin, J. (1974). Semantic feature representations for normal and aphasic language. *Brain and Language, 1*, 167–187.

SUBJECT INDEX

ABA treatment design, 99, 117–120, *118, 120*
Acquired dyslexia,
  alexia with agraphia, 165–166
  alexia without agraphia, 166
  deep dyslexia, 167–168
  developmental dyslexia comparison, 163–164
  evaluation, 169–170
    aphasia batteries subtests, 171, *171*
    Reading Comprehension Battery for
        Aphasia, 171–173, *172, 173*
  frontal alexia, 166–167
  reading processes, 164–165, *164*
  remediation targets, 175–179
    comprehension improvement, 177–178
    context cues, 178–179
    perceptual deficits, 175–176
    rate manipulation, 177, *178*
    syntactic deficits, 177
    word attack skills, 178
  treatment, 173–175, *175*
    computer use, 179–180
    planning, 173
    principles, 173–175
    tasks, 179
  underlying mechanisms, 165
Agraphia, 240–241. *See also* Aphasic writing.
Alexia with agraphia, 47, 165–166
Alexia without agraphia, 47–48, 166
Alternating treatments design, 123–124, *123, 124*
Alzheimer's disease, 2, 11, *25*
Angular gyrus, 168–169, *169*, 189
Anomias,
  classification, 187–189
  localization, 189–190. *See also* Naming
      disorders.
Anomic aphasia,
  characteristic writing deficits, *243*
  symptoms, *45*, 47
Aphasia,
  associated disorders, 50–53
    apraxia of speech, 52

dementia, 51
dysarthria, 52–53
environmental influence on language, *52*
language of confusion, 51
right hemisphere impairment, 51–52
schizophrenia, 52
classification, 38
  controversy, 38–40, 49–50
  systems, 40–43
definition debate, 34–37, 53–54
  cognitive deficit, 37–38
fluent-nonfluent, 43–44
syndromes, 44–49
  alexia with agraphia, 47
alexia without agraphia, 47–48
  anomic, *45*, 47
  aphemia, 47
  Broca's, 45, *45*
  conduction, *45*, 47
  crossed, 49
  global, 44–45, *45*
  mixed nonfluent, 47
  isolation, 45, *45*
  pure agraphia, 48
  pure word deafness, 48
  subcortical, 48–49, *50*
  transcortical motor, 45–46, *45*
  transcortical sensory, *45*, 46–47
  Wernicke's, *45*, 46
Aphasic writing, 240–242, *242*
  appraisal, 243–248
    informal measures, 246–248, *248, 249*
    standardized measures, 244–246, *245, 246,*
        247
  classification, 242–243
  prognosis, 248–254
    ability to learn, 252, *252*
    generalization, 252–253, *253*
    phonologic and lexical-semantic ability, 251
    premorbid literacy, 250
    retention, 252, *253*

Italic page numbers refer to tables and figures.

Aphasic writing, prognosis (continued)
  speech and language dissociation, 251
  willingness to practice, 253–254, 254
  willingness to write, 250–251
  treatment, 254
    computerized, 269–274, 271, 272, 273, 274, 275
    principles, 254–256
    stimulus content, 257–260
    stimulus modalities, 256–257
    traditional methods, 262–265, 263, 264, 265
    writing mechanics, 260–261, 261
    writing programs, 266–269, 266, 267, 268, 269
Aphemia, 47
Appraisal. See Patient appraisal.
Apraxia of speech, 2, 52
  aphasia differentiation, 87–88, 88
  appraisal, 71–72
Assessment,
  of naming disorders, 190–191
    stimulus selection and ordering guidelines, 191–196
  of verbal expression, 213–215
    analysis, 214–215
    functional communication tests, 214
    imitation, 213
    interview, 214
    picture description, 213–214
    process description, 214
    story retelling, 215
Ataxia, 30
Auditory comprehension, 143
  anatomy, 145–146
  aphasia classification, 41–42, 45
  assessment, 148
    Auditory Comprehension Test for Sentences, 150
    contemporary tests, 149
    discourse evaluation, 151
    early tests, 148–149
    Functional Auditory Comprehension Task, 150–151
    Revised Token Test, 150
    Token Test, 149
  impairment patterns, 144–145
  lexical-syntactic aspects, 147
  modality-stimulus influences, 146
  necessary components, 144
  peripheral auditory function, 143–144
  phoneme perception, 146
  tests, 68
Auditory comprehension deficit,
  esoteric impairments, 147–148
  treatment, 142
    alerting signals use, 155
    auditory input factors, 154
    influences, 153–155
    object-picture stimulus variables, 155–156
    principles, 151–153
    rate manipulation effects, 154–155
    sequence, 156–157, 157
    techniques, 157–160
Auditory Comprehension Test for Sentences, 150

Base-10 Programmed Response system, 113–115, 114, 156, 211
  as aphasic writing treatment method, 262–263, 263, 264
Behavioral neurology,
  brain injury sequelae, 3, 3
  epilepsy, 4–5, 4, 5
  medical management, 3–4
Behavioral data,
  importance in appraisal, 58–59
  as prognostic variable, 93–94
Biographical information,
  importance in appraisal, 56–57
  as prognostic variable, 91–92
Boston Diagnostic Aphasia Examination, 39, 62–64, 63, 65
  as aphasia classification system, 40–43, 41
    auditory comprehension, 41
    fluency, 40–41
    naming, 42
    repetition, 42
  Aphasia Severity Rating Scale, 63, 81
  writing deficits appraisal, 244–246
Brain,
  anatomy, 18–19, 18
  composition, 17
  connections, 19–20
  damage, 3–5
    epilepsy, 4–5, 4, 5
    neurobehavioral sequelae, 3, 3
  imaging, 5–8, 6, 7
  left hemisphere functions, 20–21, 21
  protection, 17–18
Broca's aphasia, 2, 3, 8, 21, 212
  brain lesion sites, 22, 46
  characteristic writing deficits, 243
  nonfluency classification, 41
  symptoms, 45, 45
  verbal expression treatment programs, 220–228
    changing criteria program, 224–228, 225
    expanding complexity or length, 223
    expanding the repertoire, 221–223
    syntax stimulation program, 223–224

Central nervous system, 16, *17*, 17–18
  cerebrum, 18–19
  connections, 19–20, *19*
  epidemiology, 25–26, *25*
  neuropathology, 23–25
    cerebral trauma, 24–25
    cerebrovascular accidents, 23–24
    diseases, 25
    tumors, 25
  protection, 17–18
Cerebral blood flow research, 28
Cerebral trauma, 24–25
  brain laceration, 24
  closed head injuries, 24
  open head injuries, 24
Cerebrovascular accidents, 23–24
  cerebral embolism, 23
  cerebral hemorrhage, 23
  cerebral thrombosis, 23
  epidemiology, 25–26, *25*
Cerebrum, 18–19, *18*
Changing criterion treatment design, 127–129,
    127, 128, 224–228, *225*
Clinical aphasiology,
  behavioral neurology, 2–5
  cognitive science, 9–11
  economics, 12–13
  neuroscience, 5–9
  principles,
    aphasiologist importance, 131
    attitudes importance, 132–133
    generalization, 138
    individual treatment importance, 134
    limitations, 133–134
    listening importance, 135–136
    modern developments, 140
    patient and family involvement, 138–139
    patient strengths, 138
    testing importance, 134–135
    treatment advisability, 139–140
    treatment goals, 131–132
    treatment stimuli, 137
    treatment structure, 136–137
  psychology, 13–14
  research history, 1–2, 11–12
Communication board, *249*
Computerized axial tomography, 5–6, *6*, 21, 27–28
Computerized treatment,
  of aphasic writing, 269–274, *271*
  visual communication system (VIC) adaptation,
    271–274, *272, 273, 274, 275*
Conduction aphasia, *88*
  characteristic writing deficits, 243
  lesions loci, *46*
  symptoms, *45*, 47

verbal expression treatment programs,
    237–239
Corpus callosum, 19, 20
Cortical deafness, 147–148
Crossed aphasia, 49
Crossover treatment design, 124–127, *125, 126*
CT scan. *See* Computerized axial tomography.
Cueing hierarchies, in naming treatment,
    197–200
  therapeutic cueing hierarchies, 200–203

Diagnosis, 80–82, 89
  aphasia versus apraxia of speech, 87–88, *88*
    dementia, 82–84, *84*
    dysarthria, 88–89
    language of confusion, 84–86, *85*
    normal language, 82
    right hemisphere communication deficits,
      86–87
    schizophrenia, 86
  case study, 89–90, *90*
Deblocking, in naming disorders treatment,
    206–207
Dementia, 51
  aphasia differentiation, 82–84, *84*
Deep dyslexia, 167–168
Developmental dyslexia, acquired dyslexia
    comparison, 163–164
Discourse analysis, 76
Dysarthria, 52–53
  aphasia differentiation, 88–89
  appraisal, 71–72

Electroencephalogram, 27
Environmental influence on language, 52
Epilepsy, 4–5, 20
Extended baseline design, *103*

Fluent aphasia, treatment techniques, 158–159
Fluent-nonfluent aphasia classification system,
    40–43, 43–44, *45*
Frontal alexia, 166–167
Functional Auditory Comprehension Task,
    150–151
Functional communication tests, 70–71

Gesture tests, in appraisal, 70
Gestural reorganization treatment program,
    218–220
  conceptual framework, 218
  methodology, 218–220

Global aphasia, 3, 158
  characteristic writing deficits, *243*
  symptoms, 44–45, *45*
  verbal expression treatment programs,
      231–235
    Florance and Deal's program, 233–234, *234*
    Visual Action Therapy, 234
Grammatical analysis, in appraisal, 74–75
Group treatment designs,
  complications, 105–108
    no-treatment group definition, 106–107
    patient variables, 105–106
    spontaneous recovery, 106
    treatment specification, 107–108
  design comparison, 111–112
  efficacy, 108–113
    early research, 108–109
    recent research, 109–111
  patient selection criteria, *105*
  single-subject designs comparison, 115–117, *115*

Helm Elicited Language Program for Syntax
    Stimulation, 223–224

Information processing deficit, treatment
    techniques, 159
Isolation aphasia, symptoms, 45, *45*

Laddering, 266–267, *266*
Language of confusion, 50–51
  aphasia differentiation, 84–86, *85*
Language Master, 202
Limited anomias, 189

Magnetic resonance imaging, 5–7, *6*, 29
Medical data,
  importance in appraisal, 57–58, *57*
  as prognostic variable, 92–93
Minnesota Test for Differential Diagnosis of
    Aphasia, 39, 65–66
  use in prognosis, 94–95
Mixed nonfluent aphasia,
  characteristic writing deficits, *243*
  symptoms, 47
Multiple baseline treatment design, *100, 102,*
      120–123, *121, 122*

Naming disorders,
  and aphasia classification, 42, *45*
  assessment, 190–191

classification, 187–188
  limited anomias, 189
  semantic anomia, 188
  word production anomia, 188
  word selection anomia, 188
comprehension deficits, 185–186
  semantic priming, 186–187
computerized treatment, 206
deblocking treatment, 206–207
environmental sounds priming, 207–208
error types, 181–182
  aphasic word associations, 183
  normal word associations, 182–183
lexical semantic and syntactic structural
    treatment, 205
localization, 189–190
multimodality drill procedure, 208–210
patient generated naming cues, 208
Schuellian treatments, 203–205
semantic field deficit,
  associations, 183–184
  boundaries, 184–185
  centrality, 185
  features, 185
  parallel production and comprehension
      deficits, 185–186
SORRT treatment program, 205–206
stimulus selection and ordering guidelines,
      191–196
  altered stimuli influence, 193
  categories influence, 193–194
  frequency influence, 191
  frequency and picturability influence, 194
  modality influences, 195–196
  objects and redundancy influence, 192–193
  operativity influence, 192
  phonemic cueing influence, 194
  single and composite pictures influence, 193
  stimulus presentation timing, 194–195
tip-of-the-tongue phenomena, 186
treatment cueing hierarchies, 197
  combining cues hierarchy, 199
  four cue hierarchy, 198–199
  hierarchy and drill combination, 202–203
  hierarchy comparison, 199–200
  Language Master hierarchy, 202
  nine step diagnostic hierarchy, 197–198
  patient created hierarchy, 200–201
  rapid movement hierarchies, 201–202
  six cue hierarchy, 198
  three cue hierarchy, 199
  three step treatment hierarchy, 201
treatment facilitation, 196–197
Nervous system,
  central nervous system, 16, *17*

composition, 17
functional organization, 16, *16*
peripheral nervous system, 16–17
Neurodiagnostics, 26–29
  cerebral blood flow, 28
  computerized axial tomography, 27–28
  electroencephalogram, 27
  isotope scanning, 27
  magnetic resonance imaging, 29
  positron emission tomography, 28–29
Neuroscience, and aphasia, 5
  anatomy and physiology, 8–9
  brain imaging, 5–8
  history, 15–16
Nonverbal intelligence measures, in appraisal,
    72–73

Object-imaging-projection instruction method,
    176
Oral expressive language tests, 69–70
Oral language. *See* Verbal expression.

PACE. *See* Promoting Aphasics' Communicative
    Effectiveness.
Patient appraisal,
  aphasic writing deficits, 243–248
    informal measures, 246–248, *248, 249*
    standardized measures, 244–246, *245, 246,*
      247
  appraisal battery, 77–78
    case study, 78–80, *79, 81*
  appraisal trends, 73–76
    communicative content and efficiency, 73–74
    discourse analysis, 76
    grammatical analysis, 74–75
    phonological analysis, 74
    pragmatic analysis, 75–76
    semantic analysis, 74
  behavioral data, 58–59
  biographical data, 56
  functional communication tests, 70–71
  general language measures, 62
    Boston Diagnostic Aphasia Examination,
      62–64, *63, 65*
    Minnesota Test for Differential Diagnosis
      of Aphasia, 65–66
    Porch Index of Communicative Ability, 65,
      66–67, *66*
    Western Aphasia Battery, 62, 64–65
  medical data, 57–58, *57*
  motor speech evaluation, 71–72
  nonverbal intelligence measures, 72–73
  psychometrics, 59–61

screening tests, 67
specific modality tests, 67–70
  auditory comprehension, 68
  gesture, 70
  oral expressive language, 69–70
  reading, 68–69
  writing, 70
speech and language data, 61–62
Peripheral nervous system, 16–17
Porch Index of Communicative Ability, 39, 65,
    66–67, *66, 79*
  use in prognosis, 95–97, *96,* 98–99
  writing deficits appraisal, 244–246, *245*
Positron emission tomography, 5–7, *7,* 28–29
Prognosis,
  of aphasic writing, 248–254
    prognostic signs, 250–251
    prognostic treatment, 251–254, *252, 253*
  behavioral profiles, 94–97
    Minnesota Test for Differential Diagnosis
      of Aphasia use, 94–95
    Porch Index of Communicative Ability use,
      95–97, *96*
  statistical prediction, 97–99
  treatment, 99–102
    ability to learn, 99–100, *99*
    generalization, 100–102, *102*
    retention, 101–102, *102*
    willingness to practice, 102, *103*
  variables, 91–94
    behavioral, 93–94
    biographical, 91–92
    medical, 92–93
Promoting Aphasics' Communicative
    Effectiveness treatment program, 160,
    216–218
  method testing, 217–218, *218*
  requirements and procedures, 216–217
    exchanging new information, 216–217
    free choice, 217
    natural feedback, 217
    turn taking, 217
Psychometrics, importance in appraisal, 59–61
  reliability, 60–61
  validity, 59–60
Pure agraphia, 48
Pure alexia, 47–48
Pure word deafness, 48, 147–148

Reading,
  angular gyrus importance, 168–169, *169*
  cognitive processes, 164–165, *164*
  evaluation measures, 170–171
    aphasia batteries subtests, 171, *171*

Reading *(continued)*
   tests, 68–69
   underlying mechanisms, 165
Reading Comprehension Battery for Aphasia,
      171–173
   controlled factors, *172*
   reliability and validity, 172
   subtests, *173*
   test construction, 171–172
Revised Token Test, 150
Right hemisphere communication deficits,
      51–52, 86–87

Schizophrenia, 52
   aphasia differentiation, 86
Schuellian treatment,
   of auditory comprehension deficit, 152–153
   of naming disorders, 203–205
Semantic anomia, 188
Semantic field,
   associations, 183–184
   boundaries, 184–185
   centrality, 185
   features, 185
   semantic priming, 186–187
Sentence comprehension, treatment techniques,
      159–160
Sequential treatment of split lists writing
      program, 267–268, *267, 268*
Severe comprehension deficit, 158
Single-subject treatment designs, 113–117
   alternating treatments design, 123–124, *123,
      124*
   Base-10 system, 113–115, *114*
   changing criterion design, 127–129, *127, 128*
   crossover design, 124–127, *125, 126*
   group treatment design comparison, 115–117,
      115
   multiple baseline design, 120–123, *121, 122*
   withdrawal design, 117–120, *118, 120*
Skateboard prosthesis, for aphasic writing, *261*
SORRT naming deficit treatment, 205–206
Split brain studies, 19, 20
   left hemisphere functions, 20–21, *21*
Spontaneous recovery, in aphasic patients, 106
Statistical procedures, in prognosis, 97–99
Stimulus selection, in aphasic writing treatment,
      256
   auditory modalities, 257
   stimulus complexity, 258–259
   stimulus length, 258
   stimulus meaningfulness, 259–260
   tactile-kinesthetic modalities, 257
   visual modalities, 256–257

Stroke. *See* Cerebrovascular accident.
Subcortical aphasia, 7, 21–22
   symptoms, 48–49, *50*

Testing. *See* Patient appraisal.
Thalamic aphasia, 21–22
Tip-of-the-tongue phenomena, 186
   computerized treatment, 206
Token Test, 149, 158–159
Transcortical motor aphasia,
   characteristic writing deficits, *243*
   lesions loci, *46*
   symptoms, 45–46, *45*
   verbal expression treatment programs,
      235–237, *236, 237*
Transcortical sensory aphasia,
   characteristic writing deficits, *243*
   lesions loci, *46*
   symptoms, *45*, 46–47
   verbal expression treatment programs,
      237–239
Traumatic brain injury, 85–86, *85*
Treatment,
   of acquired dyslexia, 173–175, *175*
   of aphasia, 108–113
      early research, 108–109
      goals, 131–132
      recent studies, 109–111
      single-subject versus group designs, 115–117,
         115
   of aphasic writing, 254
      computerized, 269–274, *271, 272, 273,
         274, 275*
      mechanics, 260–261, *261*
      principles, 254–256
      stimulus selection, 256–260
      traditional methods, 262–265, *263, 264,
         265*
      writing programs, 266–269, *266, 267,
         268, 269*
   of auditory comprehension deficit, 151–156
      manuals, 161–162
      microcomputer use, 162
      sequence, 156–157, *157*
      tasks, *161*
      techniques, 157–160
   of naming disorders, 196–197
      cueing hierarchies, 197
   techniques, 157–161
      applied pragmatics, 160–161
      attention, 157–158
      auditory comprehension tasks, *161*
      fluent aphasia, 158–159
      information processing deficit, 159

mild comprehension impairment, 160
phonemic discrimination, 158
sentence comprehension, 159–160
severe comprehension deficit, 158

Verbal expression,
  assessment, 213–215
    analysis, 214–215
    functional communication tests, 214
    imitation, 213
    interview, 214
    picture description, 213–214
    process description, 214
    story retelling, 215
  Broca's aphasia treatment programs, 220–228
    changing criteria program, 224–228, 225
    expanding complexity or length, 223
    expanding the repertoire, 221–223
    syntax stimulation program, 223–224
  conduction aphasia treatment programs,
    237–239
  general treatment programs, 216–220
    gestural reorganization, 218–220
    Promoting Aphasics' Communicative
      Effectiveness (PACE), 216–218
  global aphasia treatment programs, 231–235
    Florance and Deal's program, 233–234,
      234
    Visual Action Therapy, 234
  stimulus selection and ordering guidelines,
    215–216
    expanding complexity and length, 215–216
    expanding utterance repertoire, 216, 216

transcortical motor aphasia treatment
    programs, 235–237, 236, 237
transcortical sensory aphasia treatment
    programs, 237–239
treatment decisions influences, 211–212
  aphasia type, 212
  symptoms distribution, severity, and course,
    212–213
treatment importance, 211
Wernicke's aphasia treatment programs,
    228–231
Visual Action Therapy, 234
Visual communication system (VIC), 271–275,
    272

Wernicke's aphasia, 2, 3, 8, 21, 58, 212
  brain lesion sites, 22
  characteristic writing deficits, 243
  fluent classification, 41
  lesions loci, 46
  symptoms, 45, 46
  treatment techniques, 158–159
  visual expression treatment programs,
    228–231
Western Aphasia Battery, 62, 64–65
  as aphasia classification system, 40
    auditory comprehension, 41
    fluency 40–41
    naming, 42
    repetition, 42
  writing deficits appraisal, 244–246, 246, 247
Withdrawal treatment design, 117–120, 118, 120
Word production anomia, 118
Word selection anomia, 188

NOTES

NOTES

NOTES

NOTES

NOTES

NOTES

NOTES

NOTES

NOTES

NOTES

NOTES

NOTES

NOTES

NOTES

anterior - Broca's → expressive
(simple pics)

posterior - Wernicke's & anomic
(add content)

facilitation programs

didactic programs